Veterinary Pharmacology

An Introduction to
Veterinary Pharmacology

Frank Alexander PhD, DSc, MRCVS, FACVPT, FRSE
Emeritus Professor of Veterinary Pharmacology in the University of Edinburgh

FOURTH EDITION

Longman
London and New York

Longman Group Limited
Longman House, Burnt Mill, Harlow
Essex CM20 2JE, England
Associated companies throughout the world

Published in the United States of America
by Churchill Livingstone Inc., New York

First published 1960
Second edition 1969
Third edition 1976
Fourth edition 1985

ISBN 0-582-40904-7

British Library Cataloguing in Publication Data

An Introduction to veterinary pharmacology. — 4th ed.
  1. Veterinary pharmacology
  I. Alexander, Frank
  636.089'51   SF915

Library of Congress Cataloging in Publication Data
Main entry under title:

An Introduction to veterinary pharmacology.
  Rev. ed of: An introduction to veterinary pharmacology/
by Frank Alexander. 3rd ed. 1976.
  Includes index.
  1. Veterinary pharmacology.   I. Alexander, Frank, 1917–   . II. Alexander,
Frank, 1917–   . An introduction to veterinary pharmacology.
SF915.I53   1985   636.089'57   84-23064

Produced by Longman Group (FE) Limited
Printed in Hong Kong

Preface to the Fourth Edition

As with previous editions, the object of the fourth edition is to provide the veterinary undergraduate with a concise account of the pharmacological properties of the principal drugs used in the treatment and prevention of disease in domesticated animals. It is hoped that practising veterinarians may find the book useful. The continued growth of the subject and the imminence of the original author's retirement made it desirable to spread the burden of producing a new edition. The Editor has been fortunate in obtaining the collaboration of colleagues experienced in teaching veterinary pharmacology and is grateful to them for the time and trouble they have expended on producing their various contributions. The entire text has been revised and substantial parts completely rewritten. Wherever possible differences in the ways in which the various domesticated species metabolise and respond to drugs have been discussed. Despite efforts to make the text as concise as possible, growth has been inevitable but it is hoped that the book will continue to serve its original purpose.

Edinburgh, 1985

F.A.

Contributors

F. Alexander, Ph.D., D.Sc., M.R.C.V.S., F.A.C.V.P.T., F.R.S.E.
Emeritus Professor and former Head of Department, Department of
Veterinary Pharmacology, University of Edinburgh.

A. L. Bartlet, B.Pharm., Ph.D.
Senior Lecturer in Veterinary Pharmacology, Department of Veterinary
Pharmacology, University of Edinburgh.

S. S. Carlyle, M.A., Vet. M.B., Ph.D., M.R.C.V.S.
Lecturer in Veterinary Pharmacology, Department of Veterinary Pharmacology,
University of Edinburgh.

P. Eyre, B.Sc., Ph.D., B.V.M. & S., M.R.C.V.S., F.A.A.V.P.T.
Professor and Head of Department of Biomedical Sciences, University of Guelph,
Canada.

A. Knifton, B.Sc. Ph.D., B.V.Sc., M.R.C.V.S.
Senior Lecturer in Veterinary Pharmacology, Department of Veterinary Physiology
& Pharmacology, University of Liverpool.

R. J. Martin, Ph.D., B.V.Sc., M.R.C.V.S., Dip. Neurophysiol.
Lecturer in Veterinary Pharmacology, Department of Veterinary Pharmacology,
University of Edinburgh.

Contents

1

Introduction and general principles of drug administration

INTRODUCTION

Pharmacology may be defined as the study of the action of drugs on living tissues. It is difficult, however, to separate this from the effects produced by living tissues on drugs, as sometimes it is only after a drug has entered the body, been acted on by the tissues and the drug changed into a different substance that its characteristic pharmacological action is produced. Therefore, it is necessary to study also what happens to the drug in the body, generally termed its fate in the body. The effects produced by drugs acting on tissues are often called the pharmacodynamic actions. The actions of the tissues on the drug such as absorption, distribution, metabolism and excretion, are called the pharmacokinetics of the drug.

Veterinary pharmacology is concerned with the action of drugs on the tissues of the domesticated animals and the fate of drugs in these species. This information is essential to rational treatment of disease in these animals. Veterinary pharmacology, therefore, provides the scientific basis of veterinary therapeutics.

The action of a drug usually depends upon an adequate concentration being present in the fluids bathing the tissues or in the tissues for a time long enough to produce the effect desired. The concentration and persistence of the drug in these fluids depend upon its absorption, distribution, metabolism and clearance. All these processes involve the passage of the drug across various cell membrances.

TRANSPORT OF DRUGS ACROSS MEMBRANES

There are three main ways by which substances can cross the cell membrane: by simple diffusion, by passage through pores in the membrane, or by means of a specific mechanism. The first of these is the commonest for drugs. This is because the majority of drugs

1

are weak organic electrolytes and in the body are present as ionised and non-ionised molecules. The non-ionised molecules are lipid soluble, whereas the ionised molecules are insoluble in lipids. The cell membrane acts like a lipid membrane and since only the non-ionised molecules are soluble in lipids it follows that the non-ionised molecules will dissolve most readily in the lipids of the cell wall. Thus they will penetrate the cell membrane. Hence the rate at which most drugs penetrate a biological membrane depends principally on two physical factors; firstly the solubility of the non-ionised drug molecules in lipids, and secondly, the degree of ionisation of the parent drug.

There are small areas in the membrane which are hydrophilic. These areas or 'pores' are not simple tubes and vary in radius for different tissues. The pore radius in rat intestine will allow the passage of water and urea but not mannitol, whereas molecules up to the size of albumin can pass through pores in the glomerular capillaries. Passage through these channels is called filtration and involves the flow of water due to osmotic, hydrostatic or concentration gradients across the membrane. This mechanism, namely, filtration is commonly responsible for the transport of many small, water soluble, polar and non-polar substances.

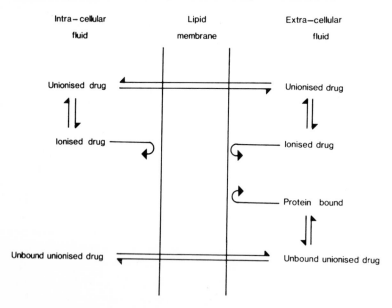

Fig. 1.1 A diagrammatic representation of various factors affecting the passage of drugs across biological membranes.

Specialised transport mechanisms are usually involved in the transfer of large, lipid insoluble, or ionised molecules across the cell membrane. This type of transport is thought to involve a part of the membrane which acts as a carrier by binding the molecule which is to be transported. The carrier transported molecule complex diffuses from one side of the membrane to the other where it releases the transported molecule and the carrier returns to its original site. Each cell appears to have a large number of specific carrier systems of which there appears to be two main types. A carrier system which operates along the concentration gradient is termed facilitated diffusion. The other type of carrier system is referred to as active transport which, in addition to the characteristics of a carrier mediated system, is capable of moving a molecule against a concentration gradient. This latter process requires energy and is inhibited by substances which interfere with energy production.

Absorption

The absorption of a drug refers to the rate and completeness with which it enters the body from the site of administration. It depends not only on the drug itself and on the factors already mentioned but also on the route by which the drug is given. The absorption of the drug depends on its solubility in water. Drugs in aqeuous solution are absorbed more quickly than those given in oil, as suspensions or as solid implants. In veterinary practice it is often convenient to give drugs by subcutaneous or intramuscular injection. Absorption from these sites varies from a few minutes in the case of substances like morphine and atropine to several weeks for the anabolic steroid trembolone. The amount and condition of connective tissue at the site and the capillary flow influence absorption, another important factor is the area of absorbing surface to which the drug is exposed. An example of the latter is shown by the fact that drugs are rapidly absorbed from large absorptive areas such as the intestinal mucosa and pulmonary endothelium. Absorption from an intramuscular injection is usually more rapid than from a subcutaneous injection, and the former route is preferred for the injection of substances which are slightly irritant and might cause pain. However, the subcutaneous space being much greater in the domesticated animals than in man allows greater volumes of fluid to be injected in these species subcutaneously without causing undue discomfort. This route can only be used for drugs which do not cause irritation otherwise a slough may be produced. The addition of Hyaluronidase to the solution injected increases absorption by increasing permeation of the connecting tissue, whereas the addition of adrenaline increases the local action of the injection by diminishing its absorption and does this by causing vaso-constriction. Trauma at the site of injection may decrease the rate of capillary flow and thus decrease absorption by releasing substances such as histamine and 5-hydroxytryptamine.

As a general rule drugs are not absorbed from the stomach although the epithelium of the rumen is permeable to many substances. The absorption of drugs given by mouth does not usually begin until they pass the pyloric sphincter. This is because the acid conditions in the stomach cause most drugs which are bases to ionise and as the ionised drug is insoluble in lipids it does not enter the cell wall. However, a lipid soluble non-electrolyte such as ethanol is rapidly absorbed through the gastric mucous-membrane. Drugs which are weak acids such as the salicylates and barbiturates which are mainly non-ionised in the gastric contents are absorbed from the stomach.

The activity of the stomach can greatly influence the rate of absorption. The quickest passage through the stomach in simple stomached animals occurs when this organ is empty and the drug given in a large volume of water. Absorption is delayed when a drug is given in a small volume of water and the stomach is full. Drugs given in a large volume of water when the stomach is full may be absorbed fairly quickly as under these conditions the fluid may pass along the lesser curvature into the duodenum and not mix with the food mass in the stomach. There is some evidence that the removal of calcium ions by the administration of a chelating agent can affect the absorption of drugs from the intestine.

The absorption of drugs given by mouth to the ruminant presents a special problem. Certain drugs such as atropine can be absorbed through the rumen epithelium, although most substances given by this route are diluted in the large volume of rumen liquor and slowly passed through the abomasum and into the intestine. It may take forty-eight hours for a single dose of a drug to leave the rumen. It is usual to give by mouth to ruminants only those drugs which are required to act within the alimentary tract, such as drugs to change the surface tension of the rumen liquor or to kill parasites in the gastro-intestinal tract.

Absorption time is reduced to a minimum when drugs are given by intravenous injections. This route is chosen therefore, when an immediate effect is desired as when certain anæsthetic agents are

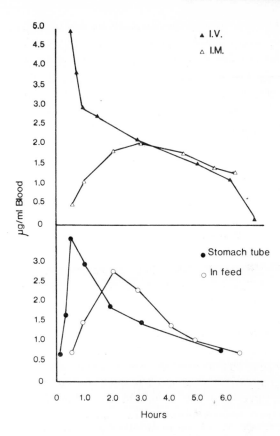

Fig. 1.2 The concentration in blood of the anti-bacterial trimethroprim after intravenous (I.V.), intramuscular (I.M.) injection, administration by stomach tube and in the feed to a pony.

given. The intravenous route also allows drugs which are irritant and therefore cannot be given subcutaneously to be administered parenterally with safety. It is essential when administering such a substance to take every precaution to ensure that none of the solution containing the drug is allowed to leak around the vein.

Volatile agents such as the various gaseous anæsthetics are usually given by inhalation. Absorption from the lungs of a volatile drug is very rapid due both to the large absorptive surface available and the good blood flow through the lungs. Drugs may also be given by local application or inserted in a suitable form into the rectum or vagina. These routes are usually employed when a local effect is desired although a few agents are absorbed systemically from these various local applications. Lipid soluble substances are more readily absorbed through the skin than are ions and lipid-insoluble substances. Skin damage increases the permeation of foreign substances through the skin, moreover, the permeability of skin varies in different areas. The thin skin over the medial aspect of the thigh is an example of a good absorptive surface. There are also differences between species in absorption through the skin.

The distribution of drugs in the body

After absorption most substances diffuse through the various fluid compartments of the body. Some drugs cannot penetrate certain cell membranes and are therefore restricted in distribution, whereas others can pass freely into all the fluid compartments. Some drugs bind to plasma or tissue proteins such as phenylbutazone, others like thiopentone enter and remain in the fat depots. Binding to plasma protein delays the entry of the drug to other tissues and the persistence in fat depots may prolong the action of a drug.

In the main drugs are distributed as follows: (a) through the extracellular fluid, i.e. bromides, thiocyanate, and iodides; (b) through the whole of the body water, i.e. urea, antipyrine; (c) fixed by cells, i.e. digitalis. Sometimes there is an obvious relationship between the distribution of a drug and its site of action, as for example, the initial high concentration of thiopentone in the brain when this barbiturate is injected intravenously.

The apparent volume of distribution of a substance can be determined by dividing the total amount of drug in the body by the concentration in the plasma. This volume may or may not correspond to an actual compartment of the body to which the drug is confined, but in the case of substances such as thiocyanate, antipyrine and plasma albumin labelled either with a dye such as Evan's blue or with radio-active iodine give values which are almost equal to the extracellular fluid volume, the total body water and the plasma volume respectively.

Drug distribute between depot-fat and extracellular water in accordance with their fat/water partition coefficient. The poor blood supply to fat causes equilibrium between the fat and blood to proceed slowly, however, once a substance has entered the depot-fat it usually persists for a long period, the insecticide dicophane, for example, can persist in the body fat for several months. A high apparent volume of distribution is often associated with a persistent action. The volatile anæsthetic methoxyfluorane which is well-known for its persistent effect has a high volume of distribution because it persists in the fat depots.

Some drugs may accumulate in various regions as a result of their dissolving in fat or binding with protein. A drug when bound to a protein cannot cross biological membranes and its pharmacological effects are reduced or abolished. Of the body proteins which bind drugs plasma albumin does so the most readily, however, the extent of this binding varies with different species, it is reversible and may be altered by hormones. The differing affinities of plasma proteins of different species may account for differences in rates of absorption, metabolism and excretion. Drugs which are bound to plasma proteins may be displaced from their binding sites by other drugs which are more strongly bound. This may have important practical consequences, for example anticoagulants such as coumarin may be displaced from plasma protein by phenylbutazone, and animals which have ingested a coumarin develop haemorrhages after phenylbutazone administration.

In general compounds which pass freely through cell membranes and enter cells pass into the brain and cerebrospinal fluid, whereas compounds which are confined to the extracellular fluid or other peripheral tissue do not enter the brain and cerebro-spinal fluid. Similarly many drugs cross the placenta by simple diffusion. It is clearly important to know whether a drug enters the brain and cerebro-spinal fluid when treating disease involving these regions, and likewise to know whether or not a drug given to the mother could enter and affect the foetus.

A popular concept of the fate in the body of a drug is the so-called two compartment model. This is shown diagramatically in

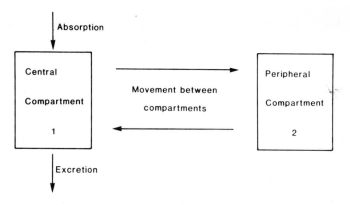

Fig. 1.3 A diagrammatic representation of the two compartment model.

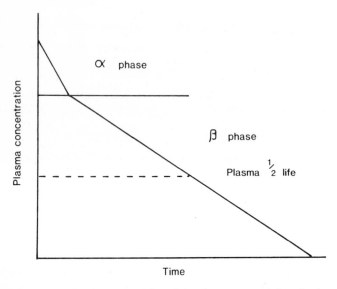

Fig. 1.4 A diagrammatic representation of the plasma concentration of a drug plotted on a semi-logarithmic scale showing the α and β phases and plasma half-life.

Figure 1.3. The concentration of the drug at a point midway down the second line is termed the plasma half-life and often represents a convenient way of comparing the rate of clearance of various drugs. This is shown in Figure 1.4.

In the two compartment model the concentration of the drug in plasma if plotted on a semi-logarithmic scale can be represented by two straight lines, the initial one being relatively short and steeply sloping and the second one a longer more gradual slope. The first line represents the mixing and initial distribution of the drug and the second line the effect on the concentration of metabolism and excretion. The concentration of the drug at a point midway down the second line is termed the plasma half-life and often represents a convenient way of comparing the rate clearance of various drugs.

Clearance of drugs

Drugs are removed from the body either unchanged or after conversion into some other substance. These conversions usually take place in the liver. The kidney and intestinal epithelium can also metabolise drugs. The unchanged drug or its metabolites usually are excreted by the kidneys, although volatile substances are excreted largely through the lungs. The bile is an excretory route for some substances, but not a very efficient one as many of these substances are re-absorbed from the small intestine. This is especially the case when the drugs are excreted as glucuronides since the intestinal bacteria produce an enzyme glucuronidase which hydrolyses the glucuronide freeing the unconjugated compound which may then be reabsorbed. A few drugs are excreted by the alimentary tract.

In most cases the removal of a drug from the body resembles a 'wash out' process. That is a constant proportion of the drug is removed in a unit of time, a similar process to washing out a bucket full of a dye by allowing water from a tap to run into the bucket and the coloured liquid to overflow. It is also called exponential clearance. An example of this is shown in Figure 1.5.

Excretion through the kidney involves three processes; a passive filtration through the glomerulus, active secretion in the tubules and passive diffusion in the tubules. The amount of drug entering the tubules in the glomerular filtrate depends not only on the rate of filtration but also on the degree of protein binding of the drug. Lipid soluble un-ionised molecules which pass in the glomerular filtrate are largely reabsorbed in the renal tubules although such molecules can pass either way through the renal tubular epithelium.

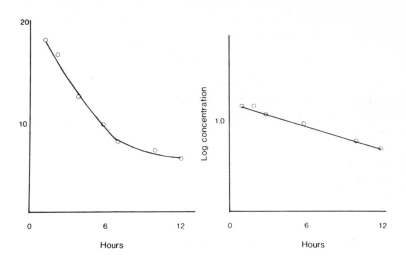

Fig. 1.5 The concentration of sulphanilamide in blood following the intravenous injection of 160 mg/kg to a sheep, plotted on an arithmetic and a semi-logarithmic scale; the linear nature of the latter curve shows the exponential form of the clearance.

When ionisation is increased, as in the case of basic drugs being excreted in an acidic urine, tubular reabsorption is diminished and more of the drug excreted in the urine. Similarly acidic drugs in an alkaline urine undergo greater ionisation and are thus less reabsorbed and more is excreted in the urine. Some drugs are actively secreted by the renal tubules even when ionised. The anion benzyl penicillin and the cation hexamethonium are examples. There is evidence of competition for secretion between various anions. The bound drug is not filtered at the glomerulus.

The excretion of drugs in milk

This route of excretion has both therapeutic and public health importance. The principles of excretion through the mammary gland are similar to those acting in the kidney, namely the diffusion of unionised lipid soluble forms of the drug diffusing through the epithelial cells of the gland. The pH of plasma and milk are important factors. Reabsorption of the unionised drug and the active secretion of drugs through the duct of the mammary gland may both occur. Since milk is usually more acidic than plasma the basic compound may be slightly more concentrated and acidic compounds less concentrated in milk than plasma. Various non-electrolytes, for example, ethanol, readily enter milk and quickly reach the same concentration as the plasma regardless of pH. Certain drugs may enter eggs and can cause taint.

Biotransformation

This term is applied to the changes which a drug undergoes within the body after absorption. These changes commonly take part in two stages. The primary stage involves reactions such as oxidation, reduction, hydrolysis, alkalation, dehalogenation etc. The second stage involves conjugation of, for example, the products of oxidation, reduction, etc. The main conjugates are with glucuronic or sulphuric acids. A few compounds are converted to their acetylate.

The principal reactions involved in biotransformation are (1) **combination with sulphuric acid**, for example phenol; (2) **combination with glucuronic acid**, for example steroid compounds; (3) **oxidation**, this is carried out by a group of enzymes which appear to be situated in the microsomes of the liver. These oxidations usually involve hydroxylation reactions; the enzymes responsible being termed hydroxylases, NADPH being an essential co-factor. Certain oxidations take place by dehydrogenation, for example ethyl alcohol is oxidised in the first instance to acetaldehyde by ethanol dehydrogenase; (4) **reduction**, for example, chloral hydrate, which is reduced to trichlorethanol. This latter compound is the substance to which choloral hydrate owes its pharmacological activity; (5) **alkylation**, the transfer of alkyl (methyl or ethyl) groups. This transformation occurs with a number of pharmacologically active substances, such as adrenaline, noradrenaline and histamine; (6) **acetylation**, certain drugs with an amino group such as sulphanilamide are acetylated by some species; (7) **dehalogenation**, this transformation occurs with a number of halogenated hydrocarbons, such as certain insecticides; (8) **hydrolysis**, a number of drugs such as procaine and various choline esters are de-esterified by esterases which are widespread in the body. Although the plasma esterases of different species are similar they may not be identical. In man, procaine is hydrolysed by a plasma esterase whereas in the horse procaine is excreted unchanged in urine.

In the main, biotransformation reactions transform the drug into a form which is more readily excreted. For example, by forming a glucuronide a drug is usually made more water soluble, hence when the glucuronide passes through the renal tubules it is less likely to be re-absorbed by entering the lipid membranes of the tubular epithelial cells whereas the more fat soluble parent compound would be absorbed at this site. The oxidation of ethanol ultimately results in the transformation of ethanol into carbon dioxide and water, substances which can be completely removed from the body, one being expired through the lungs and the other being excreted in the urine.

Species differences in biotransformations

The way in which various drugs are metabolised varies in a number of important ways in the various domesticated species. These differences are unpredictable although there are certain generalisations which can be made. **The horse** appears to be provided with a large number of enzymes capable of rapidly metabolising a large number of drugs. For example, the equine liver is a rich source of ethanol dehydrogenase. The enzymes involved in oxidising barbiturates are so efficient in the horse that pentobarbitone has a duration of action similar to that of thiopentone despite the fact that pentobarbitone is metabolised by oxidation and the action of thiopentone termined by redistribution. On the other hand, procaine which in most species is metabolised by an esterase is excreted unchanged in the urine of the horse. Chloral hydrate, a once widely used hypnotic in equine practice, only shows its characteristic action when reduced to tri-chlorethanol. The horse carries out this conversion so rapidly that when given by stomach tube the drug is converted almost as quickly as it is absorbed.

Ruminants resemble the horse in their ability to metabolise a large number of drugs. Evidence of the importance of the liver in these metabolic processes has been obtained by damaging the liver with carbon tetrachloride. A sheep with a liver thus damaged and subsequently given pentobarbitone has a greatly prolonged sleeping time produced by the administration of this drug.

Differences in the way in which species metabolise drugs can be extremely important in both toxicology and therapeutics. An important industrial chemical 2-naphthylamine causes bladder tumours in man and dogs but not in rats. The explanation of this difference lies in the fact that the carcinogen is a metabolite of 2-naphthylamine formed by man and dog whereas the rat does not form this metabolite and hence does not develop tumours. The insecticide malathion is very toxic to insects but not to mammals. Malathion itself is relatively inactive but owes its insecticidal activity to an oxidation product malaoxon. Mammals posses an esterase which can hydrolyse malathion so rapidly that it is unable to be oxidised to malaoxon, whereas insects are deficient in this esterase.

The dog appears to be unusual amongst the domesticated animals in lacking an acetylating enzyme. This is particularly noticable after the administration of a sulphonamide, a drug which is normally acetylated on the free amino group removing the antibacterial activity from the compound. Unfortunately, the lack of an acetylase makes some compounds more toxic to the dog than other species as although it lacks the acetylase it retains the power to deacetylate compounds and some drugs form a toxic compound on de-acetylation.

The cat is noteworthy in being deficient in gluconide synthesizing mechanisms, i.e., glucuronyl transferase, and a great number of drugs which are excreted as the glucuronide in most species cannot be thus treated by the cat. The cat also lacks various oxidases and many drugs metabolised by this mechanism tend to be cumulative and thus potentially toxic in the cat.

In general the young of most mammalian species lack drug metabolising enzymes. A good example of this is illustrated in the calf which if given enough pentobarbitone to produce sleep is unlikely to awaken whereas the adult cow is given a similar dose will recover in about 60 minutes.

The avian species in general have lower levels of drug oxidising enzymes than mammals. However, there are marked differences between the drug metabolising activity of the various domesticated species. Demethylase activity appears to be lower in the liver of the duck than in the turkey or chicken or goose. Moreover, geese do not appear to form glucuronides lacking glucuronyl transferase activity. Similarly, chickens have low glucuronyl transferase and high sulphate conjugating enzymes. The turkey has high activity of both glucuronyl transferase and sulphate conjugation. Both transformations take place in the liver.

In contrast to mammals conjugation with sulphuric and glucuronic acid appears to take place more readily in chickens and goslings than in mature birds of the same species. The general use of mass medication of birds to control diseases caused by mycoplasma and coccidia makes it essential to have pharmacokinetic studies and in particular work on drug metabolism carried out on the actual species to which the drugs are given.

Soon after the introduction of the sulphonamides it was shown that when the concentration of sulphonamide in plasma fell below a certain level there was no chemotherapeutic activity. This observation was important because it was the first occasion when the dosage of a drug was placed on a firm basis being correlated with the amount required to maintain the plasma concentration at a level adequate for therapeutic activity. It is, of course, only drugs which are distributed fairly uniformly throughout one of the fluid compartments of the body that such a correlation is possible. Sometimes it is possible to explain differences in the activity of a drug between different species in terms of the plasma concentration, lack of activity being associated with plasma levels too low to produce the requisite effect.

There are marked species differences in the extent of the biliary excretion of drugs. In general the dog and hen are capable of excreting a substantial proportion of certain drugs via the bile, the cat and sheep less, and the rabbit and guinea-pig very little.

Fish seem to lack the enzymes producing conjugates with glucuronic and sulphuric acid and are very susceptible to poisoning by a wide range of chemicals. This factor is especially important in consideration of effluent disposal and can give rise to poisoning in fish eating species including man. Cases of mercury poisoning in man have resulted from fish exposed to mercury in an industrial effluent being converted by micro-organisms into methyl mercury which is fat soluble. The micro-organisms when ingested by the fish permit the fish to absorb the methyl mercury which is not metabolised but stored in fat depots until ingested by another species such as man in which it causes toxic effects.

Insects do not appear to form glucuronides but form glucosides. These conjugates are presumably better adapted to the insects internal environment than the very acidic glucuronides.

Cumulation

Drugs which are slowly excreted or slowly detoxicated tend to accumulate in the body. When such substances are given at frequent intervals the amount retained in the body may be sufficient to produce signs of poisoning. This process is called cumulation.

A cumulative effect can be avoided by adjusting the maintenance dose so as to balance the rate at which the drug is inactivated or excreted.

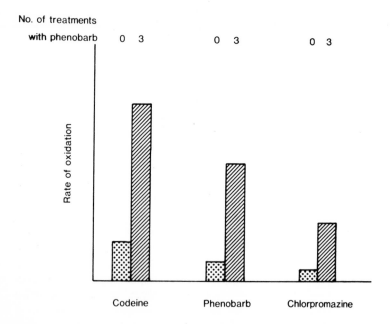

Fig. 1.6 The effect of prior treatment of phenobarbitone on the oxydation of codeine, phenobarbitone and chlorpromazine in rats. The shaded columns show the effects of three prior administrations of phenobarbitone.

Tolerance

This may be described as the state in which increasing doses are required to produce the same pharmacological or therapeutic effect. Sometimes by administering one drug, the animal becomes tolerant to a second drug; this is referred to as cross-tolerance. Although there is no ready explanation of this condition, some facts are available which may partly account for the phenomenon. It is known, for example, that prior treatment with phenobarbitone has an effect on the liver microsomes so that their oxidative enzyme activity is increased causing subsequent doses of phenobarbitone to be metabolised at an increasing rate. This increased metabolism affects not only phenobarbitone but other drugs which are metabolised by these oxidative enzymes. This is illustrated diagramatically in Figure 1.6. **Idiosyncrasy** to a drug may be said to exist when the response of an individual animal to a single dose of the drug produces an unexpected or untoward effect.

Antagonism

It is generally assumed that the specificity of activity shown by many drugs is due to their attachment to specific sites on the cells of the tissues affected. These specific sites are termed RECEPTORS. When the interaction between the drug and receptor produces activity the drug is termed an AGONIST. A drug which occupies the receptor without causing activity but denies its occupation by an agonist thus preventing the action of the agonist is called an *antagonist*. The attachment between drug and receptor depends on a variety of forces such as hydrogen bonds, hydrophobic bonds, Van der Waals forces and, exceptionally, ionic bonds. The attachment between drug and receptor is usually reversible and since ionic bonding is very strong such bonds must be rare in drug receptor attachments.

The characteristic property of receptors is their specificity. Sometimes the interaction between agonist and antagonist can be expressed by a mathematical relationship based on the assumption that agonists and antagonists compete for their recpetors in accordance with the law of mass action. This type of antagonism is called COMPETITIVE.

Antagonists can be used to classify drugs, for example, if two agonists can occupy the same receptor they should be antagonised by the same competitive antagonist. Receptors can be identified by the use of appropriate antagonists, for example, muscarinic receptors are antagonised by atropine. A competitive antagonist will produce a log dose/response curve which is parallel to the log dose/response curve produced by the agonist in the absence of the antagonist.

Some antagonists produce non-parallel log dose/response curves. This type of antagonism is called unsurmountable. Another type of antagonism is produced by drugs which have opposite actions. A drug may, for example, contract a certain plain muscle whereas another may cause the same muscle to relax. These drugs given together would be antagonistic. This is termed physiological antagonism.

Summation

This is the addition of the effect of one drug to that of one or more other drugs with similar properties, as for example, in certain mixtures of sulphonamides.

Synergism

This is a term applied to the combined action of two drugs with similar pharmacological properties, when the effect produced is greater than the sum of the effect of each drug given singly. For example, both the sulphonamides and trimethoprim have antibacterial actions, which when given together produce a much greater effect than when an equiactive dose of either drug is given separately.

Enzyme induction

When certain drugs are administered repeatedly this has the effect of increasing the activity of oxidising enzymes associated with the liver microsomes. A consequence of this increased activity of oxidases is a decrease in the activity of drugs metabolised by these enzymes. This property of increasing the activity of oxidising enzymes is usually called the enzyme inducing activity. Drugs with this property include phenobarbitone, and the insecticide dicothane. This is illustrated in Figure 1.6.

Potentiation

This is a termed applied to the enhancement of the action of one drug by another with dissimilar properties, for example, the action of of penicillin can be prolonged when probenecid is given either before or along with the penicillin. Probenecid delays the urinary excretion of penicillin.

Knowledge of a drug's absorption, distribution, metabolism and clearance are essential for the veterinary surgeon to decide by which route and how often he will need to give the substance.

SUGGESTIONS FOR FURTHER READING

Albert A 1979 Selective toxicity. London, Chapman & Hall
Brodie B B, Gillett J R 1971 Concepts on biochemical pharmacology. Handb. Exp. Pharmak. vol. XXVIII/2
Csaky T Z 1969 General pharmacology. London, Butterworths
Eneanya D I, Bianchine J R, Duran D O, Andresen B D 1981 Pharmacokinetics, drug absorption and excretion. Annual Review of Pharmacology and Toxicology 21: 31
Mandel H G, WayE L 1972 Fundamentals of drug metabolism and drug disposition. Baltimore, Williams & Wilkins
Smolen V F 1978 Bioavailability and pharmacokinetic analysis of drug responding systems. Annual Review of Pharmacology and Toxicology 18: 495–522

2

Inorganic ions affecting excitable tissues.

The principal ions involved in excitation of tissues are Na^+, K^+, Ca^{2+} and Mg^{2+}.

SODIUM AND POTASSIUM

As described in the next chapter, for probably historical reasons living tissues have a high K^+ concentration in cellular fluid and a high Na^+ in extracellular fluid. This assymmetric distribution of ions requires the expenditure of energy, and is brought about primarily by the action of specific ion 'pumps' sited in or near the cell membrane. These pumps are proteins which utilise energy from the breakdown of ATP to force Na^+ ions outwards and K^+ ions inwards across the membrane; these two processes are linked, so there is at this stage no nett charge distribution. The pumps are automatic and are actuated by the presence of Na^+ inside or K^+ outside the cell membrane. Another way of describing the process is to refer to these proteins as enzymes degrading ATP which, since they are activated by Na^+ and K^+, may be designated Na, K-ATPases; however it should be clear that the mere breaking down of ATP is not of itself particularly useful, and that this is something of a functional misrepresentation of the process.

The bulk of the cell membrane, being lipoid in nature, is not very permeable to charged particles, but there are specialised areas which in certain circumstances become highly permeable to ions, and these are referred to as 'channels'. The opening and closing of these channels may be due to changes in orientation of electrical dipoles in the membrane. In a tissue, such as nerve or muscle, at equilibrium the rate of pumping of Na^+ and K^+ is balanced by leakage of these ions down the concentration gradients thus created, and the cellular fluid concentrations are approximately Na^+ 10 mmol/l, K^+ 150 mmol/l, compared with their extracellular concentrations of 140 and 4 mmol/l respectively. In its resting state the cell membrane is much more permeable to K^+ than to Na^+; the consequent diffusion of K^+ out of the cell is therefore not accompanied by a complementary influx of Na^+, and there is thus a nett movement of positively charged particles out of the cell. The resultant potential difference across the membrane builds up until the electrical repulsion experienced by a migrating K^+ ion balances the diffusion pressure on it. This equilibrium between the chemical (potassium) gradient outwards and the positive electrical charge gradient inwards is described by the Nernst equation:

$$E = \frac{RT}{F} \ln \frac{[K^+] \text{ inside}}{[K^+] \text{ outside}}$$

R (the gas constant), T (the absolute temperature) and F (the Faraday) are all approximately constant in physiological systems, so the equation simply describes the potential difference (E) across the membrane at equilibrium as being logarithmically proportional to the ratio of K^+ concentrations on each side of it. By convention the resting potential is expressed as the inside relative to the outside; in nerve and muscle it is typically around -60 to -90 mV.

This resting potential is important in nerve and muscle cells as it provides the basis of the main means of communication between cells, and between the surface of a cell and its interior. A reduction in the potential difference which is sufficiently sudden and sufficiently large causes a rapidly developing increase in $Na+$ permeability due to the activation of Na^+-specific channels in the membrane, which results in a massive depolarisation or even a transient reversal of polarisation, since both the electrical and chemical gradients for sodium favour its inward movement. Depolarisation of the membrane also triggers the inactivation of the Na^+-specific channels and the activation of K^+-specific channels; both these processes are slower in onset and decay than the Na^+ channel activation, and between them they are largely responsible for the recovery of the resting potential and the subsequent refractory period. Meanwhile the earlier inward Na^+-current has caused the depolarisation of adjacent areas of membrane, leading to the propagation of the action potential over the entire cell surface.

It is an important property of this system that the channel inactivating processes are consequent upon membrane depolarisation itself, and do not require the passage of an action potential; if the initial depolarisation is too slow, activation does not sufficiently outstrip inactivation, and there is no action potential (a phenomenon known as 'accommodation').

Thus an increase in the resting potential (becoming more negative, moving away from the threshold potential) reduces the ease of initiation of an action potential but increases its effect once it is started; conversely small reductions in resting potential may increase the likelihood of initiating an action potential but larger reductions tend to diminish the excitability of the membrane.

Evidently changes in the external concentration of either Na^+ or K^+ will influence this series of events, but the effects of changes in K^+ concentration are of considerably greater practical importance. In the first place, as suggested above the effect on the resting potential is much more direct. Secondly, regulation of K^+ is much less well organised than that of Na^+, so that larger fluctuations may occur. Finally the amount of K^+ involved in a given proportional change is much smaller since the extracellular concentration is so much lower. Large reductions in resting potential of heart muscle (and hence in excitability and force of contraction) may follow the misguided administration of Darrow's solution, or K^+ release from traumatised tissue.

Despite the importance of Na^+ and K^+ balance to the excitability of cell membranes, the control of sodium and potassium is largely bound up with the control of extracellular fluid volume and distribution. Consideration of the factors influencing sodium and potassium metabolism is therefore deferred to the following two chapters.

CALCIUM

Calcium, in the form of the hydrated phosphate, hydroxyapatite, is the main component of the skeleton, and constitutes approximately 20% of the body dry weight and 99.9% of the total body calcium.

The vast majority of this calcium is unavailable to the rest of the body, and can largely be disregarded in a consideration of the physiology and pharmacology of calcium in normal animals, where the main control of calcium homeostasis is now thought to be exerted through the processes of absorption and excretion.

Calcium is mostly absorbed from the proximal small intestine; if large amounts of soluble calcium are present in the lumen, absorption approximates to simple diffusion, but at low dietary levels free ions are complexed near the mucosal surface and transported across the cell by a specific calcium-binding protein. The synthesis of this carrier, and hence the extent of active calcium absorption, is stimulated by metabolites of vitamin D. Absorption may be inhibited by any reduction in the luminal free ion activity. Alkaline pHs tend to cause precipitation of calcium salts, especially as carbonates and fatty acid soaps. Dietary constituents such as phytic acid may also precipitate calcium. The situation is complicated, particularly in herbivores, by the fact that from the terminal ileum onwards there is a nett movement of calcium into the gut lumen; in the horse half the total calcium efflux from the body occurs by this route. Its exact significance in calcium homeostasis is uncertain since much of it is strongly complexed to mucus and other components of the faecal mass, and may better be described as trapped than as excreted.

Controlled excretion of calcium occurs, as the major route of loss in small animals, by glomerular filtration of diffusible plasma calcium and modulation of the subsequent tubular reabsorption of the ionic fraction.

The physiological states and functions of calcium

It is generally held that metals exert biological effects by forming compounds or complexes with larger organic molecules, that insofar as these molecules are selective for particular metals they may be regarded as receptors, and that the reactive form of the metal in these processes is the free ion. In the case of sodium and potassium this last tenet does not appear to introduce any serious complications since they are mostly present in solution as free ions and their activity coefficents are around 0.9. Calcium, probably because of its double charge, is much more affected by the ionic strength of the solution. In physiological media the activity coefficient of a free ionic solution of calcium is only about 0.35; the influence of the solution's ionic strength on the *effective* concentration of Ca^{2+} (in both functional and analytical contexts) is thus considerable.

In extracellular fluid, the free Ca^{2+} coexists with a small amount of calcium which is complexed to low molecular weight compounds such as citrate, lactate and bicarbonate. Both ionic and complexed calcium diffuse freely through capillary membranes, and the concentration of this diffusible fraction, about 1.6 mmol/l, is the same in interstitial fluid and plasma. Plasma, however, contains a further fraction which is bound to plasma proteins, chiefly albumin. This normally amounts to some 0.9 mmol/l, making the total concentration up to the well known figure of 2.5 mmol/l (10 mg/dl), but the binding is very labile, and the amount of calcium in this category is heavily dependent on the concentrations of competing species, including CO_2, H^+ and Mg^{2+}, as well as the concentrations of free Ca^{2+} and protein. Since the control of plasma calcium level is exerted only on the active Ca^{2+} fraction, it should not be surprising that, on close inspection, plasma total calcium levels are by no means constant, and often fluctuate by as much as $\pm10\%$ from hour to hour.

The calcium activity at the surface of the cell is important since calcium is involved in membrane permeability changes (as it is in almost every phase of tissue excitation and response). The Na^+ and K^+ permeability changes occurring during membrane activation are reduced at high levels of Ca^{2+}; this has been explained by postulating that calcium combines with the negatively charged sites of the channel-controlling dipoles, locking them in their closed configurations. Conversely at low Ca^{2+} activities, Na^+ permeability in particular tends to increase, thus destabilising the membrane. These effects are often manifested as a raising or lowering of the excitation threshold of the tissue.

This five-fold reduction of the total 2.5 mmol/l in plasma to the approximately 0.5 mmol/l at the external surface of the cell is as nothing compared with the complex distribution and sequestration of calcium within the cell. The total calcium concentration in most tissues is not very different from that of extracellular fluid: the Ca^{2+} activity of the cytosol, on the other hand, is well below 1 micromol/l. There is thus at least a thousand-fold functional gradient across the cell membrane. In many (perhaps even all) cells changes in activity are mediated by changes in intracellular Ca^{2+} activity. Examples include the activation of phosphorylase, and hence of glycolysis, in hepatocytes by glucagon, the activation of osteoclasts by parathyroid hormone, amylase secretion by the exocrine pancreas, and the endocrine secretory activities of the pancreas, pituitary (both parts) and adrenal medulla. Of particular interest is the fact that calcium is similarly involved in the release of peripheral neurotransmitters, and in excitation–contraction coupling in muscle cells.

In all these cells Ca^{2+} appears to enter the cell during its activation through Ca^{2+}-selective channels which are different from the previously described Na^+-channels. In cardiac tissue and vascular smooth muscle, for instance, they are activated by beta-adrenergic drugs and inhibited by beta-adrenoceptor blocking drugs such as propranolol, and by 'calcium-antagonists' such as verapamil and nifedipine. The use of these drugs reveals that in cardiac pacemaking and conducting elements Ca^{2+} influx also forms a major part of the subsequent membrane depolarising current.

In most cases examined so far Ca^{2+} exerts its intracellular effects by combining with a specific binding protein, called calmodulin, which then triggers the change in the cell's activity. Skeletal muscle is exceptional in that the large majority of the rise in intracellular Ca^{2+} activity is due not to the influx of Ca^{2+} but to its release from the sarcoplasmic reticulum; furthermore the released Ca^{2+} combines with a different (but very similar) binding protein called troponin-c. Cardiac muscle is intermediate in that approximately half of the Ca^{2+} involved in its contraction is of external origin, and half is released from internal stores. Myocardial contractility is thus reduced by calcium-channel antagonists, or by low external Ca^{2+} activity (although, as we have seen, in this latter case the excitability of the membrane is increased).

Milk fever

Milk fever is generally accepted as being primarily due to hypocalcaemia. The plasma calcium levels of most domestic animals fall during the last third of pregnancy, usually by about 10–15%. In animals bred for milk production, particularly the dairy cow, there is an additional fall at the end of pregnancy associated with the onset of lactation. This seems mostly to be due to impairment of absorption from the gut and of mobilisation from reserves (probably skeletal). The exact reasons for these phenomena are not clear; the various hormonal mechanisms influencing calcium metabolism discussed below have all been implicated at one time or another, but in no case has a causative role been unequivocally demonstrated. That the cause of milk fever is not straightforward may be inferred from the fact that neither the plasma calcium level nor that of any of these hormones can be used reliably to predict the occurrence of the clinical condition.

In most cases there is a brief phase of excitement, with tetany and muscle tremor, which is probably due to the the effects of low external Ca^{2+} concentration on nerve and muscle membranes. If the plasma magnesium level is normal the falling calcium level may lead to a *relative* hypermagnesaemia; this exacerbates the hypocalcaemic failure of transmitter release at the skeletal neuromuscular junction and results in flaccid paresis. If, however, there is concomitant *hypo*magnesaemia the excitable phase may be prolonged. The hypocalcaemia also causes reductions in tone and contractility of the myocardium, as well as vascular and uterine smooth muscle. Milk fever is usually treated by administering calcium, but there is an increasing tendency to attempt dietary and hormonal prophylactic therapy in susceptible animals or herds.

Preparations of calcium

A number of common calcium compounds are insoluble in water, and this causes problems in formulating calcium for parenteral administration.

Calcium carbonate in the form of powdered limestone is very cheap and is often used for fortifying concentrates and feed additives. The calcium content is absorbed to only a very limited extent.

Calcium chloride is a highly soluble salt, indeed its deliquescence makes it rather awkward to handle. Its repulsive taste and high degree of tissue irritancy make it difficult to administer but it has been tried, dispersed in a hydroxyethylcellulose gel, as an oral prophylactic treatment of milk fever. **Calcium lactate** is also soluble, and is much more palatable as an oral preparation for small animals.

Calcium gluconate and **calcium borogluconate** are the commonest compounds of calcium for parental use. The gluconate is used in human medicine, but calcium borogluconate, prepared by dissolving boric acid in a solution of calcium gluconate, has been preferred in veterinary practice because of the greater stability of its solutions. It has been shown to be a distinct chemical compound, and it possesses chemical properties distinctly different from those of calcium gluconate, including a much greater tendency to form non-ionised calcium complexes in solution. It is thus slightly unfortunate that the *British Pharmacopoeia* (*Veterinary*) 1977 should state 'Calcium Borogluconate Injection, BP (Vet) contains calcium gluconate'. Calcium borogluconate is almost tasteless and is only slightly irritant. It only dissolves in water to any extent on heating, but the resulting solution is stable on cooling. It is usually administered to cattle as a 40% solution, containing 3% (w/v) calcium, either intravenously, in emergencies, or subcutaneously. Because of the cardiac effects of calcium intravenous injections should be given carefully and slowly. For smaller animals a 20% solution of calcium borogluconate is preferable. Various cocktails containing magnesium and phosphate as well are available if deficiencies of these are encountered or suspected.

Hormonal control of calcium metabolism

Calcium metabolism is specifically controlled in three respects: absorption from the gut, excretion or reabsorption in the urine and resorption or accretion in bone. These controls are exerted by three main hormone systems: parathyroid hormone, vitamin D and calcitonin; of these calcitonin is the most recently discovered and, paradoxically, apparently the least complex and important.

Calcitonin is a peptide produced by the C-cells of the thyroid gland (embryologically derived from ultimobranchial tissue); the main stimulus for its secretion is a rise in plasma Ca^{2+} activity. Its function is to inhibit osteoclastic resorption of bone, and it appears to be involved in minimising the transient hypercalcaemia which follows calcium ingestion by monogastric animals when its release may be triggered not directly but by gastrin released from the stomach. Despite much work on its plasma levels in parturient and lactating cattle its significance in ruminants remains doubtful. Perhaps the most interesting suggestion has been that it is in part responsible for the normal hypocalcaemia of pregnancy and thereby reduces the amount of calcium filtered and subsequently lost in the urine. It is used, with variable results, in the treatment of a number of human conditions involving excessive bone resorption, particularly Paget's disease. Several natural and synthetic preparations are available: salmon calcitonin is approximately 200 times as potent as the porcine hormone.

Parathyroid Hormone (PTH) was discovered by Collip in 1925. Like calcitonin it is a peptide hormone. It is secreted from the parathyroid glands in response to a fall in plasma Ca^{2+} activity, which most of its effects tend to reverse. PTH actually exists in plasma as a number of different fragments of the secreted molecule, with widely varying biological activities, but of considerably more uniform ability to respond to the older radioimmunoassays. It is now believed that circulating parathyroid activity is very much lower than was indicated by these assays, and that osteoclastic resorption of bone mineral (so much a feature of the early accounts of PTH's functions) requires far too high a hormone level to be a normal consequence of its secretion. At more realistic hormone-levels the main effects of PTH are the enhancement of calcium absorption from the renal tubule by a process involving the activation of adenyl cyclase, and an increase in calcium absorption from the small intestine probably mediated by its influence on vitamin D metabolism. Somewhat higher levels cause an independent phosphaturia, and levels approximately 1000 times normal cause the classical bone resorption, which normally produces a nett calciuria, since the resultant hypercalcaemia increases the filtered calcium load more than the PTH increases tubular absorption.

For many years PTH was commercially available only as a partially purified HCl-extract of bovine glands called 'Para-Thor-Mone'. This is now effectively unobtainable.

Vitamin D is the name of a dietary factor known to be involved in the prevention of rickets since the work of Hopkins and Mellanby in the early years of this century. There are two principal substances, known as **calciferol** (vitamin D_2) and **cholecalciferol** (vitamin D_3). Calciferol is formed by photochemical ring-cleavage of ergosterol in plant tissues, while cholecalciferol is similarly formed from 7-dehydrocholesterol in animal tissues. As might be expected this process occurs in the skin under the influence of the ultraviolet component of sunlight; it can contribute significantly to the body content of vitamin D, even in countries such as the United Kingdom. In most domestic animals cholecalciferol is more potent than calciferol, but the difference is only large in birds. Once present in the body vitamin D may be stored, particularly in fat and skeletal muscle, for up to 6 months.

It has become apparent during the last twenty years that vitamins D_2 and D_3 are not themselves the active agents, but the essential precursors of physiologically functional compounds which have been described as renal hormones. The two vitamins undergo similar transformations and, for convenience, the description will be limited to vitamin D_3: cholecalciferol.

Cholecalciferol is hydroxylated to form 25-hydroxycholecalciferol (**calcifediol**; 25-HCC) in the liver; some regulation occurs at this stage, since the enzyme responsible shows a degree of product inhibition. Calcifediol is the major circulating metabolite of vitamin D, and is bound to a plasma alpha$_2$-globulin; it is slightly more active than cholecalciferol and can be regarded as the transport or pro-hormone form. The aspect of vitamin D metabolism that has attracted most interest is the subsequent hydroxylation of calcifediol in the kidney, and in particular the reactions resulting in the formation of either $1\alpha,25$-dihydroxycholecalciferol (**calcitriol**; 1,25-DHCC) or 24,25-dihydroxycholecalciferol (24,25-DHCC) (Fig. 2.1).

Calcitriol has been shown to be as much as twelve times as potent as cholecalciferol. Its synthesis occurs only in the kidney, and the most clearly demonstrated stimulus of it is a low extracellular fluid Ca^{2+} activity; there is also evidence that a physiological increase in

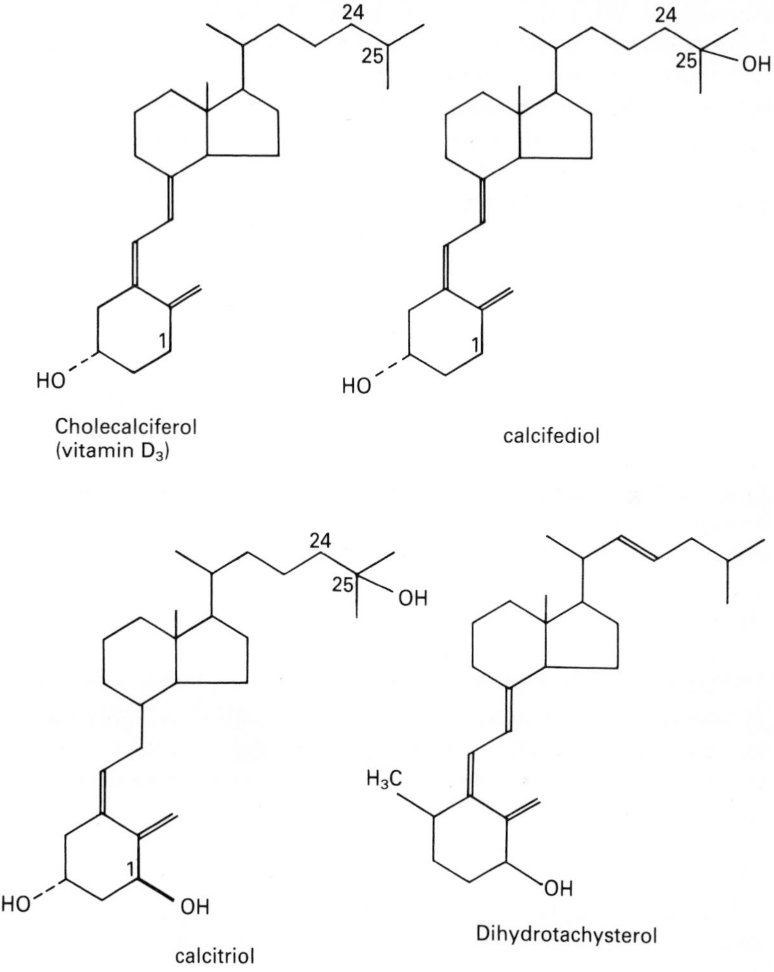

Fig. 2.1 Metabolites and analogues of vitamin D_3.

PTH secretion stimulates calcitriol synthesis. In the absence of these conditions the main reaction product is the less active 24,25-DHCC; this is thought by most workers to represent a dumping pathway, although it has been claimed specifically to enhance bone deposition of calcium.

Calcitriol is a typical steroid hormone in that it accumulates in the nuclei of target cells in the intestinal mucosa, renal cortex and osteocytes; after a delay of some hours it induces the synthesis of ribosomal RNA and hence of new protein, in this case calcium binding protein. In the gut, as has been described, this results in an increased efficiency of absorption from the lumen. In the kidney calcitriol also increases tubular reabsorption of calcium. In bone, however, the effects are more ambivalent; in calcium-deficient bone the increased gut absorption causes a nett flow of calcium into the tissue, but in normally minerallised bone calcitriol provokes a binding protein mediated resorption. There is some evidence that abnormally high plasma levels of calcifediol are especially likely to produce this effect. As with PTH, the resulting hypercalcaemia usually causes a nett increase in renal calcium excretion.

For dietary supplementation, **vitamin D** preparations, or substances containing vitamin D such as irradiated yeast or fish liver oil, are usually adequate. Vitamin D is very soluble and fairly stable in oils and alcohol; it is not soluble in water. Aqueous suspensions and dispersed solid feed-additive formulations are quite susceptible to inactivating oxidation. It is sometimes necessary to influence calcium metabolism more dramatically or immediately, and in such cases vitamin D metabolites or analogues of them may be more appropriate. **Dihydrotachysterol** (Fig. 2.1) is a closely related compound which undergoes heptic conversion; the resulting 25-hydroxydihydrotachysterol is about a four hundredth as active as calcitriol, but its production is not regulated, and it is more likely to cause hypercalcaemia through bone resorption. Toxicity may result from only slight overdosage. **1α-hydroxycholecalciferol** is easily synthesised, and is converted in the liver to calcitriol, thus by-passing the renal regulatory system; it is probably the drug of choice for the rapid activation of vitamin D dependent processes.

Vitamin D and related substances have been extensively investigated as prophylactic and therapeutic agents in the treatment of milk fever in dairy cattle. **Vitamin D_3**, as a single intramuscular dose of 10 million units in oil, has been used as a prophylactic measure; because of the need for metabolism to calcitriol followed by the induction of protein synthesis there is a 1–2 day delay before its effects are seen, which limits its usefulness in practice. **Calcifediol** and, more commonly, **1α-hydroxycholecalciferol** are more rapidly acting and more effective; the effect of dihydrotachysterol is said to be adequate for early treatment of milk fever, but too transient for reliable prophylaxis.

Finally it is pertinent to note that calciferol, in large doses, is used commercially as a rodenticide, and that a number of poisonous plants, of which the best-known is *Solanum malacoxylon*, owe their toxicity to their content of calcitriol glycosides. Overdosage with vitamin D-like substances causes bone resorption, hypercalcaemia and metastatic calcification which, if sufficiently prolonged, results in death. Of less importance is the mild conjunctivitis seen in the calves of cattle treated pre-partum with large doses of vitamin D.

MAGNESIUM

In comparison with calcium, relatively little is known about magnesium. Approximately two-thirds of the body content is in the skeleton, where it is the fourth commonest element, but its exact significance there is unknown. Most of the rest of the body magnesium is intracellular, where it is the second commonest cation after potassium; it is required for the activation of a number of enzyme systems, including that of the membrane-bound ATPase responsible for transcellular sodium and potassium gradients.

Extracellular magnesium seems to be rather similar in its distribution to calcium, although rather less closely controlled. In cattle plasma levels are approximately 0.8–1.6 mmol/l (2–4 mg/dl); of this about one third is protein bound, apparently in competitive equilibrium with the protein bound calcium. A much smaller fraction is present as active Mg^{2+}; its level appears to be controlled (or at least influenced) by the parathyroid gland. Ingested magnesium is absorbed only slowly from the gut lumen, a fact which is responsible for the efficacy of Epsom salts ($MgSO_4$) as a bulk purgative. Absorption is mostly from the upper small intestine, partly by diffusion and partly by a carrier-mediated passive process which appears to be enhanced by pharmacological doses of vitamin D and competitively obstructed by high luminal levels of Ca^{2+}. High dietary potassium levels have also been blamed for reduced magnesium absorption.

The diffusible fraction of plasma magnesium is filtered in the glomerulus and there is an active reabsorptive process located in the proximal and distal convoluted tubules; the effect of PTH on its function is not clear.

There are no very obvious specific normal functions of extracellular magnesium, but pathological or iatrogenic variations in its level can exert important effects; these are mostly the result of its relationship to calcium-sensitive processes, particularly in excitable tissues. Magnesium has effects similar to those of calcium on sodium channels in that an increased activity reduces the excitability of the membrane. A more important property of excess magnesium is its ability to act as a competitive blocker of calcium-selective channels, thus inhibiting transmitter release at synapses and reducing myocardial and smooth muscle contractility. Hypermagnesaemia may result from injudicious parenteral therapy or from administration of magnesium salts as a purge to an animal with a blocked or perforated gut; its likelihood is increased by deficient renal function. The clinical signs include skeletal neuro-muscular blockade, vasodilation and bradycardia, leading on occasion to asystolic cardiac arrest.

In view of the slow rate at which magnesium ions cross the blood-brain barrier, descriptions of the rapid anaesthetic effects of intravenous magnesium (usually as the sulphate) seem most unlikely to be true, particularly since in human volunteers experimental hypermagnesaemia produced no impairment of consciousness at all, but only complete skeletal muscle paralysis. It must be concluded that peripheral neuro-muscular blockade, rather than central nervous depression, is the explanation of the apparent anaesthesia, and that fatal doses cause death most probably as a result of respiratory paralysis and consequent asphyxia. The use of magnesium salts alone for immobilisation or euthanasia, like that of succinylcholine, must be considered both inhumane and unethical.

Magnesium deficiency is a fairly common clinical condition. Amongst young animals it is usually found in rapidly growing calves kept for too long on a whole milk (magnesium deficient) diet. In adult cattle and sheep an underlying seasonal hypomagnesaemia caused by marginal or frankly deficient intake is often converted to an overt clinical condition by some additional factor, for example the increase in potassium intake when stock are turned onto young grass. The major signs of hypomagnesaemia may be attributed to the loss of its stabilising effect on excitable membranes, and include hyperaesthesia, exaggerated tendon reflexes, convulsions and tetanic respiratory arrest. There is clinical evidence that a concurrent hypocalcaemia exacerbates the condition, partly by allowing more of the plasma magnesium to become protein-bound, and partly because it has similar effects on membrane stability itself.

Intravenous **magnesium sulphate**, usually as a 10% solution, has a rapid but transitory effect; since the solution is non-irritant, subcutaneous injection is safer. It should be appreciated that *any* manipulation of an animal in the terminal stages of hypomagnesaemia is likely to be rewarded by its sudden death from respiratory and cardiac arrest. Most of an injected dose of magnesium is taken up by the depleted skeleton, and dietary supplementation is required for a sustained response. **Magnesium oxide** (MgO), or **magnesium carbonate** ($MgCO_3$) may be added to the diet. Alternatively magnesium alloy 'bullets' may be administered by balling gun; these form a slowly absorbed depot in the rumen and work very well for up to 3–4 weeks unless the animal succeeds in regurgitating the bullet, an achievement by no means unknown.

SUGGESTIONS FOR FURTHER READING

Bowen J M, Blackmon D M, Heavner J E 1970 Effect of magnesium ions on neuromuscular transmission in the horse, steer, and dog. Journal of the American Veterinary Medical Association 157: 164–173

Fleckenstein A 1977 Specific pharmacology of calcium in myocardium, cardiac pacemakers, and vascular smooth muscle. Annual Review of Pharmacology and Toxicology 17: 149–166

Fraser D R 1980 Regulation of the metabolism of vitamin D. Physioligical Reviews 60: 551–613

Means A R, Tash J S, Chafouleas J G 1982 Physiological implications of the presence, distribution, and regulation of calmodulin in eukaryotic cells. Physiological Reviews 62: 1–39

Mullen P A 1983 Metabolic disorders of cattle: current trends in treatment and prophylaxis. In: Bogan J A, Lees P, Yoxall A T (eds) Pharmacological Basis of Large Animal Medicine, Blackwell, Oxford, p 312–326

Parsons J A 1976 Parathyroid hormone (PTH). In: Parsons J A (ed) Peptide hormones. MacMillan, New York, p 71–75

3

Distribution of body water; replacement fluids

It seems probable that the first forms of life to develop on this planet were unicellular enclosures of the seas in which they appeared, and that their internal fluid composition reflected the prevailing conditions; in particular the major cations seem to have been K^+ and Mg^{2+}. Subsequently geological and climatic influences caused a gradual change, so that the major cations became Na^+ and Ca^{2+}, and these protean life forms elected to evolve mechanisms to isolate their internal fluids from the now alien external environment. The subsequent development of multicellular organisms led to the creation of a second compartment: the extracellular fluid, which once again initially reflected the then prevailing external conditions. It is thought that continuing leaching of soil and rock has been responsible for the steadily increasing salinity of sea water, so that modern seawater is now much more concentrated than mammalian extracellular fluid. This trend, together with the occupation of progressively less hospitable ecological niches has been held responsible for the evolution of complex homeostatic mechanisms to control the extracellular fluid volume and composition. The degree of their success may be judged from the relative paucity of controls over the intracellular compartment.

The development of tissue supply systems involving the pumping of fluid round a more-or-less closed tubular system, with its attendant problems of transporting materials into and out of it necessitates the division of the extracellular fluid into vascular and interstitial compartments.

In this view of organic structure the lumina of the gastro-intestinal and renal tracts are technically outside the body; they form, however, a vital part of the fluid system as a whole, since they constitute the major areas of interaction with the external environment.

DISTRIBUTION OF BODY WATER

Estimates of the total body water content vary somewhat, but approximately 70% of the total body weight is a commonly quoted value in lean animals. This is likely to be unduly high in domestic herbivores, since a relatively large proportion of their bodyweight consists of gut contents, while in any species extreme obesity may lower the actual water content to nearer 40% of body weight. Of this 70% approximately 50% is intracellular, and of the remaining 20% extracellular water some 15% is interstitial and 5% is in the vascular compartment (the blood plasma).

The experimental measurement of total body water usually depends on the assumption that certain substances diffuse readily throughout the whole body water compartment. First amongst these is water itself, labelled to permit its measurement by replacing some of the normal hydrogen atoms with other isotopes, either tritium (^3H, detected by its feeble beta-radioactivity) or deuterium (^2H, detected by mass spectrometry). The chief problem encountered is in correcting for the loss of labelled water from the body, beginning with almost the first exhalation after administration, and continuing through the period of equilibration with the unlabelled body water. Correction usually involves extrapolating the curve of concentration of labelled in unlabelled water against time back to the time of administration (zero). Other markers used are cheaper and easier to estimate, but do not penetrate body water so quickly or completely, and hence tend to give erroneously low values. They include antipyrine and its derivatives.

Osmotic pressure and body water distribution

Although water itself passes fairly freely across most of the membranes in the body, the majority of the substances dissolved in it do not, and it is the regulation of distribution of certain solutes, that is to say their partial osmotic pressures, which largely determines the distribution of water between the main fluid compartments. The phenomenon of osmotic pressure shares many properties with that of gaseous pressure, including the facts that they are both colligative properties (i.e. depending only on the effective number of particles present and not on their chemical identity) and only obey their respective physical laws at low concentrations. A further striking similarity is the application of Avogadro's law to their quantification: in the present case it predicts the volume (22.4 l) into which a gram-molecule of an ideal solute must be dissolved to exert an osmotic pressure of one atmosphere across a perfect semi-permeable membrane.

Osmotic strengths of complex (non-ideal) solutions are conveniently expressed in terms of the osmotically equivalent molar strength of some notional ideal solute; in biological contexts usually in milli-osmoles per litre (mOsmol/l). Physiological fluids usually have an osmotic strength of about 300 mOsmol/l; from this it may be calculated that the osmotic pressure exerted by it should be three tenths of 22.4 atmospheres, or approximately 5000 mmHg. Fortunately in normal tissues the total concentration *differences*, and hence the *nett* osmotic forces across membranes, are very small, but the calculation may help to explain how strongly the distribution of solutes across membranes influences the distribution of water, as well as why the parenteral administration of hypotonic solutions is clinically undersirable.

The main osmotic determinant of the distribution of water between extracellular and intracellular compartments appears to be the active exclusion by cell membranes of Na^+, which is accompanied by the close regulation of Na^+ *concentration* ($[Na^+]$) in the extracellular fluid (ECF). This is achieved primarily in the kidney by processes more fully described in the next chapter, although the zona glomerulosa of the adrenal cortex, osmoreceptors and cells mediating sodium appetite in the hypothalamus and pressure and volume receptors at various sites in the vasculature are all also involved in the process of $[Na^+]$ regulation. When the $[Na^+]$ of the ECF falls, as, for example, in water intoxication or excessive intravenous infusion of low $[Na^+]$ fluid, the 'excess' water enters cells causing them to swell. Alternatively the exclusion of Na^+ from cells may fail, for example in tissue hypoxia, and this also causes a shift of water from the ECF into the intracellular compartment. Moderate loss of isotonic sodium solution, in haemorrhage, serum exudation from burns, or diarrhoea, is borne by the ECF alone since there is no osmotic pressure change to influence the intracellular compartment.

By contrast with this situation the distribution of water between the interstitial and vascular compartments of the ECF is not determined by electrolyte concentrations since the capillary membrane is freely permeable to virtually all small molecular weight substances (crystalloids). The colloid component, of which the plasma proteins (chiefly albumins) form the bulk, passes through the capillary membrane only to a very limited extent, and this limitation of its distribution provides a small nett osmotic force tending to draw water from the interstitial fluid into the vascular space. This colloid osmotic pressure amounts to some 25 mmHg in normal arteriolar plasma, and is thus outweighed by the hydrostatic pressure of approximately 30–35 mmHg at the arteriolar end of the capillary, so that the nett *filtration* pressure at this point in the microcirculation is some 5–10 mmHg. At the venular end of the capillary, however, the hydrostatic pressure is only some 10–12 mmHg, while the loss of crystalloid solution will have raised the colloid osmotic pressure slightly. The interstitial fluid is thus subjected to a nett *reabsorptive* osmotic pressure of about 10 mmHg.

This mechanism of interstitial fluid circulation was first proposed by Starling in 1896, and is still regarded as a useful model of tissue microcirculation. It provides, for instance, an explanation for the oedema which results from hypoproteinaemia whether due to inadequate synthesis or the consequence of excessive plasma dilution. The flow through capillaries is thought to be regulated by sphincters at the arteriolar (precapillary) and venular (postcapillary) ends, which are influenced by local tissue oxygen tension or metabolites, as well as by centrally originating sympathetic vasoconstrictor innervation.

Shock

Shock is widely believed to be largely caused by tissue hypoperfusion; this circulatory failure may be due to a large number of things, including local obstruction (thrombosis, traumatic injury), hypovolaemia (haemorrhage, diarrhoea, water or salt deprivation) and cardiac disease, but a major common factor in their effects is the sympathetic discharge which results from a falling venous return to the heart. In the early stages this induces capillary shutdown, thus directly centralising the plasma volume and increasing water withdrawal from the interstitial fluid compartment as the capillary hydrostatic pressure falls. This clearly safeguards the central arterial pressure and the perfusion of priority organs such as brain and myocardium but, equally clearly, compromises peripheral tissue perfusion. The increased tissue anoxia leads to loss of K^+ from cells and movement of Na^+ into them, partly because the intracellular Na^+,K^+-ATPase run short of high energy substrate. Another factor is the increasing intracellular acidosis: aerobic metabolism of pyruvate diminishes and lactic acid is produced instead, leading first to the displacement of K^+ from the cell by H^+

and then to generalised lactic acidosis. Probably as a direct result of the Na^+ shift, extracellular fluid is lost into cells.

An important and apparently highly unfortunate property of the capillary microcirculation now manifests itself as the precapillary sphincter, but *not* the postcapillary sphincter, responds to the pathological tissue state by relaxing. The hydrostatic filtration pressure is restored, while the absence of flow renders inoperative the colloid osmotic pressure component of Starling's model and the anoxic capillary endothelium is by now increasingly permeable to proteins anyway. The release of lysosomal enzymes further damages the endothelium and the formation of thrombi and red cell rouleaux (sludging) threatens larger areas of the vascular bed. By this stage the animal is suffering from hypovolaemia (either primary or secondary), and may be losing fluid from its circulation into its tissues faster than it is possible to administer it; this condition is often termed (slightly pessimistically) 'irreversible shock'.

FLUID THERAPY

Relatively mild water or electrolyte deficits in small animals may often be corrected by the oral or intravenous administration of crystalloid solutions. Such intravenous solutions must be sterile and pyrogen-free. and should be fairly close to normal plasma pH and osmotic pressure (gross hypertonicity tends to be better tolerated than gross hypotonicity). Common crystalloid solutions used are **sodium chloride, sodium bicarbonate, glucose** and various electrolyte mixtures based more-or-less on Sidney Ringer's investigations of extracellular fluid composition, of which the most useful are **compound sodium lactate injection** (Hartmann's solution) and **Darrow's solution**. Their compositions are given in Table 3.1.

Since Na^+ and Cl^- are largely excluded from the intracellular

Table 3.1. Approximate compositions of various fluids

Fluid	Constituent concentrations (mmol/l)					
	Na^+	K^+	Cl^-	HCO_3^-	Lactate	Glucose
Extracellular fluid	140	4	100	28	2	5
Sodium chloride injection BP	150	—	150	—	—	—
Sodium bicarbonate injection BP	170	—	—	170	—	—
Dextrose injection BP	—	—	—	—	—	280
Compound sodium lactate injection BP★	130	5	110	—	30	—
Darrow's solution	125	35	105	—	55	—

★ Also contains Ca^{2+}, 2 mmol/l.

compartment the water making up their isotonic solution is osmotically constrained to remain in the extracellular space unless or until preferential excretion of sodium by the kidney can occur. In animals with slight or moderate fluid deficits, the most important function of fluid therapy is to provide sufficient volume expansion of the extracellular fluid to restore normal renal function and hence regulation.

In discourses on fluid therapy it is conventional, for some reason, to refer to glucose by the now archaic term 'dextrose'. In a normal animal infused glucose is rapidly metabolised, unless the rate of infusion is so rapid that it saturates renal reabsorption, when it appears in the urine, and may even provoke a diuresis. The effect of a slow glucose infusion is thus that of providing free water to the animal. **Dextrose injection BP** is a 5% solution, and is approximately isotonic with plasma, but if the object of the exercise is to provide glucose as an energy source 10% or even 50% solutions may be administered with caution.

Of the solutions mentioned compound sodium lactate injection most closely resembles extracellular fluid, and can be used to replace quite extensive losses from this compartment. It is preferable to Darrow's solution which may cause a dangerous hyperkalaemia, especially if tissue damage or acidosis has resulted in high extracellular potassium levels already. The lactate contained in these solutions is metabolised in normal animals over 1–2 hours following administration; it is sometimes stated that conversion to bicarbonate is the reason for its alkalinifying effect, and the lactate concentration is expressed in terms of its potential bicarbonate yield. It is metabolically more accurate to say that its combination with H^+ to form lactic acid prior to uptake, mostly by the liver, is responsible for the effect, since a significant proportion of it may subsequently undergo gluconeogenesis rather than oxidation. Lactate is more stable than bicarbonate and shows fewer incompatibilities with other possible constituents of infusion solutions; its slow conversion helps to protect against the consequences of overdosage. However it should be evident that such solutions are contraindicated if lactic acidosis or severe liver damage is present; sodium bicarbonate solutions are more appropriate in these circumstances.

Oral electrolyte solutions

In large animals the volumes of fluid involved and the problems of handling often make intravenous fluid therapy impracticable. Subcutaneous or intraperitoneal injections must be sterile and pyrogen-free, and can be positively dangerous in animals with significant electrolyte or acid–base imbalance, since they provide additional fluid compartments into which crystalloids may diffuse, thus further distorting the extracellular fluid composition. Oral administration does not carry this risk, does not require sterility or freedom from pyrogens and has the added advantage that absorption can be selective; it is thus considerably more difficult to endanger the animal by overenthusiastic therapy, and the exact constitution of the solution is not so important.

The absorption of water and Na^+ by the small intestine is greatly enhanced by the presence of glucose and other actively absorbed nutrients such as glycine (sometimes referred to as aminoacetic acid). In one study the maximal effect of added glucose occurred at a luminal concentration of about 50 mmol/l, when absorption of Na^+ and water was twenty times the control rate. Commercial solutions usually contain glucose at approximately 100 mmol/l, together with NaCl (100 mmol/l) and varying amounts of K^+, glycine and bicarbonate precursor (lactate, citrate or acetate); Michell (1983) has compiled a useful table of their compositions.

TREATMENT OF SHOCK

The very early stages of shock are characterised by an increase in sympathetic activity and conservation of fluid (by antidiuresis), and early therapy is often directed towards augmenting these effects: crystalloid fluid therapy may improve extracellular fluid dynamics, and inotropic catecholamines may increase the cardiac output. The vasoconstrictive activity of alpha-adrenergic agonists is probably *always* unhelpful on balance, and in anything other than mild shock, current therapeutic manoeuvres are directed towards the antagonism of self-destructive endogenous responses.

Dopamine is preferred to other catecholamines for the treatment of hypovolaemic shock in man because it produces less tachycardia than noradrenaline or adrenaline for an equivalent increase in force of contraction of the myocardium. It also has a beneficial direct vasodilator effect on the renal and mesenteric vasculature, which is blocked by dopamine antagonists such as the phenothiazine tranquillisers.

Adrenal corticosteroids have had a long and controversial history in the therapy of shock. Early suggestions that they might function as vasodilators are no longer accepted and the main effect seems to be their stabilisation of lysosomal, mitochondrial and cell membranes. The administration of 5 mg/kg of **dexamethasone** to dogs suffering from experimental haemorrhagic shock largely abolished the movement of water out of the extracellular space, probably by reducing the leakage of Na^+ into cells. It is important to realise that the size of the dose necessary for this effect is very large by normal steroid therapeutic standards, at least 25 times that recommended by most of the manufacturers; it may also require supplementation with **methylprednisolone**, which appears to penetrate cells much more rapidly, for a clinically adequate response.

Expansion of plasma volume

Infusion of electrolyte solutions produces only a transient expansion of the vascular compartment: in one study of shocked human patients only 9% of a compound sodium lactate injection remained intravascular for more than a few minutes, and none of the clinical indices of circulatory efficiency changed at all. However there is some evidence that rapid intravenous injections of quite small volumes of very hypertonic sodium chloride (4 ml/kg of 2400 mOsmol/l) may produce improvements in the circulatory efficiency of severely shocked dogs which last several hours longer than their direct effects on plasma volume.

Plasma expanders are substances intended to remain within the vascular compartment, that is they do not readily cross capillary membranes. They are specifically indicated when a fluid deficit has been incurred from the vascular compartment, e.g. in severe haemorrhage, or in hypovolaemia due to loss of plasma protein; in this latter case there is a danger of overloading the interstitial fluid with an iso-oncotic infusion and an obvious theoretical advantage in the use of a hyperoncotic preparation to withdraw water from the swollen interstitial compartment.

In general terms plasma expanders should be sterile, convenient to store and administer, should not interfere with the viscosity or coagulability of blood, should persist in the circulation for a reasonable time before excretion or metabolism, and should neither be directly toxic nor provoke histamine release or an allergic response. Although all the commercially available preparations are claimed to be non-allergenic (and only comparatively rarely provoke a genuinely allergic reaction), it is by no means unknown for them to cause an anaphylactoid reaction by direct pharmacological release of histamine. Polyvinylpyrrolidone (povidone) is a synthetic substance now largely relegated to the role of a pharmaceutical dispersing agent because of its strong tendency to cause histamine release and liver damage; it also causes fibrosarcomas in rats.

Unitl recently the major plasma expanders were the **dextrans**. These are polymers of glucose formed during the metabolism of carbohydrates by a bacterium, *Leuconostoc mesenteroides*. Preparations with average molecular weights of 70 000 daltons, **dextran 70**, and 40 000 daltons, **dextran 40**, are most commonly available. There is considerable variation in the actual sizes of the molecules present; in the case of dextran 70, their molecular weights range from 25 000 to 110 000 daltons. A 4% solution of dextran 70 is approximately iso-oncotic with plasma. The usually supplied strength of 6% is therefore likely to cause a movement of water from the interstitial to the vascular compartment, in addition to the plasma expansion due to the injection volume iself. The increase in volume is normally effective for some 6–7 hours, by which time approximately 30% of a dose, comprising most of the smaller molecules, will have been excreted in the urine. The larger molecules are taken up by reticuloendothelial cells and are slowly metabolised to form water and carbon dioxide; some dextran may persist in the circulation for up to 48 hours.

Although the improvement in the microcirculation is in part due to plasma expansion, the lower molecular weight dextrans also increase capillary blood flow, apparently by coating the vessel walls and cellular elements, thus inhibiting intravascular aggregation of cells. However dextrans themselves form rather viscous solutions and the high concentrations found in the renal tubule shortly after infusion cause a large increase in luminal viscosity which has been blamed for the high incidence of renal failure following dextran infusion, seen especially in cats. Both these attributes are possessed to a much greater extent by dextran 40 than by dextran 70, as would be expected.

The higher molecular weight dextrans (110 000 daltons and larger) actually *reduce* tissue microcirculation, probably by directly increasing plasma viscosity, and are particularly liable to reduce blood coagulability, especially at total dextran dose-rates above 1–1.5 gm/kg. This is partly simply the result of dilution of the plasma clotting factors, but also because the larger molecules reduce thrombocyte and platelet activities.

Finally dextrans have occasionally produced signs of histamine release and, less commonly still, full anaphylactic reactions in human patients.

A much more recently developed plasma expander, **hetastarch** (2-hydroxyethyl starch, Volex) is also essentially a polysaccharide. Amylopectin, obtained from sorghum starch, is partially hydrolysed and then reacted with ethylene oxide until approximately 75% of the glucose residues are substituted. This reduces the rate of hydrolysis in vivo by amylases, and greatly increases the plasma half-life. The commercial preparation has an average molecular weight of approximately 400 000 daltons. Partly because of its relatively high molecular weight hetastarch does not hold as much water in the vascular compartment as does dextran 70 (14 ml/gm, as compared with 20–25 ml/gm). However the highly branched structure of amylopectin results in an almost globular molecule which is much less viscous in solution, and this property constitutes its main advantage over the dextrans; the effect of an infusion is also relatively long-lived (12–18 hours). Antigenicity is said to be low, but there is some suspicion that it may interfere with coagulation, albeit to a lesser extent than dextran 70. Approximately 40% of infused hetastarch is excreted in the urine over 24 hours, the rest is slowly metabolised in reticulo-endothelial cells.

A number of plasma expanders are derived from gelatin. **Gelatin** itself has been used since before the first world war as a plasma expander, and shows surprisingly little antigenicity; this has been attributed to its low tyrosine and tryptophan content. In view of its culinary applications it is perhaps not unexpected that a major objection to gelatin is the fact that iso-oncotic solutions tend to have a very high viscosity. The commonest derivative of gelatin is a urea-gelatin polymer called **polygeline** (Haemaccel). In the production of this the gelatin is first heat-degraded and then the peptide chains are cross-linked with urea residues to give a compound whose molecular weight averages 35 000 and ranges from 4300 to 280 000 daltons. At a concentration of 3.5% the oncotic pressure and viscosity are very similar to those of plasma. In normal animals the plasma half-life is only 4.5 hours, giving a clinically useful effect for 2–3 hours. However it persists for approximately twice this time in clinically shocked animals. About 85% of an administered dose is excreted in the urine within 48 hours, and most of the remainder appears in the faeces.

Polygeline is not toxic to the kidneys and does not interfere with tissue microcirculation or blood coagulation; its major drawback, apart from its relatively short-lived effect, is its tendency to release histamine. This effect is species-dependent and also varies between different batches of polygeline, but it is known to occur in dogs and is especially likely following rapid infusion. A number of allergic reactions have also been recorded in human patients, a fact not very clearly documented in the product's data sheet.

In summary, dextran 70 or polygeline would seem to be suitable for routine treatment, the former having a longer duration but an upper dose limit imposed by its effects on blood viscosity and co-agulation. Dextran 40 may specifically improve tissue microcirculation, while endangering renal function in some species, and hetastarch is notable for its long plasma half-life, although experience of its use in veterinary practice is still limited, compared with the other compounds.

SUGGESTIONS FOR FURTHER READING

Lorenz W, et al 1976 Histamine release in human subjects by modified gelatin (Haemaccel) and dextran: an explanation for anaphylactoid reactions observed under clinical conditions. British Journal of Anaesthesia 48: 15–165

Manning R D, Guyton A C 1982 Control of blood volume. Reviews of Physiology, Biochemistry and Pharmacology 93: 69–114

Michell A R 1983 Understanding fluid therapy. Irish Veterinary Journal 37: 94–103

Sladen G E, Dawson A M 1969 Interrelationships between the absorptions of glucose, sodium and water by the normal human jejunum. Clinical Science 36: 119–132

Thompson W L 1978 Drug therapy of shock. In: Turner P, Shand D G (eds) Recent advances in clinical pharmacology 1. Churchill Livingstone, Edinburgh, p 123–145

Velasco I T, Pontieri V, Rocha e Silva M, Lopes O U 1980 Hyperosmotic NaCl and severe haemorrhagic shock. American Journal of Physiology 239 (Heart and Circulatory Physiology 8): H664–H673

4

Drugs affecting fluid and electrolyte balance

For the most part these are drugs which, either directly or indirectly, affect the function of the kidney, since this organ bears the main responsibility for controlling the balance between intake and loss of water and the major extracellular ions. A brief account of renal function is therefore a necessary prelude. To attempt a complete and accurate representation of the presently accepted picture of fluid and electrolyte balance would be a daunting task in any circumstances; to do so within the confines of an introductory textbook of veterinary pharmacology is clearly impossible. The following account is intended only to rationalise the actions of the drugs mentioned. It is abbreviated, and it is therefore inaccurate, since so many of the phenomena to be described are still the subjects of debate and uncertainty. The reader is referred to the bibliography at the end of the chapter for fuller accounts.

NORMAL RENAL FUNCTION

Within this limited view of fluid and electrolyte balance, the kidneys can conveniently be regarded as a collection of nephrons (Fig. 4.1). The diagrammatic representation is oversimplified in that not every nephron has a medullary loop of Henle. Most of the blood supply to the kidney passes through the vascular system associated with the nephrons and this fraction (roughly 90%) is referred to as the renal blood flow. Suitable correction for the cellular components allows the calculation of the functionally more important renal plasma flow. Blood is supplied to the glomerulus from the relatively wide bore afferent arteriole and drains from it into the much narrower efferent arteriole. The blood in the glomerular capillaries is thus at a high pressure (approximately 60% of that in the aorta) and this provides the necessary energy for glomerular filtration from the plasma into the tubule lumen; about 20% of the afferent arteriolar plasma is thus accounted for, and the filtrate includes

43

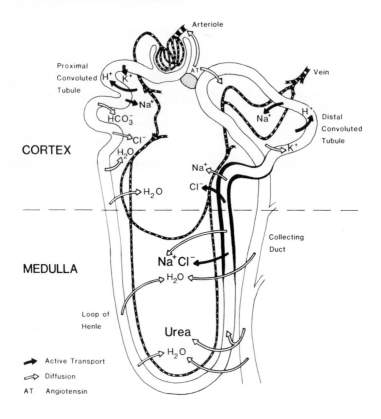

Fig. 4.1 A functional diagram of a nephron.

all plasma constituents with molecular weights of less than about 70 000 daltons. The rate of filtration is remarkably independent of the central arterial blood pressure and is probably stabilised by variations in the degree of constriction of the afferent arteriole brought about by the local effects of the renin-angiotensin system. This local control of glomerular filtration by (amongst other variables) the distal tubular Na^+ content is probably responsible for the close correspondence between filtration and absorption in the normal kidney. The precise mechanisms of this effect are much less clearly understood than are the effects of the systemic release of renin, although the initial stages are probably identical.

Renin is a proteolytic enzyme which catalyzes the cleavage of a decapeptide, angiotensin I, from the alpha$_2$ globulin known therefore as angiotensinogen. Angiotensin I is further broken down to an octapeptide, angiotensin II, by a peptidyl dipeptide hydrolase which is found in greatest amount in the lungs. It is often referred to as 'angiotensin converting enzyme', although it is also responsible for inactivating bradykinin and similar substances. Angiotensin II is an extremely potent vasoconstrictive agent, and this property probably accounts for its local effects on glomerular blood flow and filtration. At the lower levels encountered normally in the systemic circulation it probably still contributes to arteriolar tone, although its specific stimulation of thirst in the hypothalamus and of aldosterone release from the adrenal cortex, which will be referred to again later, may be of greater significance to circulatory homeostasis.

The proximal convoluted tubule

A few substances, having been filtered into the glomerulus, are then simply passed on through the tubule without more ado. Such substances can be used to determine the glomerular filtration rate, and are correspondingly valued in experimental work on the kidney. The best documented of these substances is the polysaccharide **inulin**, but the protein breakdown product **creatinine** approximates closely to this ideal behaviour in many species. **Mannitol** is the alcohol resulting from the reduction of mannose, and has similar properties which find some clinical applications.

The great majority of substances in the glomerular filtrate are reabsorbed to some extent during their passage through the tubule. In the proximal convoluted tubule some 60–80% of the filtrate is reabsorbed. From the limited viewpoint of renal pharmacology the major active processes are the reabsorption of Na^+ and K^+ and the slightly complex mechanism which results in the absorption of HCO_3^-, with other constituents, particularly Cl^- and water, being absorbed secondarily as a result of the electrical and concentration gradients thus created across the tubular membrane. In particular the permeability of the membranes to water ensures that the luminal contents remain isosmotic with the extracellular fluid. Sodium is pumped out of the tubular cells in exchange for potassium by an Na,K-ATPase similar to that found in other cells, but mostly located on the peritubular membrane, while K^+ is pumped inwards across the luminal membrane. Sodium diffusion is restricted to the luminal membrane, and this assymmetry creates a nett transtubular potential difference of about 20 mV, lumen negative. Potassium seems to be able to diffuse across both surfaces, but the nett movement is out of the lumen.

Bicarbonate penetrates the luminal membrane only very slowly, and its absorption in the proximal tubule is heavily dependent on the presence of an enzyme: **carbonic anhydrase**. This is a zinc containing enzyme whose function is to speed up the attainment of equilibrium of the reaction:

$$CO_2 + H_2O \leftrightharpoons H_2CO_3.$$

Carbonic anhydrase is capable of accelerating this reaction in either direction, according to the disequilibrium conditions obtaining. Carbonic acid, in its turn, exists in equilibrium with bicarbonate:

$$H_2CO_3 \leftrightharpoons HCO_3^- + H^+.$$

The equilibrium state of this reaction is reached very rapidly by comparison with that of the dehydration of carbonic acid, even in the presence of carbonic anhydrase, and in the renal tubular fluid the chief determinant of its position is the concentration of H^+, according to Le Chatelier's principle.

The enzyme is found within proximal tubule cells, and in association with their luminal brush borders. The activating step in

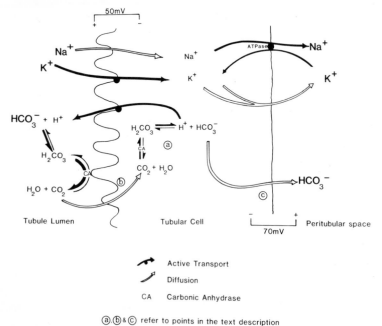

Fig. 4.2 Proximal tubular transport of sodium, potassium and bicarbonate.

the process of bicarbonate absorption is the secretion of H^+ into the tubule lumen, which is largely responsible for the favourable electrical gradient down which Na^+ diffuses into the cell. This H^+ is derived from the dissociation of carbonic acid, whose supply is facilitated by the presence of carbonic anhydrase (Fig. 4.2, a). This luminal H^+ then combines with filtered bicarbonate, that is to say it causes the equilibrium to shift towards carbonic acid, and the brush border carbonic anhydrase (which is effectively intraluminal) accelerates its dehydration to CO_2 (Fig. 4.2, b), whose concentration is low. This is because CO_2, unlike HCO_3^-, is highly diffusible through cell membranes, and once inside the cell it is rapidly taken up by carbonic anhydrase to provide the H^+ which started the cycle of events. The remaining element is the bicarbonate generated inside the tubule cell, which diffuses out across the peritubular membrane down the electrical gradient created by the Na, K-ATPase (Fig. 4.2, c).

The nett effect of all this is that sodium bicarbonate disappears from the lumen, and appears at the serosal surface of the tubule.

There are other specific absorptive processes, such as the ones which remove virtually all the glucose and amino acids, and these add to the osmotic imbalance which results in up to 80% of the water content being absorbed. However most substances in the filtrate are absorbed in the proximal tubule by passive distribution across the cell membranes as their concentrations rise; urea is a good example of these. Highly polar solutes, being less diffusible, will tend to remain in the tubule lumen, and hepatic metabolism of drugs often produces changes in their physico-chemical characteristics in this direction, thus increasing their urinary excretion. In addition, a number of organic acids are actively secreted into the proximal tubule lumen from the peritubular blood vessels, including the penicillins, probenecid, salicylates EDTA (used in heavy metal poisoning), meglumine iodipamide (used for intravenous pyelography, since it is radio-opaque) and p-amino hippuric acid, which is so completely removed from the blood that it is used as an experimental determinant of renal plasma flow. A similar secretory mechanism exists for organic bases.

The loop of Henle and collecting duct

The loop of Henle is important because it contains the main mechanisms for implementing renal water balance, and these constitute the primary sites of action of the major diuretic drugs.

Fluid entering the loop of Henle amounts to 20–40% of the glomerular filtrate. It is isosmotic with the extracellular fluid, but contains virtually no protein, amino acids, glucose, calcium, potassium or (normally) bicarbonate. It contains a variable amount of phosphates and the concentration of urea is approximately equal to that of plasma; its main osmotically active constituents are Na^+ and Cl^-.

For further details of the proposed mechanism of countercurrent osmotic gradient multiplication the reader is referred to the review by Jacobson and Kokko (1976). In brief, with reference to Figure 4.1, the descending limb is a thin-walled structure, and is permeable only to water, which diffuses out under the influence of the osmotic gradient across the wall (to be explained shortly), thus increasing the concentration of solutes inside the lumen. After the bend, as the tubule heads back towards the cortex it becomes permeable to urea. In the outer medulla the tubule becomes impermeable to water and urea, and its wall becomes thicker and shows more evidence of metabolic activity. This activity has been shown fairly conclusively to consist primarily of the active pumping of Cl^- out of the lumen into the extracellular fluid, with Na^+ being co-transported or passively following the electrical gradient thus created.

Until about 10 years ago the converse was believed: that Na^+ was pumped and Cl^- diffused. The change of opinion serves as an interesting time-marker in accounts of renal physiology and pharmacology, but is otherwise of little consequence to the practicalities of diuretic therapy; in both models NaCl is transferred from the lumen to the extracellular fluid thus creating in the outer medulla the osmotic gradient which was responsible for abstracting water from the adjacent descending limb. As the tubule runs through the cortex the process of Cl^- pumping continues until the distal convoluted segment is reached although it is no longer in such close proximity to the descending limb. The cortical part of the thick ascending limb does not, therefore, contribute much to the osmotic gradient; because the walls are still impermeable to water and urea this portion of the tubule has the important property of rendering its contents hypotonic to plasma. It is the only part of the tubule capable of this and hence is solely responsible for the production of dilute urine, that is to say, for selective water excretion.

At this point it is convenient to postpone consideration of the distal tubule, and to pass straight to the collecting duct since the interaction between this and the medullary loop of Henle forms the functional unit responsible for urinary concentration. The tubule wall remains impermeable to urea until almost the bottom of the collecting ducts, by which stage urea's luminal concentration is quite high; it therefore diffuses out at this point, forming the main inner medullary component of the osmotic gauntlet through which the descending limb of the loop of Henle runs. This phenomenon completes the description of the osmotic gradients produced by the loop of Henle, and the two remaining components of the urinary concentrating mechanism are antidiuretic hormone and the vasa recta.

Antidiuretic hormone (ADH) is an octapeptide elaborated by neurons of the supraoptic and paraventricular nuclei in the hypothalamus. These cells are sensitive to a number of influences; the longest-established experimental stimulus of their activity is a rise in carotid plasma osmolality, but they are also activated by so-called 'volume receptors' in the left atrium which appear to respond to a reduction in circulating plasma volume. Their axons terminate in the posterior pituitary, and the ADH thus released passes into the general circulation. ADH is also known as 'vasopressin', because early investigators were struck by its vasoconstrictive potency, but it is important to realize that these circulatory effects only occur at levels grossly in excess of those found in the body, and that the hormone is quite misleadingly thus designated.

Its principal normal function is selectively to increase the permeability of the terminal distal tubule and collecting duct to water. In its absence the collecting duct is virtually impermeable, and urine passes from the distal tubule to the renal pelvis almost unchanged; in its presence water is drawn through the duct wall by the high medullary osmotic pressure, and the urine is thus concentrated.

The final element in the concentrating system is its blood supply: the vasa recta branch from the peritubular vessels, and follow the course of the loops of Henle into the medulla and back out again. Their walls are permeable and the contents therefore equilibrate with the interstitial fluid. Clearly the rate of flow in the vasa recta is crucial to the function of the system, since if it is too low insufficient of the absorbed solutes and water will be reclaimed, while if it is too high too much will be removed and the osmotic gradient will be dissipated.

The distal convoluted tubule

The activity of the early portion of the distal tubule resembles that of the adjacent loop of Henle, and the continued abstraction of NaCl makes its contents more dilute. The main part of this segment and the early collecting duct behave very similarly to the proximal tubule, with two important exceptions.

Although the tubular cells contain carbonic anhydrase, there is none associated with their brush borders. Thus H^+ secreted in exchange for absorbed Na^+ is trapped in the lumen. For the same reason, although HCO_3^- is normally virtually completely removed in the proximal tubule, any which does arrive in the distal tubule (due to alkalosis or pharmacological interference) is not readily absorbed.

The second characteristic of the distal tubule cells is the presence in their peritubular membrane of a Na,K-ATPase which is both physiologically and pharmacologically different from that in the proximal tubule. Physiologically it differs in that its synthesis is induced by circulating adrenal hormones; about half is induced by glucocorticoids, but the other half is due to the effects of the specific minerallocorticoid **aldosterone**. This is released from the zona glomerulosa indirectly in response to tubular Na^+ content, *via* plasma angiotensin II, as indicated earlier, but also directly as a result of a rise in plasma K^+ concentration. The aldosterone combines with cytosol receptors in the distal tubule cells provoking nuclear transcription of RNA and consequent synthesis of new enzyme.

In the absence of absorbable luminal bicarbonate, Na^+ absorption is balanced by diffusion into the tubule of K^+ or by H^+ secretion in acidosis. The exact balance of contribution seems to reflect their respective intracellular availabilities, but aldosterone-mediated sodium absorption nearly always causes a significant loss of potassium, in fact potassium balance is much more dependent on aldosterone than is that of sodium. Adrenal corticosteroids have similar effects on sodium–potassium balance in intestinal absorption and exocrine secretory processes.

Tubular acid–base balance

It may be seen that Na^+ reabsorption depends in part upon H^+ secretion into the lumen. The maximal gradient that this pump mechanism can maintain is about a thousandfold, which is a difference across the membrane of 3 pH units; further Na^+ absorption (or H^+ secretion) is only possible if there are substances present in the lumen which can combine with H^+, thus lowering its concentration. These substances are known as buffers. Bicarbonate is an obvious example, but its conversion to carbonic acid and absorption only restores the *status quo* of the plasma. Excretion of an acid load requires additional buffers to be present in the filtrate, and one of these, especially important in acidosis, is phosphate. The pK (pH giving 50% dissociation) of the equilibrium:

$$HPO_4^{2-} \rightleftharpoons H_2PO_4^-$$

is about 6.8, so that it is an effective buffer down to approximately pH 5.8. In terms of a chemically balanced equation, the H^+ which combines with the HPO_4^{2-} can be regarded as displacing an equivalent amount of Na^+, which is then absorbed. Organic acids such as creatinine and lactate have lower pKs (approximately 5 and 4 respectively); they are correspondingly less able to buffer H^+ and hence spare Na^+.

When the pH of the filtrate falls below 6 for more than a few days the distal tubule cells start to break glutamine down to glutamic acid and ammonia. The free ammonia diffuses readily into the lumen where it combines with H^+ to form NH_4^+, which is trapped by its lack of lipid solubility, thus allowing further hydrogen ion secretion to occur.

DIURETICS

Osmotic diuretics

Diuresis is defined as an increase in urine volume; although, as will be seen, virtually all diuretic drugs can be thought of as inducing an osmotic diuresis, the term is normally reserved for those substances which are themselves not absorbed from the tubule and thus hold an osmotically equivalent amount of water in the lumen against the absorptive gradients. Chief amongst these is **mannitol** (referred to earlier), although the necessity for intravenous administration limits its usefulness. **Isosorbide** behaves similarly, but has the advantage of being absorbed by mouth in monogastric species. This is more than mere convenience since the concomitant plasma expansion is also much reduced.

Urinary acidifying drugs

These are nowadays of only slight interest as diuretics. They consist essentially of salts with a metabolisable cation and a fixed anion, and are typified by **ammonium chloride**. When absorbed, either orally or parenterally, the equilibrium:

$$NH_4^+ \rightleftharpoons NH_3 + H^+$$

is driven to the right by hepatic uptake of ammonia and its incorporation into urea. In effect the original NH_4Cl is thus quantitatively converted into HCl, and the resulting excretion of this unwelcome acid load increases the urine volume. The effect is often small and transient, and the side-effects unpleasant. However ammonium chloride and **mandelic acid** are sometimes used to acidify the urine as part of the treatment of lower urinary tract infections.

Carbonic anhydrase inhibitors

These drugs owe their existence to the discovery, in the 1950s, that the acidosis and polyuria which frequently followed sulphonamide therapy were due to the inhibition of kidney carbonic anhydrase. The subsequent search for sulphonamides with enhanced carbonic anhydrase inhibition led eventually to the marketing of acetazolamide, which is probably the commonest member of the group.

Acetazolamide (Fig. 4.3, Diamox) is active by either oral or parenteral routes. In monogastric animals plasma levels are maximal within 1–2 hours of ingestion and most of it is excreted, via the kidneys, within 24 hours. From the introductory account of renal function it will be apparent that the main effect of carbonic anhydrase inhibition is to interfere with the absorption of bicarbonate from the proximal tubule, by reducing the supply of H^+ to the membrane pump and by reducing the rate of absorption of carbonic acid from the lumen; filtered bicarbonate is thus trapped in the

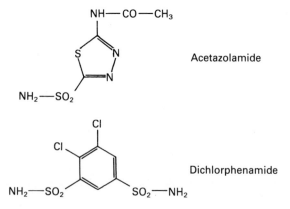

Fig. 4.3 Diuretics which inhibit carbonic anhydrase.

urine, together with an electrically equivalent amount of Na^+ and an osmotically equivalent amount of water. Once the filtrate has left the proximal tubule the ability of the kidney to deal with bicarbonate is strictly limited, and it becomes, in effect, an osmotic diuretic. The result is an increased volume of alkaline urine containing sodium bicarbonate, and a corresponding metabolic acidosis.

This response is limited in magnitude and duration for two reasons. In the first place the major sites or urine concentration are quite unaffected by the drug, and hence tend to counteract the effect as soon as the loss of fluid is perceived. Secondly the acidosis is caused by a deficiency of bicarbonate which is reflected in a reduced filtered bicarbonate load, and consists of an increase in the availability of H^+ which tends to circumvent the inhibition of intracellular carbonic anhydrase. Repeated dosing with acetazolamide thus rarely results in a commensurate extension of the response. A less common problem with acetazolamide is that, like most diuretics which interfere with sodium movement, it also reduces calcium absorption, and this fact, together with the increased urine bicarbonate content can lead to urolithiasis.

Acetazolamide inhibits the carbonic anhydrase mediated movement of bicarbonate across membranes throughout the body, and thereby reduces the secretion of bicarbonate-based fluids such as parotid saliva, pancreatic juice and, particularly, aqueous humour. These affects are not self-limiting, as are those in the kidney tubule, and carbonic anhydrase inhibitors are important drugs in the treatment of glaucoma.

Some other drugs in this group, such as **dichlorphenamide** (Fig. 4.3, Daranide), cause the excretion of chloride as well as bicarbonate, and are more potent diuretics; this is probably because they possess some of the properties of the next group of drugs.

Thiazides

These were, in their turn, developed from the carbonic anhydrase inhibitors. They are much more potent diuretics, although showing only weak carbonic anhydrase inhibition, and they have largely usurped the position of the older drugs. The first of them was **chlorothiazide**, but this was soon improved by saturation of its heterocyclic ring to form **hydrochlorothiazide** (Fig. 4.4, Vetidrex etc.), which is a more potent diuretic still, although an even weaker carbonic anhydrase inhibitor. Since then a large number of thiazides

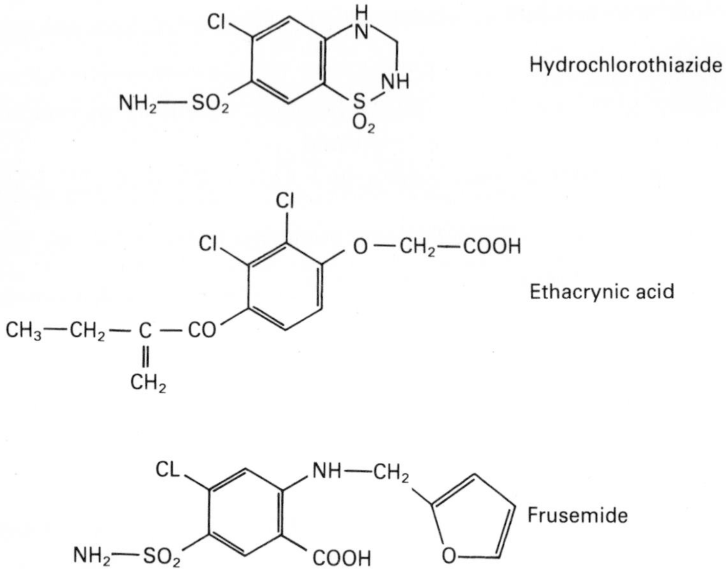

Fig. 4.4 Potent diuretics which primarily affect the loop of Henle.

have been developed, patented, advertised and sold, but some comfort may be derived from the knowledge that apart from simple variations in potency, and hence dose-rate, the differences between them are negligible. Hydrochlorothiazide is much the commonest thiazide in veterinary therapeutics.

The major effect of the thiazide diuretics is to inhibit the chloride pump, and hence the absorption of NaCl from the cortical portion of the thick ascending limb of the loop of Henle; most of the important properties of these drugs stem from this action. Because this is the only part of the tubule capable of causing nett resorption of solute from the urine, the solute content of the resulting diuresis is high. Indeed if hydrochlorothiazide is administered to a sheep with an acetazolamide induced diuresis, *both* the flow-rate and the osmolality of the urine usually increase markedly. Oedema in cases of cardiac disease is predominantly due to salt retention by the kidneys in an unsuccessful attempt (teleologically speaking) to improve the circulation, and thiazides are particularly useful in these circumstances.

The thiazides are neither susceptible nor especially conducive to acid–base disturbances; however their action leaves subsequent tubular function relatively unaffected, and the resulting large increase

in luminal sodium content leads to compensatory aldosterone secretion, sodium resorption and potassium loss in the distal tubule.
Although this seems rarely to cause problems in veterinary practice,
it remains a potential hazard of longterm thiazide therapy, particularly when used in conjunction with digitalis glycosides, whose toxicity is increased by hypokalaemia. The danger may be reduced by
dietary supplementation, or by the use of potassium-sparing diuretics. Other side effects include interference with glucose metabolism, which may occasionally precipitate diabetes mellitus, and a
reduction in uric acid excretion. Calcium excretion is usually reduced, although the reason for this is not known.

The thiazides are active by mouth as well as by parenteral administration; their effects are fairly slow in onset, even after intravenous injection, and usually persist for about 12 hours. With
repeated dosage the response often diminishes, but it is not self-
limiting as is the case with carbonic anhydrase inhibitors. The thiazides do not appear to be metabolised to any significant extent and
are mostly excreted in the urine. They are probably the most generally useful of the diuretic drugs.

In man the thiazides are occasionally found useful in the treatment of diabetes insipidus, their oral activity making them convenient if not very efficaceous. The mechanism of this unexpected
property has been the subject of much unconvincing speculation,
but it seems possible that the blocking of solute absorption in the
cortical loop of Henle may lead to enhanced solute-mediated water
absorption in the distal tubule and collecting duct.

Loop diuretics

The chief members of this group are ethacrynic acid, frusemide and
bumetanide. They have as their main effect the inhibition of Cl⁻
pumping throughout the whole length of the thick ascending limb
of the loop of Henle, thus paralysing the kidney's ability both to
concentrate and to dilute the urine; they do not appear to have any
significant effect on proximal and distal tubular function. Their
effects are exerted from the luminal surface of the loop cells; because they are extensively bound to plasma proteins relatively little
is filtered in the glomerulus, and they rely on the proximal tubule's
organic acid secretory mechanism for access to their site of action.
Substances which block this mechanism, for example probenecid,
can therefore reduce their efficacy.

Although their mode of action was not fully understood during the period of their popularity, the **organomercurials** were in fact mostly effective by virtue of their interference with chloride pumping in the loop of Henle. The organic acid part of compounds such as **mersalyl** ensured secretion into the tubule lumen, and diuresis was probably due to the local release of small amounts of inorganic mercury ions on thiol groups in the tubular cell enzyme systems.

The various serious toxic effects of mercurial compounds led to the investigation of substances potentially capable of complexing thiol groups for diuretic activity, and the first major success was **ethacrynic acid** (Fig. 4.4). This organic acid has a more rapid and potent diuretic effect than the organomercurials, and is active orally as well as parenterally. Although approximately one third of an administered dose is metabolised in the liver, the remainder is secreted into the kidney tubule lumen, where its inhibition of Cl^- pumping produces a very large volume of urine whose composition and osmolality tend towards those of the glomerular filtrate. Ethacrynic acid can produce a diuresis so severe that clinical dehydration and acute circulatory collapse may follow its injudicious use. In comparison with this effect other postulated actions of ethacrynic acid, such as altering the distribution of renal blood flow and antagonising ADH, are of minor significance.

Although the compensatory reactions of the distal tubule can hardly begin to cope with this gross insult to normal renal function, prolonged therapy may result in potassium depletion; however this is not as great as it would be from an equivalent thiazide-induced diuresis. These distortions of fluid and electrolyte balance are the most serious hazards normally attendant on the use of loop diuretics; non-renal side-effects, which include gastro-intestinal disturbances following oral dosage and (rarely) ototoxicity, are relatively unimportant.

Frusemide (Lasix) is much the commonest member of this group of drugs. Its formular (Fig. 4.4) is interestingly reminiscent of the carbonic anhydrase inhibitors, and this is believed to account for the slightly greater loss of bicarbonate than is occasioned by ethacrynic acid. Otherwise their general pharmacological properties are virtually identical. Frusemide is rapidly active by oral or parenteral routes of administration; diuresis starts within a few minutes of intravenous injection and the peak effect occurs at 2–3 hours. This rapidity of action is very useful in emergency diuresis, for example in pulmonary oedema following cardiac failure or over-transfusion. A clinical advantage of frusemide over ethacrynic acid is that it is easier to control the degree of diuresis by varying the dose-rate.

Bumetanide is a diuretic very similar to frusemide, but approximately 50 times as potent. In ponies both bumetanide and ethacrynic acid appear to have a marginally smaller effect on water output than on solute output as compared with frusemide. However in general the loop diuretics are better suited to the rapid removal of fluid than to prolonged removal of solute, in comparison with the thiazides.

'Potassium-sparing' diuretics

These drugs are so named because they interfere with the function of the distal tubule and collecting duct, inhibiting the absorption of Na^+ by various means, and so reducing K^+ loss at these sites. This process is not a major part of the total renal absorptive effort and the resultant diuresis is correspondingly feeble. However they are useful in conjunction with longterm diuretic therapy, especially with thiazides, to obstruct the physiological antagonistic response to natriuresis and reduce the risk of hypokalaemia. Indeed they may lead to potassium accumulation, particularly in herbivores, which have a high potassium intake; it follows that these drugs should not be combined with potassium supplementation.

Spironolactone (Fig. 4.5, Aldactone) is an analogue of aldosterone, and acts as a competitive antagonist at its cytoplasmic receptors, thus blocking the aldosterone-stimulated synthesis of Na, K – ATPase. In support of this model, there is a delay of 2–3 days

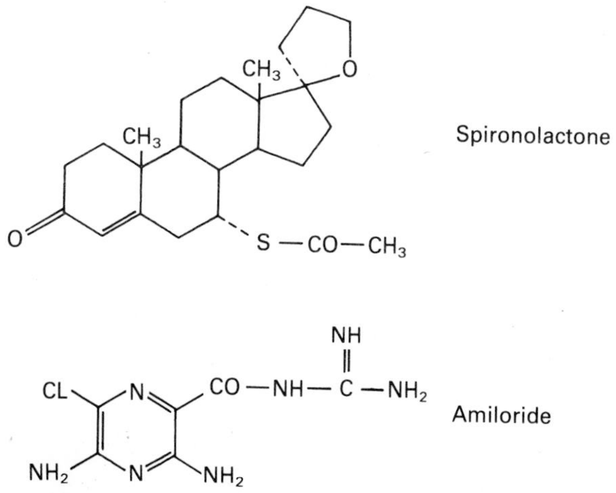

Fig. 4.5 'Potassium-sparing' diuretics.

between administration and maximal effect, the drug is ineffective in the presence of low plasma levels of aldosterone, and it can be antagonised by high doses of the hormone. It is also apparent from such studies that a significant proportion of the Na^+-pumping activity in the distal tubule is independent of aldosterone. Spironolactone is practically insoluble in water and fixed oils, and is only available for oral use.

Triamterine acts by directly inhibiting the aldosterone-sensitive ATPase; it thus achieves much the same effect as spironolactone and with a similar time course, although it is not dependent on the presence of aldosterone for its effect. Like spironolactone it is practically insoluble in common solvents.

Amiloride (Fig. 4.5) has a somewhat different site of action in that it appears to block the Na^+ channels in the luminal membrane, thus depriving the peritubular membrane of its supply of Na^+ rather than obstructing its ability to deal with it. Na^+ permeability is thus reduced throughout the distal tubule and collecting duct and even, to some extent, in the proximal tubule as well. It is also much quicker acting than the other drugs in this group. Although only marketed in tablet form the hydrochloride is adequately soluble in water, and its intravenous injection into sheep sharply reduces the urinary potassium content within a few minutes.

Captopril is a drug which inhibits the angiotensin converting enzyme, and thus reduces the secretion of aldosterone. Its durietic effects are very weak, and it is more commonly used as an anti-hypertensive agent, when its concomitant inhibition of bradykinin breakdown may also be implicated. However it enhances the action of direct natriuretic agents and reduces potassium loss.

Xanthine diuretics

The various naturally occurring and synthetic xanthines stimulate the CNS, increase cardiac efficiency and cause a diuresis which to some extent is due to a direct effect on the kidney. **Theophylline** is the most potent of the natural xanthines, and this ranking correlates with their abilities to inhibit phosphodiesterase and hence increase cellular cyclic AMP levels. Exactly how this causes a reduction in sodium and chloride absorption in the tubule is not clear, but in any case the diuresis is weak and evanescent.

Physiological diuretics

It is occasionally desirable to provoke diuresis in order to increase urinary flow or volume, e.g. in the treatment of cystitis or to avoid tubular precipitation of acetylated sulphonamides, rather than with the intention of reducing body fluid volume. In such cases increasing **water** intake may suffice: doses of 100 ml/kg body weight by stomach tube to large animals have been found satisfactory. In small animals, increasing the **sodium chloride** or **bicarbonate** content of the diet may achieve the same result more easily, provided that renal function is unimpaired.

ANTIDURETICS

These are usually only required in cases of diabetes insipidus, a condition which exists in two forms. In *nephrogenic* diabetes the kidney does not respond to antidiuretic hormone, although pituitary secretion may be normal. Further assault by antidiuretic hormone or its analogues is not often very productive, and therapy with **thiazides** is indicated.

In *primary* diabetes posterior pituitary secretion of antidiuretic hormone is deficient for some reason, but the kidney is usually fully sensitive to it. **Chlorpropamide** is a drug mainly used to stimulate insulin secretion in diabetes mellitus, but it has similar effects on the posterior pituitary, if hormone is there to be released. **Antidiuretic hormone** itself can be administered by intravenous injection or by nasal insufflation (very poorly tolerated by most small animals), but its effect is very short-lived as it has a plasma half-life of about 10 minutes.

Pitressin tannate is a crude pituitary extract which can be injected subcutaneously or intramuscularly as a suspension in oil; it is longer-lasting than ADH but tends to provoke an immune reaction which may leave the animal worse off than ever. It is not currently commercially available.

Desmopressin, or l-deamino, 8-D-arginine vasopressin, is a close synthetic analogue of the natural hormone with a much longer biological half-life and reduced pressor activity. Twice-daily dosage is said to be effective and well tolerated in man; however it still has to be given parenterally.

SUGGESTIONS FOR FURTHER READING

Brater D C 1983 Pharmacodynamic considerations in the use of diuretics. Annual Reviews of Pharmacology and Toxicology 23: 45–62

Jacobson H R, Kokko J P 1976 Diuretics: sites and mechanisms of action. Annual Review of Pharmacology and Toxicology 16: 201–214

Lote C J 1982 Principles of renal physiology. Croom-Helm, London

Michell A R 1980 The kidney: regulation and disturbances of body fluids. In: Yoxall A T, Hird J F (eds) Physiological Basis of Small Animal Medicine, Blackwell, Oxford, ch 4, p 71–126

5

Drugs affecting tissue metabolism

THYROID HORMONES

The thyroid hormones **thyroxine** and **liothyronine** (Fig. 5.1) are present in the thyroid gland incorporated in the glycoprotein thyroglobulin. The first stage in their synthesis involves the active uptake of I^- from the plasma, its oxidation, probably to I^+, and the iodination of tyrosine residues in the thyroglobulin peptide chain. These residues are then converted *in situ* into the hormones, which are then only released for secretion by the breakdown of the thyroglobulin. Both synthesis of the thyroglobulin and secretion of the thyroid hormones are enhanced by thyroid stimulating hormone (TSH) whose release from the anterior pituitary is, in its turn, subjected to negative feedback control by plasma thyroid hormone levels. Secretion of hormone from the normal gland is reduced in iodine deficiency, and this depression is relieved by iodine supplementation. Paradoxically in thyroid hypersecretory states an increased iodine intake reduces secretion to normal for a while, but

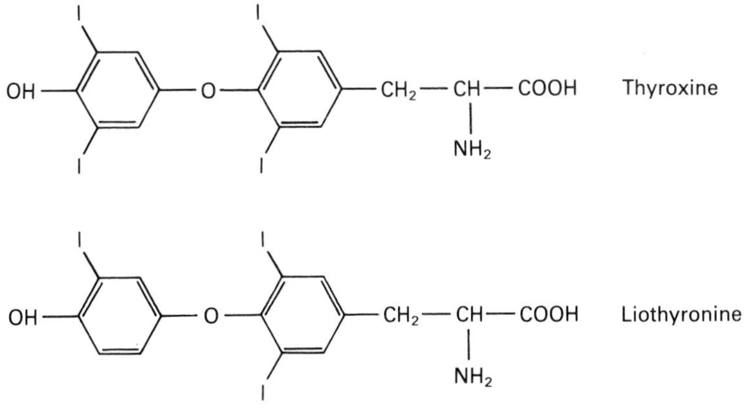

Fig. 5.1 Thyroxine and liothyronine.

it returns to its previous level over a period of a week or two. The gland normally secretes thyroxine and liothyronine in a ratio of about 4 : 1, but raised TSH levels and iodine deficiency increase the proportion of liothyronine.

In man these hormones have long-lasting effects due, apparently, to the presence of plasma proteins which bind them. Circulating thyroxine is tightly bound; its effects take some days to develop fully, and it has a biological half-life of about 7 days. Liothyronine is less tightly bound, and hence quicker and shorter acting; its effects are seen within a few hours, and its half-life is usually 2–3 days. Although the pharmacokinetics of thyroid hormones in small animals are generally held to conform to this pattern, there are preliminary American reports that their half-lives may only be around 12 and 6 hours respectively. The dose-intervals recommended are corresponding short: once or twice daily for thyroxine and three times daily for liothyronine; these findings are summarised in Rosychuk (1982). Both compounds are conjugated in the liver and then excreted in the bile.

On a molar basis thyroxine has only about a quarter of the potency of liothyronine. Approximately 30% of circulating thyroxine is deiodinated peripherally to liothyronine and this latter substance therefore accounts for 80% of thyroid hormone activity. The fact that liothyronine can maintain hypothyroid dogs at metabolic normality with plasma thyroxine levels of zero lends further support to the suggestion that thyroxine is normally only a circulating pro-hormone, and that the true active thyroid principal is liothyronine; however receptors specific for thyroxine have been found in cell nuclei, so that its role may be more complicated than this.

Nearly all the effects of thyroid hormones are thought to be mediated by specific effects on protein synthesis. They are vitally concerned in tissue differentiation and maturation. In foetal and newborn animals thyroid deficiency leads to inadequate development of the CNS, which can only be remedied by early replacement therapy. Thyroid deficiency also leads to failure of growth of skin and hair and increased protein leakage from capillaries; these are usually much more responsive to treatment. The calorigenic effects of thyroid hormones are often explained in terms of their ability to uncouple oxidative phosphorylation, but this only occurs at gross overdosage. The hormones are required for the maintenance of normal cellular metabolic activity and body temperature; moderate overdosage results in hyperthermia. A number of the metabolic effects of thyroid hormones are probably due to their ability to stimulate synthesis of beta-adrenoceptors. The most important consequences of this are seen in the heart as tachycardia and arrhythmia which in severe thyrotoxicosis can lead to heart failure. Other effects which may be adrenoceptor-mediated are increases in lipolysis and gluconeogenesis, although the latter may be masked by the general increase in metabolic rate.

To some extent the iodination of tyrosine and other amino acids can occur *in vitro*, and the resulting compounds show activity similar to that of thyroid hormones, but the use of substances such as iodinated casein for inappropriate purposes such as improving milk yield (it provokes a very disadvantageous change in the feed conversion efficiency) is now considered obsolete. Of similar status is the use of dessicated extracts of thyroid gland; both thyroxine and liothyronine are readily and cheaply available as pure synthetic compounds which are much more satisfactory than the unstable and variable natural products. There are attractions in the rapid direct effects of liothyronine, but its evanescence can be a clinical disadvantage, and its suppression of thyroxine secretion may lead to further derangement of thyroid function; for normal purposes therefore thyroxine is the drug of choice in hypothyroid conditions.

Anti-thyroid substances, by contrast, are much less used nowadays, although some naturally occurring ones are of toxicological interest. Goitrogens are found in a number of animal feedstuffs, the best known being L-5-vinyl-2-thioxazolidine, which is released from ingested brassicae. A diet consisting mostly of turnips, cabbage or kale may not only inhibit the cow's thyroid, but may even result in a sufficiently high level of toxin in the milk to produce goitre in children drinking it. Synthetic goitrogens such as **propylthiouracil** (PTU) and the longer-acting **methimazole** inhibit thyroid hormone synthesis by blocking iodine uptake in the gland, and reduce the effect of released thyroxine by interfering with peripheral deiodination. Since nearly all cases of hyperthyroidism are due to neoplasia the most sensible approach is surgical removal, but antithyroid drugs may be of some use in treating cases which are inoperable for any reason. They can also be used as preoperative prophylactics against thyroid crisis provoked by surgical trauma, but adding **potassium iodide** to the diet for a week or so before surgery to normalise thyroid activity is preferable. **Propranolol** may also be useful in blocking the beta-adrenoceptor mediated effects on the heart, unless actual congestive failure is present or threatened.

Although antithyroid substances have been used as routine feed additives in meat-producing animals, 'growth promotion' is hardly an expression appropriate to their effect, since they actually reduce the rate of weight gain, increase the carcass fat content (mostly subcutaneous, which in pigs may reduce its value) and, naturally since fat has the highest energy-content of all tissues, tend to worsen the feed conversion efficiency. Their use for this purpose is not recommended or widespread.

CARBOHYDRATE METABOLISM

The two most important derangements of carbohydrate metabolism requiring therapeutic intervention are diabetes mellitus, mostly in dogs, and ketosis, mostly in sheep and cattle; both consist essentially of a cellular deficiency of glucose.

Diabetes mellitus

In the case of diabetes the deficiency is caused by a failure of glucose uptake by peripheral cells, due to an absolute or relative lack of insulin, or by a failure of the cells to respond to it. Insulin is a protein hormone consisting of 51 amino acids arranged in two cross-linked chains. A larger molecule called proinsulin is synthesised in the beta cells of the pancreatic islets of Langerhans; the chains are split off from it and stored as a crystalline complex whose composition approximates to 6 molecules of insulin and 2 of zinc. When the beta cells are stimulated the remaining fragment of proinsulin is secreted along with the insulin, and occasionally becomes the subject of an undesirable autoimmune response.

Insulin is released into the portal blood supply, and the hepatic cells are exposed to a higher concentration than are the peripheral tissues since up to 50% of it is removed during this first passage through the liver. Overall, the plasma half-life of insulin is only a few minutes since it rapidly binds to sensitive tissues and then exerts its metabolic effects for several hours. The release of insulin is generally stimulated by a rise in the glucose concentration of the plasma perfusing the pancreas, as might be expected from its major effect of enhancing the movement of glucose into cells by increasing carrier-mediated transport across the membrane. However insulin release is influenced by a number of other factors as well. Several amino acids directly stimulate insulin secretion, and insulin in its turn stimulates amino acid uptake by cell membranes, as well as stimulating ribosomal protein synthesis and reducing intracellular catabolism of amino acids. Insulin release is increased by a rise in plasma free fatty acid (FFA) concentration and, once again, it increases the uptake of FFA by fat cells and tips the balance of their metabolism towards lipogenesis. All these effects tend to reduce plasma glucose and FFA levels and hence exert a negative feedback on insulin secretion.

The relationship of insulin with other hormones acting on carbohydrate metabolism is highly complex, and is exemplified by the effects of **glucagon**, which is released from the islet *alpha* cells in response to a fall in plasma glucose or FFA concentration, or to sympathetic stimulation. Glucagon decreases cellular glucose and FFA uptake and increases gluconeogenesis and lipolysis, thus raising the plasma glucose and FFA levels (removing the stimulus to its release) and opposing the action of insulin; in addition glucagon stimulates the release of adrenaline and growth hormone, both of which similarly oppose the metabolic effects of insulin. It is thus slightly unexpected that glucagon also stimulates the release of insulin; it would seem that the ratio of glucagon to insulin is the important variable controlling carbohydrate metabolism. In postprandial absorptive states both levels rise, whereas in stress conditions glucagon concentration rises and that of insulin falls.

Clinical cases of diabetes can be classified according to the plasma insulin and glucose levels. In type I diabetes plasma insulin is low or absent and hyperglycaemia is always present; the condition corresponds to the human classification of 'juvenile onset' diabetes. Type II diabetes is characterised by normal or high insulin levels and hyperglycaemia; this corresponds to the human 'maturity onset' classification. In neither type is the plasma insulin level responsive to induced changes in plasma glucose level. It has been suggested that damage to islet beta cells (by, for example, autoimmunity or over-stimulation) may lead to the production of defective insulin and hence to type II diabetes; eventually the cells suffer from 'exhaustion atrophy', and so the condition progresses to type I. If indeed this be the case it is perhaps worth noting that a more usual response of endocrine tissue to excessive stimulation is not atrophy but hypertrophy. However the theory does offer a possible explanation of the so-called 'chemical' diabetes which is characterised by relatively normal plasma insulin and glucose levels but an abnormally slow *response* to hyperglycaemia. This condition has been classified as type III (Kaneko et al, 1978), and is thought to represent the earliest detectable stages in the development of diabetes.

The numbering system is thus inversely related to the proposed chronological sequence.

This view of diabetes deals only with insulin production and its immediate effects, but it should be evident that factors other than simply insulin may well be involved in clinical diabetes; for instance it has been postulated that increased glucagon secretion may be necessary for the production of hyperglycaemia, and excessive production of growth hormone rapidly leads to a diabetes-like metabolic derangement.

Most of the effects of diabetes mellitus can be attributed to the unavailability of glucose to peripheral tissues. Liver cells form a partial exception to this generalisation: although glucose uptake occurs in the absence of insulin, the process is more rapid in its presence. A more complete exception is the brain, most of whose cells do not need insulin at all for glucose uptake; this is perhaps just as well since in most species and at most stages of postnatal development they show a marked preference for glucose over other substrates. However the cells of the hypothalamic satiety centre do need insulin for glucose uptake, and in consequence diabetic animals often show an increased appetite.

Despite this, the increased gluconeogenesis from amino acids leads to muscle wasting; fatty tissue is also lost since lipogenesis is reduced. Increased beta-oxidation of fatty acids leads to excess production of acetyl coenzyme A (acetylCoA) which the simultaneous shortage of citric acid cycle intermediates (particularly oxaloacetate) diverts to the synthesis of ketone bodies such as acetoacetic and betahydroxybutyric acids. These produce metabolic acidosis; their urinary excretion causes loss of Na^+ and K^+ and compounds the osmotic diuresis occasioned by the glomerular filtration of glucose at a rate exceeding the tubular maximum for its reabsorption. The cellular metabolic relationships are discussed further in the following section of this chapter, and are summarised in Figure 5.3.

Arteriolar and capillary endothelial cells are also affected by the disordered carbohydrate metabolism, showing evidence of microaneurysms and atheromatous changes, leading in many cases to retinal haemorrhages and to kidney and cardiac disease. Gangrene of the extremities is another common result of this diabetic microangiopathy. The condition is thought to be caused by high levels of growth hormone, and it is often not improved much by controlling the plasma glucose level.

Diabetic neuropathies and cataracts, however, are thought to be due directly to the hyperglycaemia; at any rate reducing glucose levels halts their progress and in the case of neuropathy may even allow some recovery.

Preparations of insulin and therapy of diabetes mellitus

Because of the linkage of insulin secretion to absorption from the gut and its preferential initial distribution to the liver it is impossible perfectly to mimic physiological normality, and hence completely to alleviate diabetes mellitus, by intermittent systemically administered doses of insulin; nonetheless this remains the commonest therapeutic measure. Various preparations of insulin have been formulated; they all require the owner's intelligent cooperation in their administration as well as in the dietary management necessary to minimise the degree and variation of insulin requirement. Insulin is obtained from bovine or porcine pancreas. Modern preparations are highly purified and immune responses to them are rare; when these occur, however, they may sometimes be relieved by changing the species of origin.

Soluble insulin injection is an acidic solution of crystalline insulin containing small amounts of zinc. It is usually given subcutaneously or intramuscularly, when its effects are seen in about 30 minutes, reach a maximum at 4 hours and effectively last 6–8 hours. Intravenous administration gives a faster onset. **Neutral insulin** injection is very similar, but the solution is brought approximately to pH 7 with acetate buffer. The solution is slightly more stable at room temperature, and has a slightly more rapid onset of action.

The inconvenience of giving injections of soluble insulin several times a day and the resulting large fluctuations in carbohydrate metabolism led to the development of less soluble depot preparations, using either protein complexes or zinc salts. Not surprisingly, the proteins occasionally cause hypersensitivity reactions and these formulations are now not regarded very favourably. **Protamine zinc insulin** is prepared from insulin and an excess of protamine with a little zinc and phosphate buffer. The preparation must not be given intravenously and soluble insulin should not be mixed with it since it is complexed to an unpredictable extent by the free protamine. Its effects last from 4 to about 30 hours after injection. **Isophane insulin** is very similar except that the minimum necessary amount of protamine is added to the insulin, and the suspension is opaque rather than merely turbid. It is slightly more rapidly acting. **Globin zinc insulin** is an unbuffered complex of globin and insulin with rather similar properties to those of isophane insulin.

Of considerably greater importance are the various **insulin zinc suspensions** which contain increased amounts of zinc. They are prepared in the absence of phosphate, which precipitates zinc, and are buffered with acetate; they should not, therefore, be mixed with protamine or isophane insulin. The suspension may be either **amorphous** (with particles of maximum dimension less than 2 μm) or **crystalline** (particles between 10 and 40 μm). Amorphous ('semilente') insulin is effective between 1 and 12–16 hours after injection, with a peak at around 6 hours, while crystalline ('ultralente') insulin is effective between 4 and 30–36 hours, with its peak effect at 10–18 hours. The two forms are freely mixable to give intermediate durations of effect. Bovine crystalline insulin zinc is also mixed with porcine soluble insulin, in the proportions 3 : 1, to give **biphasic insulin injection** with both rapid onset and long duration. None of these insulin zinc preparations are suitable for intravenous use.

Oral hypoglycaemic drugs

These are drugs which tend to reduce the plasma glucose concentration (Fig. 5.2). They are mostly used in human practice for treating maturity onset (type II) diabetes; they have not found much

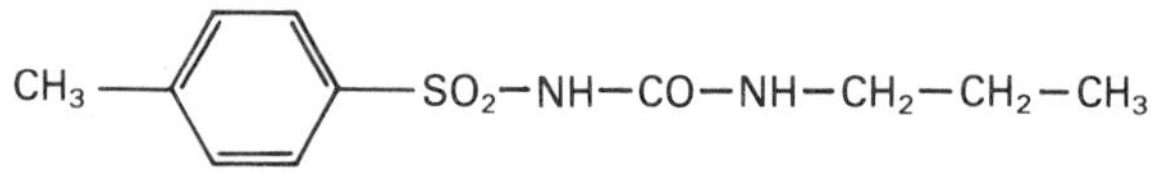

$$CH_3 - \langle \bigcirc \rangle - SO_2-NH-CO-NH-CH_2-CH_2-CH_3$$

Tolbutamide

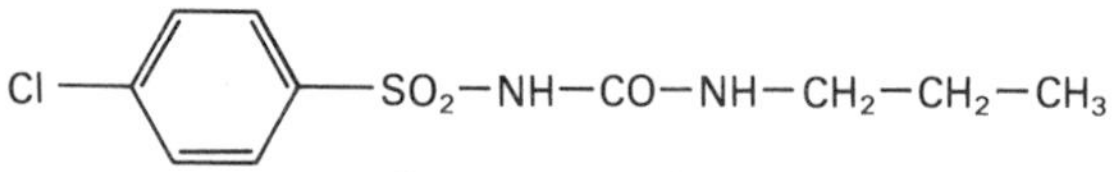

$$Cl - \langle \bigcirc \rangle - SO_2-NH-CO-NH-CH_2-CH_2-CH_3$$

Chlorpropamide

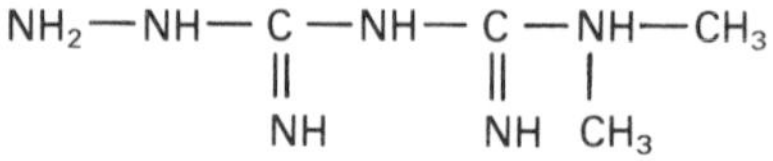

$$NH_2-NH-\underset{\underset{NH}{\|}}{C}-NH-\underset{\underset{NH}{\|}}{C}-\underset{\underset{CH_3}{|}}{N}H-CH_3$$

Metformin

Fig. 5.2 Oral hypoglycaemic drugs.

application in veterinary treatment of diabetes, although Kaneko et al (1978) suggest that they may be of value combined with dietary management in type III cases.

The sulphonylureas seem primarily to augment insulin release from the beta cells, although they probably also enhance its peripheral effects; at all events they depend upon the existence of some competent islet tissue. They tend to cause obesity, and they can cause actual hypoglycaemia, which may be severe and prolonged. Their effects are potentiated by non-steroidal anti-inflammatory drugs such as aspirin and phenylbutazone, and by sulphonamides. **Tolbutamide** has a very short duration of effect since it is mostly rapidly inactivated by metabolism in the liver; it is thus contraindicated in liver disease but relatively safe in renal disease. **Chlorpropamide**, by contrast, is not much metabolised: it therefore has a longer half-life, but may produce signs of overdosage through accumulation in cases of renal insufficiency.

The biguanides do not seem to interact with insulin's release, but they probably augment its effects; they reduce hepatic output and intestinal absorption of glucose and increase its peripheral uptake. They do not cause hypoglycaemia in normal animals although they may produce a number of other toxic effects, including lactic acidaemia; this is especially common and severe in human patients treated with **phenformin**, and is a much less frequent complication of therapy with **metformin**.

Ketosis

This condition is also known as acetonaemia in cattle; in this species it usually occurs during the immediately post-parturient increase in milk production but it may also occur, as it usually does in sheep, in the last third of gestation when it is also known as pregnancy toxaemia. It is usually caused by the demand for glucose outstripping the supply, so that the glucose-utilising tissues effectively starve; the condition is thus functionally indistinguishable from the ketosis engendered by starvation in any animal. In many cattle the first and economically most important consequence of ketosis is a reduction in milk production, which often cures the condition, but in high-yielding cows the hormonal stimulus to lactation may prove too strong for this eminently sensible inhibition. More severe ketosis causes inappetance, and from this point onwards the animal is trapped since the worse its condition becomes the less food it takes

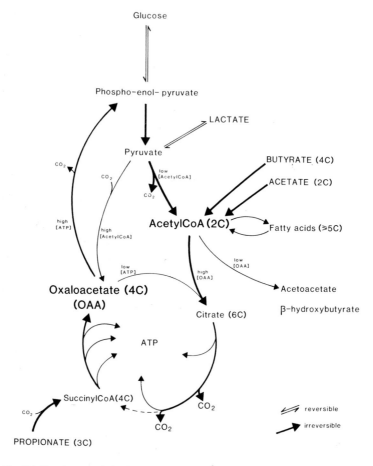

Fig. 5.3 Ruminant carbohydrate metabolism.

in. In sheep the condition usually results from an unreasonable persistence in the attempt to maintain twin foetuses.

Ruminant animals ingest very little carbohydrate (and much of what they do is rapidly appropriated by the ruminal microflora). They derive their materials and energy mostly from volatile fatty acids produced by rumen fermentation; the commonest acids are acetic, butyric and propionic. As can be seen in figure 5.3, the first two are converted into acetylCoA and then mostly either broken down to produce energy in the citric acid cycle after combination with oxaloacetate, or converted to fat. To all normal intents and purposes only propionate is capable of generating glucose; if propionate is not present in the diet or produced from it by rumen fermentation, then gluconeogenesis and hence the synthesis of lactose and glucose-derived aminoacids is blocked.

Another important aspect of this system is the fact that none of the other fatty acids can be used to synthesise oxaloacetate, without which acetylCoA, whether from fatty acid oxidation or from glycolysis, cannot be broken down. Thus when hepatic cellular oxaloacetate levels fall the citric acid cycle grinds to a halt and the liver's main supply of energy (and this wholly inadequate) arises during the beta-oxidation of fatty acids; the resulting excess of acetylCoA is turned into acetoacetate and thence into beta-hydroxybutyrate. These ketone bodies cannot support gluconeogenesis and, although they can supply the *energy* requirements of extrahepatic tissues (up to 75% in brain), adaptation to their utilisation is often too slow to keep pace with the deteriorating situation. Furthermore since their synthesis is a consequence of the liver's reliance for energy on beta-oxidation, they are produced in gross excess and thus cause acidosis and urinary loss of water and cations.

Treatment of ketosis

In moderate cases the remedy for ketosis is simply to restore the balance of gluconeogenesis and energy production in the animal's metabolism. The most direct way of achieving this is by intravenous injection of glucose, and this gives rapid but transient relief of the condition.

Oral therapy is more practicable in farm animals; glucose is clearly useless by this route, but a number of substances are preferentially glucogeneogenic, chief amongst which is **propionate**, usually administered as the sodium salt, but sodium or calcium **lactate** is also suitable. **Propylene glycol** and **glycerol** are fermented to propionate by rumen microflora, and thus constitute less direct remedies. This may be important in severely ketotic patients, which may also require intravenous administration of glucose and alkalinising fluids such as **sodium bicarbonate** or **compound sodium lactate** to achieve a sufficiently rapid and adequate response.

Single intramuscular injections of glucocorticoids such as **betamethasone** or anabolic steroids such as **trienbolone acetate** are an attractively easy alternative in practice, and seem to produce reasonable results. Their success is slightly unexpected since corticosteroids themselves increase the tendency towards lipolysis and fatty acid breakdown, while the hyperglycaemia which is the chief rationale for their use is partly due to their anti-insulin effect on cellular uptake of glucose. However they also increase gluconeogenesis from aminoacids and the synthesis of oxaloacetate from pyruvate. It is likely that part of the clinical response also stems from their euphoric effects (including stimulation of appetite) and the reduction in milk production that they cause. Corticosteroids are certainly much less effective in ketotic ewes unless they also induce abortion.

VITAMIN E AND SELENIUM

Vitamin E is the classical name for a factor in plant oils which was found to be required by rats for the production of live young; it received this name simply because vitamins A, B, C and D had been discovered already. Although the original material used was wheatgerm oil the major natural source now is soya bean oil. 'Vitamin E' is actually a family of several closely related alcohols known as tocopherols. Of these **alpha-tocopherol** is much the most important; it is twice as active as any of the others and it is the only one absorbed to any extent from the diet. Older literature on dietary levels and nutritional requirements which did not take account of these facts is thus largely invalidated.

The activities of naturally derived vitamin E preparations and of the various synthesised tocopherols are still often expressed in international units, although their use was officially discontinued many years ago; 1 IU is the activity of 1 mg of dl-alpha-tocopherylacetate. The tocopherols are insoluble in water, but highly soluble in oils. They are rapidly inactivated by heat, light and oxygen, but can be stabilised by the addition of antioxidants. At the biochemical level vitamin E is involved in reactions characterised by the formation of free radicals, where it seems to act as a buffer or intermediary. This role is very similar to that of selenium, and the two are intimately associated in the function of a number of tissues, especially in skeletal and cardiac muscle. Tocopherol is also involved in the safe metabolism of polyunsaturated fatty acids, and an increase in the dietary content of them leads to an increased vitamin requirement.

Selenium shows chemical properties similar to those of sulphur, including a variable valency; most of selenium's biological functions are carried out by the Se^{2-} ion, while selenite (SeO_3^{2-}) is the most toxic form. The reduction of selenate to selenite in alkaline dry soils and its subsequent uptake by plants (in some cases active accumulation as selenoaminoacids) constitutes a serious hazard to grazing livestock in parts of America, but is outside the scope of the present chapter.

Selenium is a component of a number of proteins, including glutathione peroxidase which protects red blood cells against damage from the high intracellular oxygen tension by facilitating the controlled reduction of H_2O_2. The level of this enzyme in red cells is a useful guide to the selenium status of the animal. Selenoproteins are also involved in cytochrome electron transfer, and a selenium-containing haemoprotein appears to form part of skeletal and cardiac muscle energy transfer systems.

In mammals skeletal and cardiac **nutritional myopathies** are due to selenium and vitamin E deficiencies. In the USA the condition is associated with feeding low-selenium hay and is best treated by supplementation with selenium. In Europe myopathies are often associated with feeding badly cured hay or young grass containing high levels of polyunsaturated fatty acids, and usually respond better to vitamin E. Mulberry heart in pigs appears to be primarily a selenium deficiency.

In poultry vitamin E deficiency alone causes encephalomalacia, while uncomplicated selenium deficiency leads to poor growth and reduced fertility. A deficiency of both results in vascular wall damage, and seems to be the cause of an exudative diathesis, especially in the pectoral muscles.

There is a growing belief that marginal selenium deficiency is widespread, and a corresponding increase in the popularity of supplementing feedstuffs with selenium. Top-dressing deficient pasture with selenium is relatively ineffectual by comparison.

Overdosage with tocopherol can cause skeletal muscle weakness and disturbances of reproductive function, while among the most sensitive signs of selenium toxicity are infertility, degeneration and fibrosis of striated muscle and polioencephalomalacia. These toxic effects can occur at feed or water selenium concentrations of 5–20 nmol/g, and it is particularly noteworthy that they may very easily be mistaken for the signs of deficiency.

VITAMIN K AND OTHER FACTORS AFFECTING BLOOD CLOTTING

Vitamin K was discovered in 1929 when chicks fed on a fat-free diet developed subcutaneous haemorrhages and prolonged blood coagulation times. The factor responsible for preventing this syndrome was shown to be fat soluble and naturally present in liver and in green plant tissues; its absence leads to a failure of prothrombin synthesis. It was given the letter K from the German word 'Koagulation'. Several different compounds exist under this name, and their trivial nomenclature has been confused by differing American and British conventions; the nomenclature employed in this account follows the international standard system.

Phylloquinone (vitamin K_1, phytomenadione, phytonadione) was isolated from plant material, and is slightly more active in most systems than **menaquinone** (vitamin K_2) which is found in animal materials and is synthesised by bacteria. Both are naphthaquinones with an isoprenoid sidechain. **Menadione** (vitamin K_3, menaphthone) lacks this sidechain; it is prepared synthetically and is itself virtually inactive. Prenylation of menadione to form menaquinone occurs slowly in the livers of most animals, although the rate in birds is usually greater than in mammals. None of these compounds are significantly water soluble, and both the quinones are dependent on normal bile secretion and fat digestion for their adequate absorption; menadione appears to be absorbed independently of biliary function. Vitamin K deficiency is only likely to occur in chronic disorders of the intestine such as diarrhoea and malabsorption, or following prolonged disruption of its microflora by, for example, the oral use of broad spectrum antibiotics.

In bacteria vitamin K acts as an electron carrier, as does the closely related ubiquinone in mitochondrial oxidative respiration, but in mammals and birds its principal function is to catalyze the γ-carboxylation of the first ten glutamate residues in the N-terminal portion of the hepatic prothrombin precursor. This post-ribosomal modification to prothrombin (clotting factor II) enables it to bind Ca^{2+} (factor IV) in the plasma clotting process. Vitamin K is similarly required for the formation of factors VII, IX and X. Vitamin K dependent γ-carboxylation of some proteins unconnected with blood clotting has been reported; in particular the existence of a low molecular weight protein apparently involved in initiating the minerallisation of the foetal skeleton may explain the teratogenicity of some vitamin K antagonists.

The precise mechanism of action of vitamin K is still unclear, but it is probably reduced to the hydroquinone before it can catalyze the addition of CO_2 to the glutamate residue. In the process it is itself converted into an inactive epoxide whose reactivation depends upon reduction to the original quinone by a specific enzyme.

This vitamin K epoxide reductase is inhibited by a number of compounds, mostly derived from 4-hydroxycoumarol, which thus block the supply of reduced vitamin K and hence of clotting factors. **Dicoumarol** was the first of them to be discovered, as the causative agent of a haemorrhagic condition seen in cattle fed spoiled sweet clover silage. Similar compounds such as **warfarin** are used as anticoagulants in human practice to avert threatened thrombosis, and they have been similarly employed in the treatment of navicular disease in horses; interestingly, clinically effective doses sometimes did not alter the plasma clotting time, although they always reduced blood viscosity. However it is their use as rodenticides, and subsequent unintended poisoning of cats and dogs, that constitutes their main veterinary significance. Such cases are relatively rare with warfarin because single doses do not deplete vitamin K levels significantly, and repeated ingestions are required to cause toxicity.

So-called 'super-mice' owe their impressive title simply to the possession of a dominant autosomal gene which reduces the susceptibility of their vitamin K epoxide reductase to hydroxycoumarol antagonists, usually by a factor of 50–200 times. This mutation also exists in rats; in both cases the possessor's dietary requirement for vitamin K is increased approximately twentyfold.

Preparations of vitamin K and its antagonists

Phylloquinone is available in tablets and capsules, or as a colloidal suspension in water for parenteral use; it is fairly stable to heat and air, but is inactivated by light. Its intravenous injection can reduce the clotting time in animals poisoned with warfarin within 15 minutes. This route of administration should be reserved for real emergencies since there is a high incidence of anaphylactoid and haemolytic reactions; subcutaneous or oral administration is considerably safer in less urgent cases.

Various menadione derivatives, such as **menadione sodium bisulphite** are water-soluble, and hence more easily formulated. They are still light-sensitive, and are more irritant to tissues. They are adequate for dietary supplementation, but conversion to the active vitamin is insufficiently rapid to be of much benefit in most cases of poisoning with hydroxycoumarol anticoagulants.

Warfarin, usually as the sodium salt, is effective after regular parenteral or oral administration for more than 2–3 days. In plasma it is almost entirely bound to albumin, and has a half-life of 30–40 hours. Other drugs which bind to albumin frequently cause some slight displacement of bound warfarin and hence a large rise in its plasma free concentration; barbiturates, salicylates and phenylbutazone are particularly likely to produce this effect. However the duration of warfarin's inhibition of vitamin K epoxide reductase is relatively short, and thus phylloquinone replacement therapy is only required for 4–6 days. More recent vitamin K antagonists, especially indanediones such as **diphenadione** are more effective as rodenticides since their inhibition lasts for 3–4 weeks, and they may produce toxic signs following a single dose. Animals inadvertently poisoned with these compounds need a correspondingly prolonged period of therapy. Diphenadione has also been used as a systemic vampiricide in Southern American cattle; presumably the bat's blood coagulatory mechanisms are more sensitive to the drug than are those of its host.

Directly acting anticoagulants

The vitamin K antagonists are ineffective *in vitro*; the compounds considered in this section are all directly effective in blocking coagulation. Most of them do so by binding Ca^{2+}, and hence by blocking the activation of both extrinsic and intrinsic clotting systems.

Ethylenediaminetetraacetate (**EDTA**) and citrate both form soluble complexes and so only alter the ionic calcium fraction, but **oxalate** precipitates the calcium and so removes it from the plasma completely. When citrate is used as an adjunct to blood transfusion care must be taken that it is not administered to the recipient in quantities sufficient to produce generalised anticoagulant effects.

Heparin is a strong acidic (anionic) mucopolysaccharide found in mast cells; commercial preparations are mostly extracted from bovine lung and porcine intestinal mucosa, and are available as sodium, potassium and various other salts. Its physiological role is unknown since its major effects are on plasma, where it has not been detected in normal animals. Heparin accelerates the action of a protease inhibitor called antithrombin III which inactivates not only thrombin but also a number of other clotting factors, and this property of heparin appears to form the basis of its anticoagulant effects, which are virtually immediate and occur both in vivo and *in vitro*. Heparin is not absorbed from the gut and for therapeutic purposes is best given by slow intravenous infusion, but for low-dose therapy it can be injected subcutaneously or into fat. It should not be injected into muscle, where it tends to cause haematomas.

Heparin also causes the release of lipoprotein lipase from blood vessel endothelium, and this results in a lowering of plasma lipid content. Systemic use of heparin has few other effects on blood clinical chemistry, but the use of relatively large amounts *in vitro* may alter the cationic composition of a sample.

The half-life of heparin in the circulation is dose-dependent, but is normally only a few hours. It can be antagonised by **protamine sulphate**, a strongly basic protein isolated from fish roes which complexes heparin. It should, however, be used with caution since it is itself anticoagulant in overdosage.

IRON AND COPPER

There are many similarities between the properties and functions of iron and copper. They are both transition metals, capable of several valency states and highly prone to complex formation. They are found at the active centres of a number of enzymes concerned with oxidation–reduction and electron transfer reactions, most notably in the cytochrome system. Iron is also a vital component of haemoglobin and myoglobin. Their free ions are highly toxic and virtually never occur in normal circumstances. The two metals also have many common features from the pharmacological and therapeutic points of view.

Metabolism of iron

Iron is absorbed by a mechanism in the proximal duodenum which involves the binding of ionic iron to receptors, and which is saturable. The receptors also bind chromium, manganese, cobalt and zinc; these metals therefore all inhibit each others' active absorption. Large doses of iron are absorbed throughout the small intestine by a slower non-specific process, which is not saturable. Once absorbed into mucosal cells iron is loosely chelated to small molecules, probably mostly aminoacids and monosaccharides. Such substances in the gut lumen also enhance the non-specific uptake of iron, whereas compounds forming stable chelates, particularly hydrophilic ones such as EDTA and phosphates (both organic and inorganic), tend to reduce iron absorption.

Inside the mucosal cell iron may be taken up by *ferritin* or passed to the serosal surface where it combines mostly with *transferrin*. An increase in chelated iron in the cytosol directly activates ribosomal synthesis of apoferritin, a complex protein with a molecular weight of about 450 000 daltons which is capable of storing 4500 atoms of ferric iron (over half its own weight) as the oxyhydroxide. Ferritin catalyses the oxidation of Fe^{2+} to Fe^{3+} itself. In the gut this mechanism functions to block iron absorption since the ferritin is lost into the lumen when the mucosal cells are shed from the tips of the villi; the extent of this trapping mechanism is limited by the rate of ferritin synthesis.

The combined effect of these absorptive processes and the 'mucosal block' by ferritin is that between 6 and 25% of dietary iron is absorbed into the body. This is of clinical significance because of the negligible extent of iron excretion: the average life of an iron atom in a man is approximately 8 years and the rate of turnover is much the same in domestic animals.

In most other cells ferritin serves more simply as a readily available reserve of iron and its level is normally maintained so that each molecule contains about 3000 atoms. Cells take up transferrin-bound iron from extracellular fluid by a process of micropinocytosis. The iron is released to cytosol chelators and thence to ferritin-storage, and the transferrin is returned to the exterior. Redistribution of iron follows the reverse pattern with the important difference that the conversion of Fe^{2+} to Fe^{3+} prior to binding by transferrin is not autocatalyzed, but is brought about by the copper-containing protein *caeruloplasmin*. Small parenterally administered doses of iron are taken up mostly by iron-requiring tissues, especially bone marrow but also hepatocytes, where the ferritin-iron is maintained in an available state. As the dose is increased its fate changes in that an increasing proportion is taken up by hepatic Kupffer cells, where the ferritin is rapidly converted to the insoluble and unmetabolisable *haemosiderin*, giving rise to the typical histological signs of iron overload.

In summary then, iron balance is only controlled by its intestinal absorption. Parenteral administration bypasses this control, and overdosage by either route is at best wasteful and may lead to toxic accumulation.

Preparations of iron

Ferrous (Fe^{2+}) salts are better absorbed orally than ferric (Fe^{3+}) ones since the solubilities of the two ions at pH 8 are 10^{-2} and 10^{-18} mol/l respectively. Complex preparations offer no significant advantages over simple **ferrous sulphate**; this is particularly true of 'slow release' compounds which are merely less completely absorbed and whose claimed safety is thus more economically achieved by a reduced dose of the sulphate. Most ferrous salts have a relatively mild or pleasant taste; the evil reputation of iron tonic mixtures is due partly to the use of ferric salts, and partly to the largely punitive inclusion of bitters such as quinine.

The commonest parenteral preparation of iron is **iron dextran**. This chelate must be given by careful deep intramuscular injection, and may produce tissue staining, especially if it leaks out from the injection site. It occasionally produces an anaphylactic reaction; this is most frequently seen in horses.

Acute iron toxicity is difficult to treat since even strong complexing agents such as EDTA do not sequester iron firmly enough to prevent toxicity. **Desferrioxamine** is a useful specific iron chelator in human practice, but is extremely expensive.

Copper metabolism

Copper is absorbed from the intestine to a small extent by an active process. The bulk of absorbed copper is taken into mucosal cells chelated to aminoacids, and is then complexed to a small molecular weight sulphur-containing protein known as *metallothionein*, which probably serves the dual role of providing a slow-release reserve for subsequent translocation and of limiting absorption in the same way as ferritin does for iron. Metallothionein also binds zinc and cadmium and competition for absorption between these metals is probably exerted at this point.

Absorption of copper is severely restricted by the presence of high levels of molybdenum and sulphate in the diet due to the formation of insoluble copper-thiomolybdate complexes. Although molybdenum is an essential trace element its main clinical significance stems from the ability of high-molybdenum ('teart') soils to precipitate secondary copper deficiency. Primary copper deficiency is usually associated with chalk or old red sandstone soils.

Copper is transferred from the intestine to the liver bound to plasma albumin, crosses the hepatocyte membrane bound to aminoacids, and is stored chelated to metallothionein and other molecules. As with iron overload, excess copper accumulates in the liver, and excretion is very slow, being mostly in bile. Redistribution to other organs is accomplished by *caeruloplasmin*, which thus appears to be a genuinely dual-purpose molecule. The plasma concentration of caeruloplasmin correlates well with the animal's overall copper status, and its estimation is less prone to contamination-errors than is that of copper itself.

A lack of caeruloplasmin leads to an inadequate supply of iron to bone marrow and hence to hypochromic anaemia. Many of the other effects of copper deficiency can also be attributed to the absence of specific copper-containing proteins. The lack of *mono-amine oxidase* reduces desmosine synthesis; subsequent failure of elastin and collagen cross-linkages may result in aortic rupture or osteoporosis. Poor coat pigmentation due to reduced synthesis of melanin can be ascribed to inadequate levels of *tyrosinase*. Both the offspring and milk of animals kept on low copper or high molybdenum pastures are likely to be deficient in copper, and young lambs may either be born with or develop 'swayback' due to a failure of CNS myelination. This is probably caused by the effect of inadequate levels of *cytochrome oxidase* on phospholipid metabolism.

Preparations of copper

Copper sulphate is cheap and has been used as an oral supplement; absorption is usually approximately 10% of the dose. Its high solubility limits its usefulness as a pasture top-dressing. Cupric oxide can be given orally to ruminants to provide a slowly dissolving depot, either as a glass bolus which stays in the reticulum, or as short needles which lodge in the abomasal wall.

Parenteral administration of copper bypasses the intestinal block, and increases the risk of poisoning by overdosage. Intravenous copper sulphate has been used in cattle but if the plasma binding capacity is saturated the free copper ions resulting are extremely toxic. Consequently it is probably safer to administer complexed formulations of copper, usually by subcutaneous injection. Of these **copper diethylamine oxyquinoline sulphonate** releases its copper most rapidly. It is thus the most efficacious in relieving deficiency, and the least likely to produce a local reaction; it is, however, the most prone to producing signs of acute toxicity. **Calcium copper EDTA** (or **edetate**) and **copper methionate** are about equally effective, but the latter more frequently causes local reactions.

Copper toxicity

Ruminants are more susceptible to copper poisoning than other domestic animals, and sheep are particularly sensitive. Acute copper toxicity usually occurs when excess copper is ingested, often as a result of top-dressing pasture with copper salts or with manure from pigs fed high levels of copper as a growth promoter. In severe cases many affected animals die from the immediate gastroenteritis and consequent circulatory collapse before appreciable amounts of copper have been absorbed. Chronic toxicity occurs with a lower intake of copper. This may result from over-supplementation or from industrial contamination of pasture; in addition some fodder plants, for example *Trifolium* and *Lupinus* species, concentrate copper from the soil. The signs of chronic toxicity are also sudden in onset since the excess copper is stored in the liver until some factor, such as liver fluke infestation or, eventually, the hepatic level of copper itself, provokes its massive release, causing further liver damage as well as considerable haemolysis.

Treatment of animals showing clinical signs is rarely successful, but prophylactic therapy with copper chelating compounds such as **calcium EDTA** may be helpful. **D-penicillamine** both chelates copper and enhances its urinary excretion (the L-isomer is toxic, being a potent pyridoxine antagonist). At a more economically realistic level, feeding **molybdenum** and **sulphate** supplemented diets may inhibit further absorption of copper from contaminated feedstuffs.

SUGGESTIONS FOR FURTHER READING

Buck W B 1978 Copper/molybdenum toxicity in animals. In: Oehme F W (ed) Toxicity of heavy metals in the environment, part I. Dekker, New York, ch 22, p 491–513

Harr J R 1978 Biological effects of selenium. In: Oehme F W (ed) Toxicity of heavy metals in the environment, part I. Dekker, New York, p 393–426

Herbert V, Das K C 1976 The role of vitamin B_{12} and folic acid in haemato- and other cell-poiesis. Vitamins and Hormones 34: 3–30

Kaneko J J, Mattheeuws D, Rottiers R P, Vermeulen A 1977 Glucose tolerance and insulin response in diabetes mellitus of dogs. Journal of Small Animal Practice 18: 85–94

Mullen P A 1983 Metabolic disorders of cattle: current trends in treatment and prophylaxis. In: Bogan J A, Lees P, Yoxall A T (eds) Pharmacological basis of large animal medicine. Blackwood, Oxford, p 326–332

Munro H N, Linder M L 1978 Ferritin: structure, biosynthesis, and role in iron metabolism. Physiological Reviews 58: 317–396

Rice D A, Blanchflower W J, McMurray C H 1981 Reproduction of nutritional degenerative myopathy in the post ruminant calf. Veterinary Record 109: 161–162

Rosychuk R A W 1982 Thyroid hormones and antithyroid drugs. Veterinary Clinics of North America: Small Animal Practice 12: 111–148

Suttle N F 1981 Comparison between parenterally administered copper complexes of their ability to alleviate hypocupraemia in sheep and cattle. Veterinary Record 109: 304–307

6

The pharmacology of cholinoceptive and adrenoceptive mechanisms

INTRODUCTION

Effector organs are supplied with motor nerves which may be classified as cholinergic or adrenergic according to whether transmission at the neuro-effector junctions is mediated by acetylcholine or noradrenaline. With a few exceptions, the somatic motor and parasympathetic nerves are cholinergic and sympathetic nerves adrenergic.

The terms cholinoceptive and adrenoceptive were introduced by Sir Henry Dale to denote sensitivity to acetycholine or noradrenaline. The cholinoceptive or adrenoceptive nature of effector cells is due to the presence of specific receptors for acetylcholine or noradrenaline, known as cholinoceptors or adrenoceptors, respectively. The combination of a drug with adrenoceptors will produce or abolish sympathomimetic effects. Drugs which combine with cholinoceptors mimic or antagonise parasympathetic effects, produce stimulant effects like nicotine, or block transmission in ganglia and in many instances at the skeletal neuromuscular junction. Pesticides which act on cholinoceptive mechanisms in insects or helminths are considered in a later chapter.

Autonomic and somatic motor nerves

The autonomic nervous system may be defined as that part of the peripheral nervous system which regulates the activities of glands, plain muscle and heart. It comprises all the efferent fibres in peripheral nerves with the exception of those in the motor nerve supply to the voluntary muscles. Autonomic fibres leave the central nervous system in some of the cranial and spinal nerves. The autonomic fibres in the motor roots of the thoracic and upper lumbar spinal nerves constitute the pre-ganglionic sympathetic nerves. The outflow of autonomic fibres from the cranial and sacral regions of the nervous system constitute the parasympathetic nerves. Most of the viscera are supplied with sympathetic and parasympathetic nerves. This is not invariably so however, some of the viscera being supplied with sympathetic fibres only. For example, there is no parasympathetic innervation of the systemic blood vessels, errector pili (hair muscles), sweat glands, adrenal gland, or plain muscle in the upper eyelid and nictitating membrane.

Table 6.1 Some sympathetic and parasympathetic effects of autonomic nerve stimulation.

Organ	Sympathetic	Parasympathetic
Heart	Acceleration. Impulse formation and conduction accelerated. Increased contractility.	Cardiac slowing and reduced A-V conduction.
Blood vessels	Widespread constriction, vasodilatation in myocardium and voluntary muscles.	—
Plain muscle:		
Iris	Contraction of radial muscle (mydriasis)	Contraction of circular muscle (miosis)
Ciliary		Contraction (accommodation of lens for near vision)
Bronchial	Relaxation	Contraction
Hair muscles (errector pili)	Contraction	—
Alimentary tract	Inhibition of motility	Increased motility
Gall bladder	Relaxation	Contraction
Spleen	Contraction	—
Bladder (fundus)	Relaxation	Contraction
(sphincter)	Contraction	Relaxation
Vas deferens, Seminal vesicle & prostate glands	Contraction	
Uterus	Relaxation or contraction	—
Glands:		
Sweat	Secretion	—
Salivary	Secretion (viscid)	Secretion
Gastric		Secretion
Liver	Glycogenolysis	Increased bile flow
Pancreas		Secretion
Bronchial		Secretion
Adrenal medulla	Adrenaline secretion	—

Although the effect of stimulating the sympathetic supply to an organ is often the opposite of that to parasympathetic stimulation (Table 6.1), it should not be supposed that the sympathetic and parasympathetic nervous systems simply act antagonistically. For example, the dilator and constrictor muscles of the pupil are kept in a state of tonic contraction by sympathetic and parasympathetic nerves, respectively. In dim light the pupil dilates because of reduced activity in the parasympathetic supply. In a frightened animal the pupil dilates even in bright light, due to increased activity in the sympathetic nerve fibres.

The autonomic nerve fibres emerging from the cerebro-spinal axis are medullated, and they pass to a ganglion where they synapse with other neurones (Fig. 6.1). The non-medullated axons of the ganglion cells constitute the post-ganglionic nerves which pass on to the effector cells (glands, plain muscle and heart). Thus all autonomic impulses have to be transmitted across a ganglionic synapse if they are to be effective. In a typical sympathetic nerve the pre-ganglionic fibres are short and synapse in a ganglion near to the vertebral column. A pre-ganglionic fibre may synapse with a large

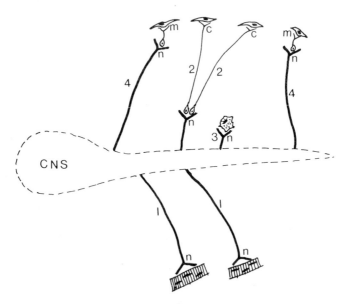

Fig. 6.1 Illustration of different pathways of efferent nerves. Motor nerves to voluntary muscle (1). Sympathetic nerves to plain muscle, heart or gland cells (2), or adrenal medulla (3). Parasympathetic nerves to heart, plain muscle or gland cells (4). Chemical transmission at synapses or neuro-effector junctions mediated by catecholamine (C) or acetylcholine (nicotine effect, N; muscarine effect, M).

number of ganglion cells. Thus the central location of the sympathetic ganglia favours the distribution of the nerve impulse over a large area of the body, and sympathetic nerves are the efferent pathway for reflexes which affect activity in widely distributed effector organs, e.g. blood vessels, sweat glands and hair muscles. In contrast, most parasympathetic ganglia are peripheral in location, often within the tissue of the innervated organ. Thus parasympathetic activity is localised and usually affects a single organ.

Central control

Autonomic reflexes such as micturition, defaecation or ejaculation may be produced after transection of the spinal cord, and peristalsis occurs in the isolated intestine. In an intact animal, however, autonomic activity is under the control of higher centres. The medulla contains the vagal, vomiting, respiratory, vasomotor, cardio-accelerator and cardio-inhibitory centres, from which descending fibres synapse with the neurones of the pre-ganglionic autonomic nerves. The activity of the centres in the medulla is under the influences of nuclei in the hypothalamus, which also have connections with higher centres and the pituitary. The activity of the sympathetic nervous system is controlled by neurones in the posterior region of the hypothalamus, and the parasympathetic by anterior nuclei.

Humoral transmission

In 1904, Elliot noted the similarities between the effects of sympathetic nerve stimulation and adrenaline, and that the effector cells still responded to adrenaline after the sympathetic nerves had been cut and allowed to degenerate. He suggested that sympathetic impulses might release an adrenaline-like substance from the nerve terminals. In 1907, Dixon found that the alkaloid muscarine mimicked the responses to vagal stimulation, and suggested that a muscarine-like substance acted as a chemical transmitter of vagal impulses. Nevertheless, many still held to the view that the nerve impulse was carried over to the effector cells electrically, until Loewi (1921) demonstrated the chemical nature of transmission.

Loewi isolated two frog hearts, the first preparation with the extrinsic nerves attached and the second without. Each preparation was attached to a Straub canula filled with a little Ringer solution. When the vagus or sympathetic nerves were stimulated the rate and strength of the contractions in the first preparation were reduced or increased, respectively. Ringer in the canula attached to the first heart was withdrawn by pipette and tested on the second heart. If the vagus nerve was stimulated during withdrawal of Ringer, then it acquired the ability to inhibit the spontaneous contractions in the second preparation. Similarly, when the sympathetic nerve was stimulated as the Ringer was transferred to the second preparation, the beats in the second heart speeded up and became stronger. Loewi concluded that the nerves did not influence the heart directly, but that chemical substances liberated from the terminals of the two nerves, which he provisionally called 'vagusstoff' and 'acceleranstoff', modified the function of the heart.

The action of the vagusstoff on frog heart was antagonised by atropine. Loewi and Navratil (1926) recognised the close similarity between acetylcholine and the vagusstoff, both being inactivated in the heart by an ester-splitting enzyme (cholinesterase) which was inhibited by physostigmine.

Dale and his collaborators established that acetylcholine was the chemical mediator at the parasympathetic nerve endings, autonomic ganglia and motor nerve endings. The perfusates collected from these structures during periods of nerve stimulation contracted the dorsal muscle of the leech or frog rectus abdominus muscle, reduced the arterial blood pressure of the cat and inhibited the frog heart. When the acetylcholine in the perfusate was assayed on each of these test objects, a consistent estimate was obtained. Furthermore, the action of the perfusate was potentiated by physostigmine and blocked by atropine or d-tubocurarine.

Cannon confirmed that an adrenaline-like substance transmitted sympathetic nerve impulses at neuro-effector junctions. He found that following sympathetic denervation, an organ developed a high sensitivity to adrenaline. It could then be used to detect the small amount of adrenaline-like substance released into the circulation when the sympathetic nerve supply to a distant organ was stimulated. For example, stimulation of the sympathetic hepatic nerves released an adrenaline-like substance which contracted the denervated nictitating membrane.

CHOLINOCEPTIVE MECHANISMS

Cholinergic nerves and the synthesis and release of acetycholine

Cholinergic nerves contain an enzyme, choline acetylase, which is capable of acetylating choline very rapidly. In the nerve terminals acetylcholine is stored in synaptic vesicles, which are small intracellular bodies about 0.05 μ in diameter (Fig. 6.2). When an action potential invades the nerve terminal acetycholine is released by exocytosis, many of the synaptic vesicles fusing with the neurilemma and discharging their contents at the neuro-effector junctions.

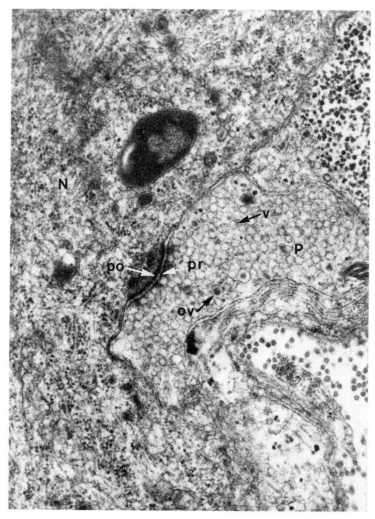

Fig. 6.2 Electron micrograph of an axosomatic synapse from a frog sympathetic ganglion, showing a presynaptic axon (P) in contact with the soma of a neuron (N). The presynaptic axon contains numerous round synaptic vesicles (v) and a few larger vesicles (ov) with osmophilic cores. Presynaptic (pr) and postsynaptic (po) membranes are separated by the synaptic cleft. Magnification x 39 975. (*By courtesy of Dr S S Kempson and Mr Derek Penman.*)

The dual action of acetylcholine

Dale (1914) noted the similarity between the pharmacological actions of acetylcholine and the alkaloid muscarine. For example, both substances stimulated the secretions of the exocrine glands, produced contraction in plain muscles, slowed and weakened the heart beat and dilated arterioles. These effects were antagonised by atropine. Most of the muscarine-like actions of acetylcholine are parasympathomimetic, in that they mimic the responses to stimulation of the parasympathetic nerves (Table 6.1). In addition to parasympathomimetic actions, the muscarine-like actions include responses of certain effector organs which are without a parasympathetic nerve supply, e.g. the dilatation of arterioles and the contractions of the nictitating membrane and splenic capsule.

When acetycholine is given intramuscularly or subcutaneously it produces little effect owing to its rapid hydrolysis by cholinesterase in the tissue. Intravenous injection of acetylcholine produces short lasting effects including a bradycardia and decrease in the arterial blood pressure. Dale discovered that acetylcholine had a dual action (Fig. 6.3), for when the muscarine-like actions has been abolished by atropine, the injection of acetylcholine at an increased dose produced responses which resembled those of the alkaloid nicotine. Thus after atropine, an intravenous injection of acetylcholine stimulated the sympathetic ganglia and adrenal medulla producing widespread vasoconstriction and an increase in the arterial blood pressure.

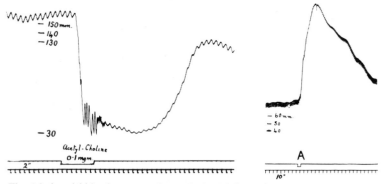

Fig. 6.3 Arterial blood pressure of anaesthetised (left) and spinal (right) preparations of cats. Left: after acetylcholine (0.1 mg) the blood pressure was reduced due to vasodilatation and bradycardia (muscarine effects).
Right: acetylcholine (5 mg) after atropine (1 mg) produced a rise in blood pressure due to stimulation of the sympathetic ganglia and adrenal medulla (nicotine effects). (*After* Dale 1914 *Journal of Pharmacology* 6: 152.)

Nicotine-like effects are produced by acetylcholine acting at cholinoceptors in the neurones of the sympathetic and parasympathetic ganglia, the motor endplates of voluntary muscle and the chromaffin cells of the adrenal medulla (Fig. 6.1).

Choline esters

The cationic group of the choline esters (Fig. 6.4) is essential for muscarine and nicotine-like activity, and it is generally considered that it enters into salt formation with an anionic group on the cholinoceptors. Trimethylation of the nitrogen is optimal for activity, and both the muscarine- and nicotine-like actions of the molecule are reduced when hydrogen atoms or ethyl groups are substituted for the methyl groups on the nitrogen. Choline has little pharmacological activity, however, and it seems probable that the greater activity of the esters is due to the carbonyl group being adsorbed on a positively charged portion of the cholinoceptor.

Acetyl-β-methylcholine does not produce nicotine actions but is about half as potent as acetylcholine in producing muscarine actions. It is remarkable that such a small change in the acetylcholine molecule should produce a substance with muscarine-like activity only. It may be that only minor differences in structure exist between the receptors mediating muscarine- and nicotine-like effects.

The methylation of the β-carbon atom in acetycholine also makes the molecule a poor substrate for plasma cholinesterase. Thus acetyl-β-methylcholine given intravenously produces a more marked bradycardia than acetylcholine. This action of acetyl-β-methylcholine has been used to control attacks of paroxysmal tachycardia.

Carbachol is carbamoyl choline. It has strong nicotine activity, weak muscarine activity and resists hydrolysis by cholinesterase. It has been given subcutaneously for purging the horse or to relieve post-operative retention of urine. This is hazardous as too much carbachol will be painful and produce bronchospasm and excessive cardiac slowing.

Alkaloids with acetylcholine-like activity

Each of these alkaloids (Fig. 6.4) exhibits a different ratio of potencies in producing muscarine- and nicotine-like effects. Moreover, the cholinoceptors mediating muscarine-like effects are heterogeneous (see gallamine), as also are nicotine receptors (see hexamethonium). Thus alkaloids which combine with cholinoceptors produce a variety of effects. Most alkaloids are relatively resistant to enzymatic inactivation, and this may give a misleading impression of an increase in potency as compared to acetylcholine.

Muscarine Muscarine is the active constituent of a mushroom, *Amanita muscaria*, which is not uncommonly a source of poisoning

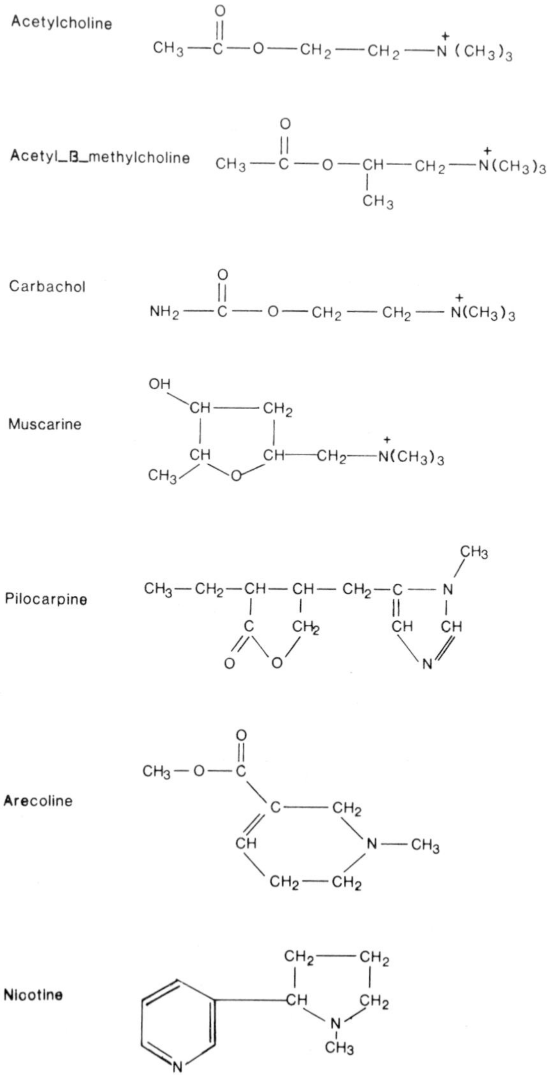

Fig. 6.4 The chemical relationships of cholinomimetic agents.

in Europe and North America. It is absorbed from the alimentary tract and mostly excreted unchanged in the urine. Muscarine is a deadly poison, producing bradycardia, vasodilatation, hypotension, bronchial constriction, miosis, salivation, increased peristalsis and urination. Atropine, the specific antidote, prevents death.

Arecoline This substance is a constituent of betel nuts, and has muscarine- and nicotine-actions. In the east, betel nuts are chewed as their sialogogue action is considered an aid to digestion.

Arecoline was used in dogs to expel *Echinococcus granulosus*, a tapeworm which is a human health hazard. Following oral administration, arecoline is effectively cleared from portal blood during a single pass through the hepatic circulation. Hence arecoline is unlikely to produce untoward effects following oral administration, other than stimulation of the alimentary tract. This is excessive in the cat, in which species arecoline is contra-indicated.

Pilocarpine This alkaloid is present in the leaves of *Pilocarpus jaborandi*, a small tree indigenous to South and Central America and the West Indies. Pilocarpine has strong muscarine and weak nicotine activities, and is especially effective in stimulating the secretions of exocrine glands and constricting the pupil. A solution of pilcarpine nitrate (0.25–2.0% w/v) is applied to the eye to reduce the intraocular pressure during glaucoma, or to reverse the mydriatic and cycloplegic actions of an atropine-like drug.

Nicotine Nicotine produces pharmacological actions which are different to those of muscarine. In small doses, nicotine stimulates the sympathetic and parasympathetic ganglia, the adrenal medulla, the chemoceptors in the carotid and aortic bodies and the motor endplates in striated muscle. Nicotine also produces central effects, stimulating the respiratory, vagal, vomitting and vasomotor centres in the medulla and the supraoptic nucleus in the hypothalamus. Antidiuretic hormone is released from the pituitary in response to the stimulation of the supraoptic nucleus. Large doses of nicotine desensitise and block the cholinoceptors in these effectors, and for example, block ganglionic transmission and relax voluntary muscle.

Nicotine base penetrates mucous membranes and skin, and its salts are readily absorbed from the alimentary tract. In cases of poisoning, nicotine produces biphasic effects, the stimulant action of the alkaloid being followed on by a blockade of the cholinoceptors in the effector organs. Early signs of poisoning include salivation, respiratory stimulation, colic and vomiting. The arterial blood pressure is increased as the alkaloid stimulates the sympathetic ganglia and the adrenal medulla. Fasciculation occurs in voluntary muscle as the nicotine excites the motor endplates, and this leads to incoordination and weakness in the limbs. The depressant effects of nicotine quickly supervene, and death from respiratory failure may occur within a few minutes. Nicotine depresses the activity of the respiratory centre, desensitises the chemoceptors to the normal physiological stimuli and produces weakness or paralysis in the respiratory muscles. There is no specific antidote, but if artificial respiration is started promptly animals will often survive as nicotine is fairly rapidly metabolised.

Other alkaloids seem to produce certain nicotine-like effects only. For example *coniine*, the alkaloid in hemlock (*Conium maculatum*), produces an ascending paralysis in the voluntary muscles and respiratory arrest. It was used in ancient Greece to kill criminals. *Lobeline*, an alkaloid from lobelia, stimulates the chemoceptors and medullary centres, and produces respiratory stimulation, nausea and vomiting. In smokers, lobeline produces an aversion for tobacco, each smoke being accompanied by nausea and vomiting after treatment with the drug.

Nicotine sulphate solution is sometimes used to kill red mites and other external parasites of poultry. It is applied as a perch paint, the parasites inhabiting crevices in the poultry house and infesting the birds at roost. Nicotine sulphate should not be used for this purpose when the poultry house has been freshly limed. The lime liberates the volatile base which poisons birds at roost, as it is inhaled and absorbed through skin. Nicotine sulphate was formerly used as an anthelmintic in sheep and poultry. Although nicotine is no longer used for this purpose, two widely used anthelmintics, levamisole and pyrantel, combine with nicotine receptors in roundworms to produce paralysis.

Cholinesterase

The structure of cholinesterase resembles that of the cholinoceptor, in that there are two binding sites for the substrate. The cationic head of acetycholine enters into salt formation with an anionic site in the enzyme, while the electrophilic carbon of the carbonyl group of acetylcholine combines with an esteratic site. The possible mechanism of the fission of the ester linkage in acetylcholine, at the active centre of the esteratic site of cholinesterase, is shown in Figure 6.5.

In vertebrates, there are two distinct cholinesterases with different patterns of substrate specificity. One enzyme is very active in hydrolysing acetylcholine, even at low substrate concentrations,

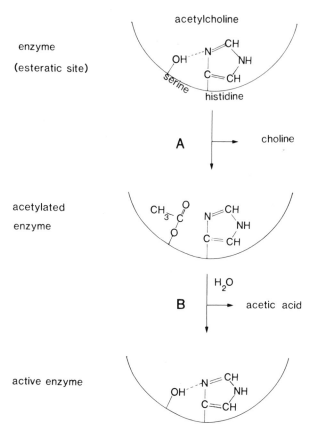

Fig. 6.5 Illustration of the fission of acetylcholine at the esteratic site of cholinesterase. (A) The reaction between enzyme and substrate results in acetylation of a serine residue in the enzyme and liberation of choline. (B) The acetylated enzyme is rapidly hydrolysed with the regeneration of the active form of the enzyme and liberation of acetic acid. The imidazole group of a histidine residue in the enzyme acts as a proton acceptor, thereby facilitating these reactions.

but exhibits little activity when incubated with butyrylcholine or benzoylcholine. This enzyme is called true- or acetylcholinesterase, both names acknowledging its role in the hydrolysis of acetylcholine released at nerve endings. Acetylcholinesterase activity is present in the grey matter of the central nervous system, peripheral nerves, motor endplates and erythrocytes. The second enzyme, pseudo- or butyryl-cholinesterase, hydrolyses butyrylcholine at a faster rate than acetylcholine. Butyrylcholinesterase activity is present in the liver, plasma, skin and the mucosa of

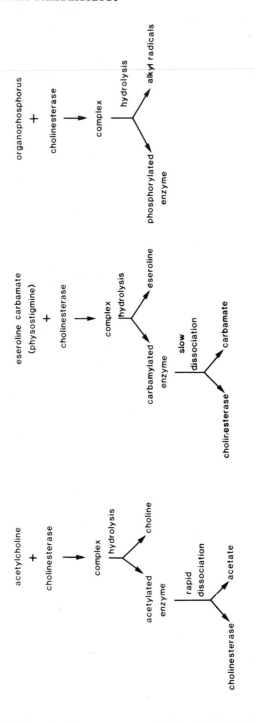

Fig. 6.6 Diagrammatic summary of the reaction of cholinesterase with its substrate or inhibitors.

the alimentary tract. Butyrylcholinesterase hydrolyses procaine, suxamethonium and atropine, and possibly esters of dietary or microbial origin following their absorption from the gastrointestinal tract.

The cholinesterases in invertebrates have substrate and inhibitor specificities which differ from those of the vertebrate enzymes. Organophosphorus compounds which selectively inhibit the cholinesterases in insects or helminths have a useful application as pesticides.

Anticholinesterases

Potent inhibitors of cholinesterase, which reduce the activity of the enzyme by 50% at a concentration of 1 μmol/l or less, produce pharmacological effects which may be likened to those arising from sustained stimulation of cholinergic nerves. There are three kinds of anticholinesterase drugs in common use. Certain bases combine only with the anionic site of the enzyme, e.g. edrophonium. These drugs rapidly combine and dissociate from the enzyme, producing effects of short duration. The other kinds of anticholinesterases are esters of carbamic acid or organophosphorus compounds. These inhibitors are bound to both the anionic and esteratic sites in the enzyme, and hydrolysed (Fig. 6.6). The acid which is liberated in the hydrolysis reacts with the esteratic site of the enzyme. Carbamylated cholinesterase dissociates at about one millionth of the rate of the acetylated enzyme. Thus physostigmine inhibits the enzymatic hydrolysis of acetylcholine competitively, producing pharmacological effects which subside within a few hours. In contrast, phosphorylated cholinesterase is a very stable complex. Following administration of an organophosphorus compound to an animal, the activity of cholinesterase only recovers as the enzyme is replenished by biosynthesis, which may take several days.

Physostigmine (eserine) is obtained from the Calabar bean. It inhibits cholinesterase competitively, and potentiates the effects of cholinergic nerve stimulation or injected acetycholine for a few hours. It is ineffective in tissues in which the parasympathetic nerves have been cut and allowed to degenerate.

Physostigmine readily passes the blood–brain barrier, and parenteral administration of a large dose may inhibit the respiratory centre. It is well absorbed from the conjunctiva and a solution (0.1–1.0% w/v) is used for its miotic action or in the treatment of glaucoma.

Neo-stigmine (Prostigmine) is a synthetic analogue of physostigmine (Fig. 6.7). It contains a quaternary ammonium group which is almost fully ionised at physiological pH. Thus the blood–barrier is relatively impermeable to neostigmine, which is safer than physostigmine following parenteral administration. Neostigmine bromide is given by injection or orally.

Physostigmine

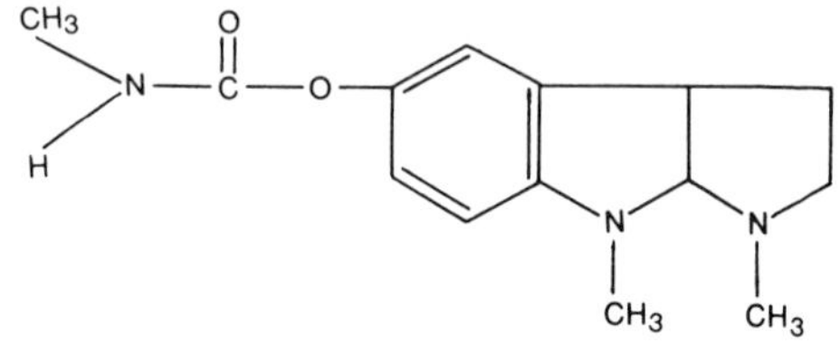

Neostigmine

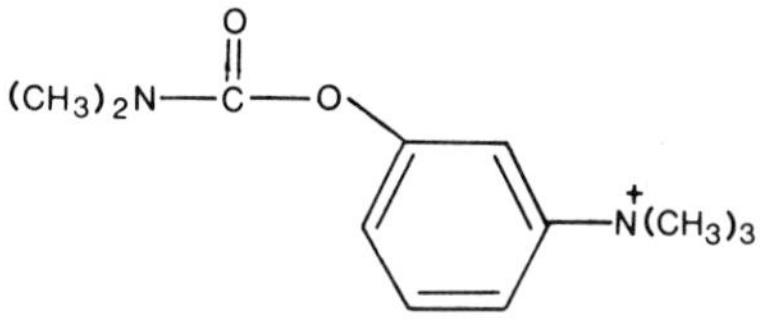

Edrophonium

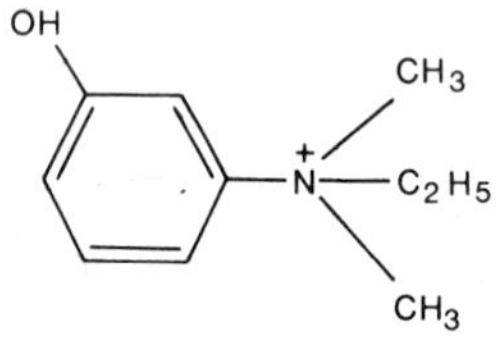

Pyridostigmine

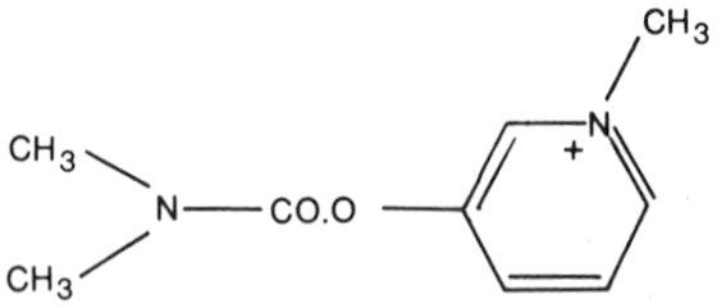

Ecothiopate

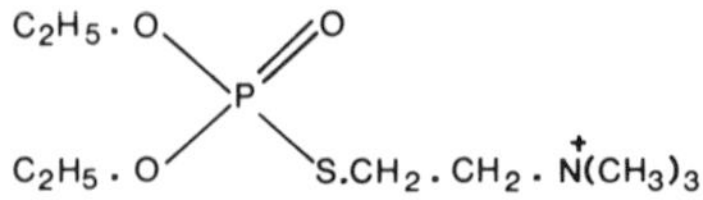

Fig. 6.7 Chemical structures of anticholinesterases.

In addition to being a potent anticholinesterase, neostigmine is a weak agonist at nicotine receptors. Thus the influence of neostigmine on cholinergic transmission is particularly marked where liberated acetylcholine has a nicotine-like action on the effector cells. Neostigmine is used to reverse the effects of competitive neuromuscular blocking drugs (e.g. d-tubocurarine), and to improve neuromuscular transmission in myasthenia gravis. When the dose of neostigmine is relatively high, it is given together with atropine which antagonises the unwanted muscarine effects.

Myasthenia gravis is a condition marked by great weakness and fatiguability of the voluntary muscles, possibly due to a reduction in the number of cholinoceptors at the motor endplates. This is suggested by a reduction in binding of alpha α-bungarotoxin at the neuromuscular junction in myasthenia gravis. Alpha-bungarotoxin binds specifically and irreversibly to cholinoceptors.

Pyridostigmine (Mestinon) has a longer duration of action than neostigmine, and is sometimes preferred for the treatment of myasthenia gravis. It is similar to neostigmine.

Edrophonium (Tensilon) produces very prompt effects which subside after five minutes. It is useful in the diagnosis of myasthenia gravis.

Ecothiopate (Phospholine) is applied to the conjunctiva as a long lasting miotic. It is an organophosphorus compound which produces an irreversible inhibition of cholinesterase, and a single application to the eye lowers the intraocular pressure for about a week. The drug contracts the ciliary muscles which pull on the trabeculum, opening up this sieve-like structure through which the aqueous fluid drains from the eye. The spasm of the ciliary muscle is painful.

Anticholinesterase poisoning

Although the anticholinesterases used in therapeutics mostly inhibit the enzyme reversibly, the irreversible inhibitors will also be considered as the organophosphorus compounds are widely used as pesticides and produce cases of poisoning. Death due to failure of respiration is caused by a combination of effects of these drugs. The anticholinesterases depress the respiratory centre, produce pulmonary oedema and bronchospasm by augmenting the effects of parasympathetic nerves, and cause powerful fasciculation or neuromuscular blockade in the respiratory muscles. The central and muscarine-like effects of the unmetabolised acetylcholine can be antagonised by atropine.

For the organophosphorus compounds, additional protection from the nicotine-like effects can sometimes be obtained by prompt administration of *pralidoxime* (PAM), a cholinesterase reactivator. The reactivation of the cholinesterase is often successful if the enzyme has been complexed with the inhibitor recently. In the longer term, the enzyme-inhibitor complex undergoes a process termed 'aging' with the loss of an alkyl group. The complex cannot be reactivated once it has 'aged'. Furthermore, certain organophosphorus compounds (e.g. schradan) produce a phosphorylated enzyme which cannot be reactivated even when newly formed. Treatment with pralidoxime may overcome the effect of an anticholinesterase at the neuromuscular junction. However, is should be considered additional to the requirement for atropine.

The reversible anticholinesterases such as physostigmine and neostigmine are relatively specific inhibitors of cholinesterase. However, organophosphorus compounds inhibit the activity of a number of hydrolytic enzymes including trypsin and thrombin. Some organophosphorus compounds produce a delayed neurotoxicity which seems unrelated to cholinesterase inhibition. Axons become demyelinated in the medulla, spinal cord and sciatic nerve, and a flaccid paralysis develops in the extremities. The condition is untreatable.

Ganglion blocking drugs

Transmission of the nerve impulse at sympathetic and parasympathetic ganglia is mediated by acetylcholine. The impulse releases acetylcholine from the terminals of the pre-ganglionic fibres. The acetylcholine combines with nicotine receptors in the membranes of the postganglionic neurones, changing their permeability to Na and K and producing a depolarisation. When the depolarisation of the postganglionic neurone reaches a critical level it gives rise to an impulse, which is propagated along the post-ganglionic fibre to the neuro-effector junction.

Ganglionic transmission is blocked by any drug which antagonises the nicotine actions of acetylcholine. Many of these drugs also produce neuromuscular blockade, but others block the ganglionic action of acetylcholine selectively. For example, hexamethonium is a competitive antagonist of acetylcholine in autonomic ganglia, and produces very little effect at the neuromuscular junction. This observation suggests that nicotine receptors are not all identical. However, none of the ganglion blocking drugs presently available discriminates between the sympathetic and parasympathetic ganglia.

Other drugs which selectively antagonise the ganglionic action of acetylcholine include pempidine and pentolinium, which were formerly used for the reduction of blood pressure. The blockade of sympathetic ganglia produces vasodilation and postural hypotension, as changes in posture are no longer accompanied by the reflex autonomic adjustment of vasoconstrictor tone. The blockade of parasympathetic ganglia gives rise to much inconvenience, as accommodation is paralysed, the secretion of saliva and juices of the gastro-intestinal tract are inhibited, and retention of urine and constipation occur.

Although preganglionic impulses are normally transmitted via the nicotine receptors of ganglion cells, muscarine also stimulates these cells. Muscarine receptors are only a small component of the cholinoceptive mechanism of the ganglia, but under certain circumstances their sensitivity is increased so that they become instrumental in mediating synpatic transmission. This happens when successive injections of nicotine are made into the circulation of the superior cervical ganglion of the cat. Ganglionic transmission is blocked by the nicotine and then restored in the continued presence of the drug, transmission in the presence of nicotine being readily blocked by atropine (Trendelenburg, 1966a). This example illustrates how resistance to a drug (nicotine) may develop as the nature of the receptors controlling a function changes.

The skeletal neuromuscular junction

The cell bodies of the lower motor neurones lie in the anterior horns of the grey matter of the spinal cord and in the motor nuclei of the cranial nerves. Their axons constitute the somatic motor nerves, which pass out from the CNS to striated muscles without interruption. The motor nerves branch extensively in the musculature, and lose their myelin sheath as they approach neuromuscular junctions. At the nerve terminal there are a number of swellings filled with synaptic vesicles, which lie in clefts in the muscle fibre membrane (Fig. 6.8). The membrane lining the clefts is cholinoceptive, and its area is greatly increased by the folding of the membrane. The narrow junctional gap is lined with cholinesterase, which is bound to both the pre- and post-junctional membranes.

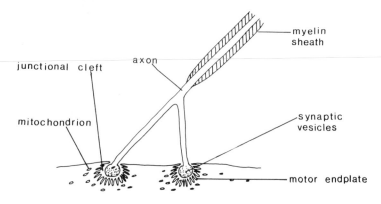

Fig. 6.8 Illustration of the neuromuscular junction. The synaptic vesicles in the nerve terminals are filled with acetylcholine, and the motor endplates are cholinoceptive. Acetylcholinesterase is bound to the nerve terminals and motor endplates.

When action potentials invade a nerve ending, there is an influx of Ca^{++} ions into the axoplasm. The Ca^{++} causes many of the synaptic vesicles to secrete their content of acetylcholine into the junctional gap by a process which resembles exocytosis. The acetylcholine diffuses across the junctional gap and combines with cholinoceptors. This increases the permeability of the cholinoceptive region of the membrane (motor endplate) to small ions, and it is depolarised.

In mammalian species, the striated muscle fibres are focally innervated, each fibre being supplied by a single nerve and having one motor endplate in the membrane. In birds and reptiles, however, many of the striated muscle fibres are innervated by 80 or more nerves, with a correspondingly large numbers of cholinoceptive areas in the membrane of each fibre. An avian muscle such as the biventer-cervicis contains both focally- and multipily-innervated fibres. There are a few mammalian muscles (extraocular and oesophageal) in which multiply-innervated fibres are found. The coupling of the depolarisation of the motor endplate to muscular contraction is different in focally- and multiply-innervated muscle fibres.

In a focally-innervated fibre, the depolarisation of the endplate under the influence of acetylcholine increases until the potential difference between the endplate and the surrounding membrane (still in the resting state) is sufficient to make current flow into the endplate. This specifically increases permeability to Na^+ in the membrane adjacent to the endplate. This event is propagated as an action potential throughout the membrane and into the interior of the fibre via the system of T-tubules, and a rapid release of Ca^{++} from the sarcoplasmic reticulum and a twitch ensue. In multiply-innervated fibres, the synchronous depolarisation of all the motor endplates sometimes activates the contractile mechanism without the propagation of an action potential. The release of Ca^{++} under the influence of motor endplate depolarisation is much slower than that in response to an action potential, and the outcome is a contracture. Focally- and multiply-innervated muscle fibres are sometimes described as 'twitch' and 'tonic' fibres, respectively.

In innervated striped muscle, only the motor endplate region of the sarcolemma is cholinoceptive. It is difficult to demonstrate the action of acetylcholine in mammalian voluntary muscle, as each constituent fibre is focally innervated with cholinesterase bound to the surface of the motor endplate. However, if acetylcholine is given by close intra-arterial injection, enough arrives at the cholinoceptors to produce a brief contraction. The multiply innervated fibres in avian and amphibian muscles are more sensitive to drugs which stimulate cholinoceptors. For example, in vitro preparations of the frog rectus abdominus or chick semispinalis muscles contract when acetylcholine is added to the bathing solution. Following exposure to an anticholinesterase, these preparations become sensitive enough for the bioassay of acetylcholine.

Blockade of neuromuscular transmission

Curare The South American Indians used curare as an arrow tip poison. It is a resinous extract prepared from the bark and leaves of various species of *Strychnos* and *Chondrodendron*, which produces death from paralysis of the respiratory muscles. The active constituents of the poison are quaternary bases which are not absorbed from the alimentary tract, so that animals killed with curare could be eaten with safety.

In 1857, Claude Bernard examined the action of curare. He used a frog nerve-muscle preparation, stimulating the muscle directly from electrodes placed on the muscle or indirectly from electrodes on the nerve. When the nerve was bathed with curare solution the muscle continued to respond to both direct and indirect stimulation, showing that the poison had no adverse effect on the nerve. Following application of curare to the muscle however, only direct stimulation produced a contraction in the preparation. The response to a direct stimulus showed that the muscle was unaffected by curare, and Bernard had to explain the abolition of the response to the indirect stimulus in the absence of an effect on the muscle or the nerve trunk. He concluded that curare produced paralysis by an action at the nerve ending. This was remarkably near the truth, as curare is now known to be competitive antagonist of the action of acetylcholine at the motor endplates. This may be demonstrated using the isolated rectus abdominus muscle of the frog.

Competitive and depolarising blocking drugs

Drugs which antagonise the action of acetylcholine at motor endplates are used as adjuncts to general anaesthesia for the production of muscular relaxation. They readily produce paralysis of all the voluntary muscles, and attempts to relax the abdominal muscles selectively involve a risk of paralysis of the respiratory muscles. Thus the anaesthetist using a neuromuscular blocking drug must be prepared to give artificial respiration. The drugs used clinically for producing muscular relaxation antagonise acetylcholine either competitively or by depolarisation of the motor endplates.

Competitive neuromuscular blocking drugs (d-tubocurarine, gallamine, pancuronium, fazadinium) combine reversibly with cholinoceptors in the endplates without affecting permeability to small ions. They compete with acetylcholine for occupation of the cholinoceptors, protecting the endplate from the depolarising action of acetylcholine. The outcome is a flaccid paralysis. This kind of neuromuscular block can be surmounted by an anticholinesterase drug. For example, neostigmine inhibits cholinesterase activity at the neuromuscular junction, and prolongs the effect of acetylcholine released at the motor nerve ending. This allows the transmitter to compete more effectively with a competitive antagonist for cholinoceptive sites in the endplate, and neuromuscular transmission is restored (Fig. 6.9).

Neuromuscular transmission can also be blocked by a drug which produces depolarisation at the endplates, e.g. suxamethonium. Acetylcholine released at motor nerve endings cannot depolarise cholinoceptive sites in the motor endplate when these have already been depolarised by suxamethonium. Thus under the influences of suxamethonium, the skeletal muscles are paralysed but not necessarily relaxed as the depolarisation of the motor endplates produces fasciculation or contracture in the muscles. In mammalian species,

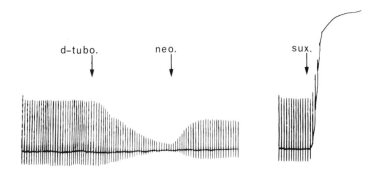

Fig. 6.9 Contractions of isolated biventer cervicis muscle produced by supramaximal nerve stimulation at a frequency of 8/min. Left: antagonism of neuromuscular transmission by d-tubocurarine (5 μg/ml) and its reversal by neostigmine (0.5 μg/ml). Right: neuromuscular block and contracture produced by suxamethonium (0.5 μg/ml).

suxamethonium produces fasciculation in the muscles followed by flaccid paralysis. In species with multiply-innervated muscle fibres, suxamethonium produces a contracture in the skeletal muscles and so is contra-indicated in avians (Fig. 6.9). The anticholinesterases which are antidotes for competitive neuromuscular blocking drugs, potentiate the effect of depolarising agents. This is because of summation of the depolarising actions of acetylcholine and the blocking agent at the motor endplates.

The neuromuscular blocking drugs do not affect consciousness or produce analgesia, and there is a danger that a paralysed animal may regain consciousness during surgery. Unfortunately, the muscle relaxants block ganglionic transmission, so that reflexes which are useful in the assessment of depth of anaesthesia may be absent in a paralysed animal. The Cruelty to Animals Act (1876) requires that the special permission of the Secretary of State must be given before any experiment with a curare-like substance is carried out in an animal.

d-Tubocurarine chloride This is an alkaloid constituent of curare (Fig. 6.10). It is given intravenously during surgery to produce adequate relaxation of the voluntary muscles without deepening the plane of anaesthesia. Tubocurarine blocks transmission in autonomic ganglia and so causes a tachycardia and reduction in arterial blood pressure. The drug is a quaternary base which releases histamine from tissues, particularly in the dog. The histamine causes bronchospasm and further reduction in the arterial blood pressure. There seems to be some variation in the response to d-tubocurarine,

Tubocurarine

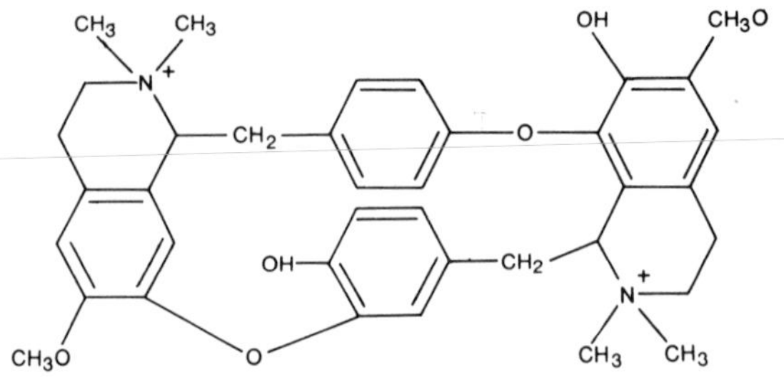

Gallamine

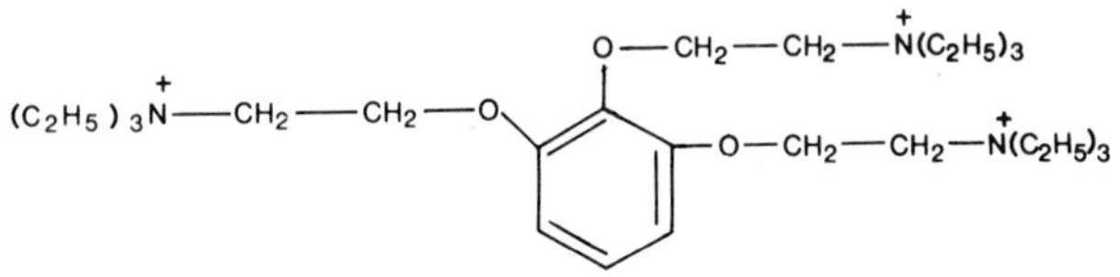

Pancuronium

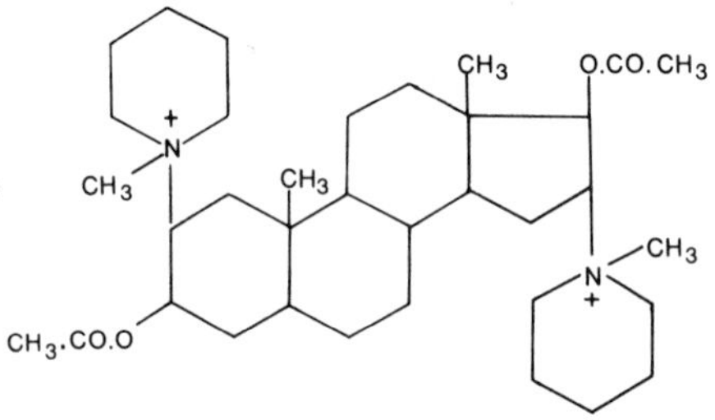

Suxamethonium

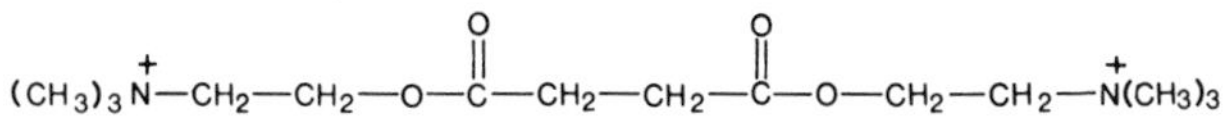

Fig. 6.10 Chemical structures of muscle relaxants.

and some anaesthetics advise administration of a small dose to assess the animal's response before using the drug for muscular relaxation.

Tubocurarine is injected slowly so that the effect can be assessed during administration. It produces weakness in the voluntary muscles which progresses to paralysis, this effect first becoming apparent in the muscles of the face and neck and spreading to the limbs, abdomen, intercostal muscles and diaphragm. The maximum effect of the drug is produced 3–5 minutes following intravenous administration. Means of artificial respiration must be available in case the respiratory muscles should be paralysed, and if an overdose of the drug is given neostigmine should be injected intravenously to restore spontaneous respiration. The neostigmine should be preceded by atropine, which blocks the unwanted parasymapthomimetic effects of the anticholinesterase. The dose of neostigmine is critical, as too much of the drug may produce neuromuscular blockade by depolarisation in the motor endplates. The effect of d-tubocurarine subsides after 30–40 minutes. Although the drug is partly metabolised in the liver, most of it is excreted unchanged in the urine and bile.

Ether anaesthesia or premedication with a phenothiazine ataractic drug potentiates the effect of d-tubocurarine and other competitive neuromuscular blocking drugs, necessitating some reduction in their dosage. Large doses of streptomycin also potentiate the effect of the competitive blocking agents.

Gallamine triethiodide (Flaxedil) Gallamine, like d-tubocurarine, is a competitive neuromuscular blocking drug which is given to anaesthetised animals for relaxation of the voluntary muscles. Small doses of gallamine are given intravenously until the desired effect is obtained. The muscle relaxant effect is produced in about a minute of giving the drug and lasts 20–30 minutes. Gallamine is less potent than tubocurarine as a histamine liberator and ganglion blocking agent. Indeed, the arterial blood pressure is frequently raised following gallamine. This is because gallamine antagonises acetylcholine acting on cardiac muscle. Gallamine is unexpectedly potent in blocking the action of acetylcholine in the heart, and produces a marked tachycardia which outlasts the muscle relaxant effect of the drug. Many other muscarine actions of acetylcholine seem not to be antagonised by gallamine, however, so the drug cannot be described as atropine-like. Gallamine is contraindicated in any animal with cardiac insufficiency or hypertension, and has been reported to cause arrhythmias when used as an adjunct to cyclopropane. For the most part gallamine is not metabolised and is cleared from the body by urinary excretion. In the dog, biliary excretion does not provide an alternative route for the clearance of gallamine as it does for d-tubocurarine. Thus gallamine is contraindicated in subjects will renal failure. It is also best avoided in obstetrics, as it diffuses across the placenta.

Pancuronium bromide (Pavulon) The potency of pancuronium as a competitive muscular relaxant is about 5 times that of d-tubocurarine or 10 times that of gallamine. Muscular relaxation starts 1–3 minutes after an intravenous injection of pancuronium, lasts approximately 45 minutes and may be antagonised by neostigmine or pyridostigmine together with atropine. Pancuronium antagonises the action of acetylcholine on the heart, producing a tachycardia and increasing the arterial blood pressure. It is not a potent histamine liberator. Pancuronium is excreted in the bile and urine, and is satisfactory in animals with renal insufficiency. It diffuses across the placenta.

Fazadinium bromide (Fazadon). Fazadinium is a competitive neuromuscular blocking drug which produces short lasting muscular relaxation in the dog (about 20 minutes), which is prolonged by halothane anaesthesia. In both dogs and cats, fazadinium produces retching and vomiting and so is best used following intubation. This drug tends to lower the arterial blood pressure, and probably blocks transmission in autonomic ganglia.

Suxamethonium chloride (succinylcholine, Anectine, Brevadil). The motor endplates in voluntary muscle are depolarised by suxamethonium. In mammalian species, intravenous injection of the drug is followed in about 30 seconds by a short period of painful muscular fasciculation and then by muscular relaxation, which lasts about 20 minutes in the dog and 3–5 minutes in the horse or cat. The relaxation of the musculature is often accompanied by apnoea or respiratory arrest. The brevity of the action of suxamethonium is due to its hydrolysis by pseudocholinesterase activity in plasma, and when this is low apnoea may be very prolonged. Thus suxamethonium is used in species (horse, dog) with a high pseudocholinesterase activity in plasma, and is not recommended for use in ruminants where the activity of this plasma enzyme is extremely low. Unfortunately, the occasional horse or dog may have an atypical or low peseudo-cholinesterase activity in the plasma, and this gives rise to a very prolonged response to suxamethonium. This idiosyncrasy may be alleviated by infusion of blood or freeze dried plasma with a high pseudo-cholinesterase activity. The drug cannot be used for muscular relaxation in avians, as the tonic fibres in the musculature respond with sustained contracture.

Suxamethonium does not dull consciousness or produce analgesia, and it should only be given to animals which have been anaesthetised. The drug may be given by intravenous infusion if a prolonged period of muscular relaxation is required. When the effect of suxamethonium is sustained by infusion or injection of a large dose, the nature of the antagonism of acetylcholine at the motor endplates changes gradually from depolarisation to competitive block. If the respiration stops, the anaesthetist should give artificial respiration until spontaneous respiration is restored. There may be a dilemma regarding the administration of an anticholinesterase drug, because although this will antagonise a competitive blockade of acetylcholine at the motor endplates it will intensify a depolarisation block. The nature of the effect of suxamethonium may be diagnosed by injecting the short acting anticholinesterase edrophonium intravenously. If this produces improvement for a few minutes, indicating that the action of suxamethonium has become competitibe, neostigmine may be given.

An intravenous injection of suxamethonium is sometimes given to an anaesthetised animal to aid the passage of an endotracheal tube. The drug produces a brief relaxation of the laryngeal muscles which is sufficient for this purpose.

Suxamethonium has a biphasic action in autonomic ganglia, stimulating the postganglionic nerves and then blocking ganglionic transmission. Thus it may produce or abolish many sympathomimetic or parasympathomimetic effects. An intravenous injection of suxamethonium produces bronchospasm, bracycardia and salivary and bronchial secretions. Premedication with atropine blocks these effects. Infusion of suxamethonium may lead to tachycardia and a rise in blood pressure.

Suxamethonium increases the concentration of potassium in plasma, possibly in consequence of the muscular fasciculation. Thus suxamethonium is contraindicated in animals with cardiac insufficiency, as the combination of hyperkalaemia and vagal stimulation is likely to cause a cardiac arrhythmia.

Anticholinesterases, procaine and narcotic analgesics have the reputation of enhancing the effect of suxamethonium. Alkaline solutions of suxamethonium are unstable, and suxamethonium should not be mixed with the sodium salt of a barbiturate.

Atropine sulphate

A number of common solanaceous plants including *Atropa belladonna* (deadly nightshade), *Datura stramonium* (thornapple) and *Hyoscyamus niger* (henbane) contain the alkaloids 1-hyoscyamine and 1-hyoscine. During extraction, 1-hyoscyamine is transformed into a racemate of d- and 1-hyoscyamine, which is known as atropine.

Atropine is well absorbed from the alimentary tract and may be given by mouth in tablets or a mixture containing tincture of belladonna. Atropine is more frequently given by injection, however,

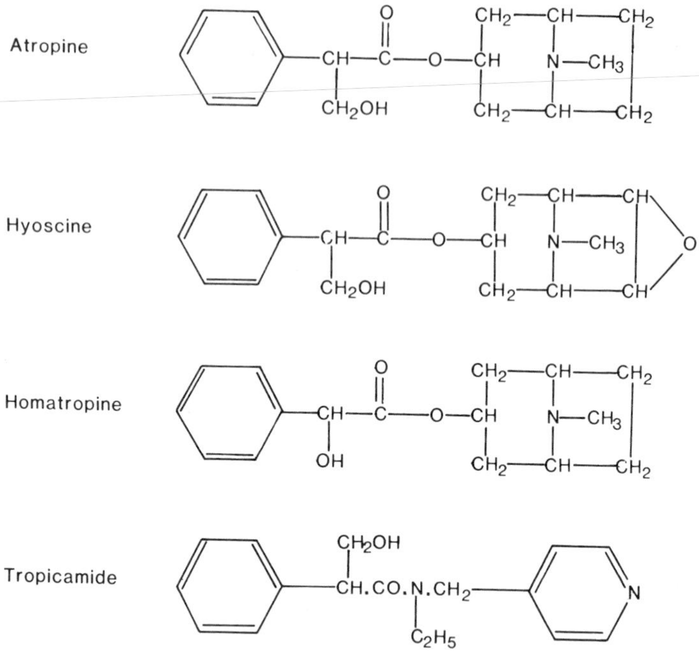

Fig. 6.11 Chemical structures of atropine-like drugs.

when its action takes effect in about 5 minutes and begins to subside after 2–3 hours.

Atropine is metabolised in the liver, only a small amount of the
drug being excreted unchanged in the urine. It can be difficult to
atropinise a rabbit. This is because the plasma and tissues of some
rabbits contains atropinesterase, an enzyme which hydrolyses the
ester linkage in atropine (Fig. 6.11). The presence of this enzyme
in rabbits is genetically determined.

Atropine combines reversibly with the cholinoceptors in plain
muscle, heart muscle and gland cells, without stimulating them.
Thus it is a competitive antagonist of all the muscarine-like effects
produced by choline esters, anticholinesterases or certain alkaloids.
It also antagonises most of the effects which are produced by stimulation of parasympathetic nerves. However, vasodilatation in the
salivary glands in response to stimulation of the chorda tympani,
contraction of the fundus of the bladder in response to pelvic nerve
stimulation and contraction of the fowl rectum in response to stimulation of Remak's nerve are all unaffected by atropine. Thus these
parasympathetic nerves may not be cholinergic.

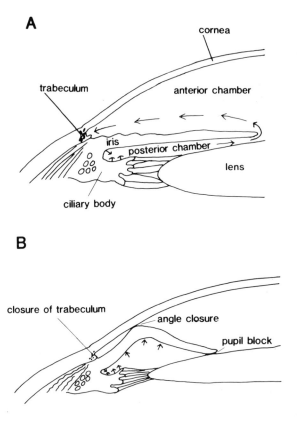

Fig. 6.12 Influence of atropine on the circulation of aqueous humor in the eye. (A) The arrows depict the secretion of aqueous by the epithelium of the ciliary body, and its passage through the pupil into the anterior chamber. The aqueous drains from the eye through a sieve-like structure, the trabeculum. (B) Under the influence of atropine, the pupil dilates and the ciliary muscles relax. Dilatation of the pupil blocks a narrow filtration angle, and may impair the passage of aqueous through the pupil. Relaxation of the ciliary muscles leads to closure of the trabeculum. In some subjects, these changes produce an abrupt rise in intraoccular pressure.

Atropine antagonises autonomic reflexes in which the efferent pathway is a parasympathetic nerve, and constriction of the pupil in bright light is abolished by the drug because of paralysis of the sphincter muscle in the iris. The mydriasis produced by atropine is accompanied by a dangerous rise in intraocular pressure in an animal predisposed to narrow-angle glaucoma. This is due to the iris blocking the filtration angle in the anterior chamber of the eye (Fig. 6.12). Atropine relaxes the ciliary muscle so that the lens is focused for distant vision and accommodation is blocked.

Other autonomic reflexes antagonised by atropine include micturition, peristalsis and salivation. Atropine diminishes the secretions of all the glands which are under the control of the parasympathetic nervous system. Thus the lachrymal, bronchial, pancreatic and gastro-intestinal secretions are reduced, although the reduction in secretion of HCl by the oxyntic cells is insufficient to have much effect on the pH in the stomach. In man and cat, atropine inhibits sweating. This is the outcome of a pharmacological curiosity. Although the sweat glands are innervated by sympathetic fibres in these species, these are cholinergic.

The effect of atropine often depends upon the prevailing parasympathetic tone, or the presence or absence of a cholinomimetic drug. For example, atropine has little effect on the bronchioles unless the parasympathetic tone is high or the animal affected by a muscarine-like drug. In these circumstances, atropine reduces the tone in the plain muscle and produces a dilatation of the bronchioles. Vagal tone in the heart is antagonised by atropine, producing an increase in the heart rate and speeding up conduction in the bundle of His.

Atropine first stimulates the CNS from the motor cortex to the medulla, and then produces depression. In the early stages of atropine poisoning, an animal is restless and excited with dilated pupils, dry mouth and hyperpyrexia. A sedative will control the excitement, and unabsorbed alkaloid may be precipitated in the stomach by a mixture containing tannins. In the later stages of poisoning, the CNS is depressed and artificial respiration and possibly an analeptic drug may be required. The peripheral effect of atropine are not lethal, and may be relieved by physostigmine.

Hyoscine hydrobromide (scopolamine) antagonises the muscarine effects of acetylcholine, and produces peripheral effects which are similar to those of atropine. However, hyoscine and atropine produce different effects in the CNS. In dog and man, hyoscine is a central depressant. A dog is sedated following treatment with hyoscine and restless after atropine. In cattle, hyoscine may produce excitement.

Tropicamide (Mydriacyl) and *homatropine hydrobromide* are short acting atropine-like drugs which are used for their ocular effects. Application of a solution of tropicamide to the eye produces a dilatation of the pupil within 15 minutes and lasting about 8 hours. The effects of homatropine in the eye last about 24 hours. Physostigmine reverses the mydriasis and cycloplegia produced by these drugs.

Uses of atropine-like drugs

Atropine is used as a premedicant before administering a general anaesthetic. It prevents excessive salivation and bronchial secretion, thus facilitating gaseous exchange across the pulmonary epithelium and reducing the incidence of postoperative pneumonia.

Atropine is a specific antidote for poisoning produced by an anticholinesterase or parasympathomimetic drug. A prolonged effect is required in the treatment of poisoning with an organophosphorus compound, and atropine sulphate is given intramuscularly 3 times a day until symptoms subside.

Atropine-like drugs are used for their effects on the gastro-intestinal tract: a reduction in gastric secretions, hypermobility, muscle spasm and colic. Tincture of belladonna is sometimes compounded with an absorbent in a preparation intended to stop diarrhoea.

In ophthalmology, atropine is used to dilate the pupil and paralyse accommodation. The pupillary reflex may not fully recover for over a week after atropine. Thus shorter acting drugs such as tropicamide are often preferred, especially if an eye is predisposed to narrow-angle glaucoma. Atropine does not produce mydriasis in avians, because the irides consist of striped muscle in these species.

The central depressant and anti-emetic effects of the hyoscine are useful in the prevention of travel sickness in humans. Although there seems to be no evidence for the efficacy of hyoscine in the dog, it has been used to allay travel sickness in this species.

Drugs and toxins which block the release of acetylcholine from nerves

Magnesium ions antagonise the effects of calcium, which couples the action potentials in nerve and striped muscle to acetylcholine release and muscular contraction, respectively. Thus solutions of magnesium sulphate injected intravenously block neuromuscular transmission, and calcium borogluconate is usually effective in surmounting the effect of magnesium.

A local anaesthetic drug given at high concentration in the region of the nerve terminal may prevent the release of acetylcholine by blocking the passage of action potentials in nerve fibres before they invade the nerve endings. Procaine and certain other local anaesthetics also antagonise the action of acetylcholine at the motor endplates, and this effect contributes to the ensuing neuromuscular block. Tetrodotoxin, obtained from the puffer fish or California newt, is more specific in preventing the sodium conductance that underlies action potentials in nerve and striated muscle. It seems to be without effect in plain muscle.

The anaerobic organism *Clostridium botulinum* produces a number of toxins which react with nerve terminals preventing the release of acetylcholine. Botulinum toxin paralyses skeletal muscle and inhibits parasympathetic nerves, producing a dilatation of the pupil and a paralysis of accomodation, impairment of gastro-intestinal activity and urinary retention. Cases of human poisoning occur occasionally from the ingestion of contaminated canned meat or fish. As little as 1μg of the toxin may be fatal in man, and artificial respiration may have to be given for several days or weeks. Carrion and stagnant water provide an anaerobic environment for the organism, and botulism in wild birds is very widespread.

The venom of the Taiwan banded krait contains two polypeptides, α- and β-bungarotoxin, which block cholinergic transmission by different mechanisms. Alpha-bungarotoxin binds selectively and irreversibly to cholinoceptors and antagonises the action of acetylcholine at motor endplates. Beta-bungarotoxin disperses the synaptic vesicles and acetylcholine from nerve endings. The venom of the black widow spider depletes synaptic vesicles and neurotransmitter from both adrenergic and cholinergic nerves.

ADRENOCEPTIVE MECHANISMS

Adrenaline and noradrenaline

The adrenergic neurones of the sympathetic nervous system and the chromaffin cells of the adrenal medulla contain enzymes which synthesise noradrenaline from L-tyrosine. In chromaffin cells, noradrenaline is methylated to adrenaline, the hormone of the adrenal medulla. In adrenergic neurones, biosynthesis mostly proceeds no further than noradrenaline, the sympathetic transmitter.

Adrenergic nerve endings and adrenal medullary cells contain dense core vesicles in which adrenaline and noradrenaline are stored together with adenosine triphosphate (ATP) and chromagranin, a soluble protein. When action potentials invade the nerve endings or acetylcholine is released from the splanchnic nerves in the adrenal medulla, the contents of the vesicles are released extracellularly by a process resembling exocytosis.

Inactivation of catecholamines

Adrenaline and noradrenaline are inactivated in the body by uptake mechanisms which sequester the amines intracellularly, and by enzymes which methylate or deaminate the amines (Fig. 6.13).

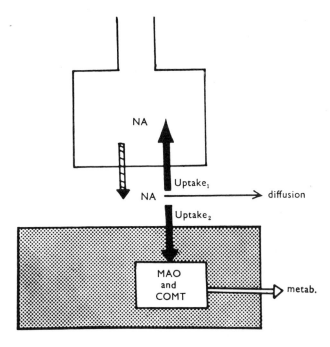

Fig. 6.13 Mechanisms for inactivation of noradrenaline at adrenergic nerve terminals (After Iversen *British Journal of Pharmacology* 1971 41: 580.)

Iversen (1963) found that an isolated heart abstracted noradrenaline from the perfusion fluid very rapidly, and that the uptake was reduced by more than 95% in preparations made from immunosympathectomised animals. Noradrenaline is taken up actively by a sodium dependent mechanism in the adrenergic nerve endings in the preparation (Uptake 1). Following Uptake 1, noradrenaline is taken up by the intraneuronal storage vesicles so that it can be released again by action potentials. Uptake 1 has no affinity for isoprenaline and is inhibited by cocaine.

Another mediated uptake of catecholamines takes place in certain non-neuronal cells. In the heart, Uptake 2 is a low affinity system which transports exogenous catecholamines into myocardial cells.

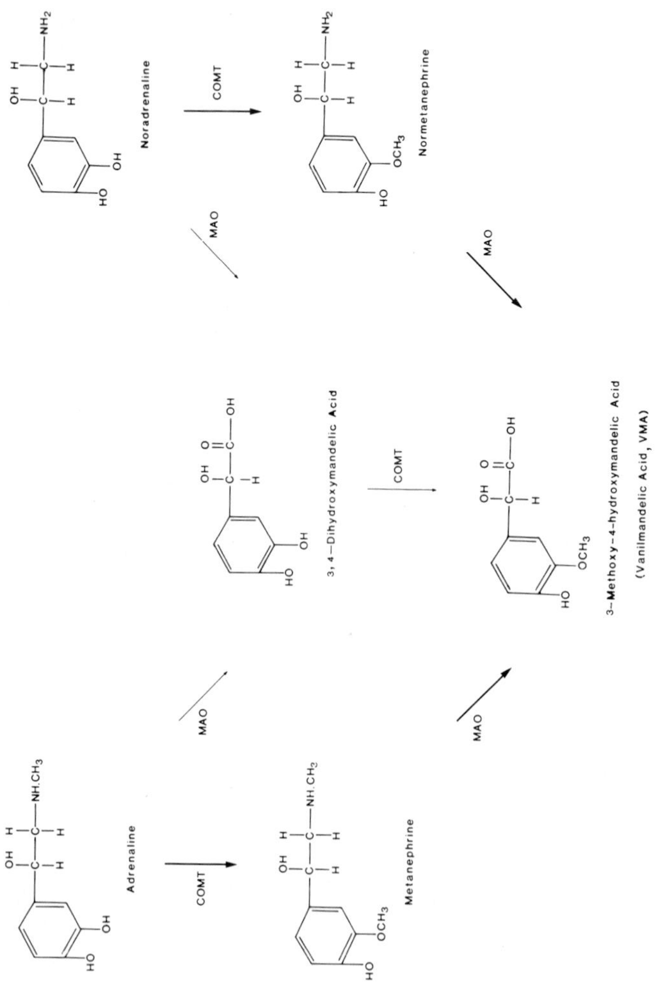

Fig. 6.14 Metabolism of adrenaline and noradrenaline by catechol-O-methyltransferase (COMT) and monoamine oxidase (MAO).

Uptake 2 is followed by extensive enzymatic destruction of the catecholamines. Isoprenaline has a greater affinity than noradrenaline for Uptake 2. Corticosterone is a potent and selective inhibitor of Uptake 2.

The role of catechol-O-methyl-transferase (COMT) in the metabolism of adrenaline and noradrenaline was discovered by Axelrod. This enzyme methylates the 3-hydroxyl group of catechols, and transforms noradrenaline into normetanephrine which does not produce sympathomimetic effects (Fig. 6.14). COMT is widely distributed in tissues and metabolises catecholamines rapidly and extensively. Monoamine oxidase (MAO) is a mitochondrial enzyme, present in all tissues except blood. It oxidatively deaminated monoamines in which the amine group is attached to an unsubstituted methylene group. Mitochondria are plentiful in nerve endings, and MAO seems to control the amounts of catecholamines in adrenergic nerve endings. When MAO activity is inhibited by iproniazid, the amounts of catecholamines in the brain and heart are increased.

Urine contains small amounts of catecholamines together with larger amounts of their metabolites. The principle urinary metabolite, 3-methoxy-4-hydroxymandelic acid (VMA), is produced when either adrenaline or noradrenaline is metabolised by both COMT and MAO. The urinary excretion of these substances is increased following exercise or stress.

Actions of adrenaline

Adrenaline mimics all the effects produced by stimulation of the sympathetic nervous system. Sympathomimetic effects seem to prepare the animal for fight or flight. Pharmacologically they can be separated into two classes, β-effects which can be blocked by propanolol and α-effects blocked by phenoxybenzamine.

β-effects include the metabolic effects of the amine. Adrenaline stimulates the breakdown of glycogen in liver and muscle and in consequence increases the concentrations of glucose and lactate in the blood. It also stimulates lipolysis, breaking down adipose tissue with the release of free fatty acids and glycerol. These β-effects are the outcome of adrenaline increasing the activity of an enzyme, adenylate cyclase. The product of adenylate cyclase activity, cyclic adenosine monophosphate (cyclic AMP), acts as an intracellular messenger. Cyclic AMP increases the activities of phosphorylase and lipase, which produce glycogenolysis and lipolysis, respectively.

Theophylline produces β-effects such as relaxation of the

bronchioles and stimulation of the heart. It also inhibits phospho-diesterase, an enzyme which destroys intracellular cyclic AMP. Thus the role of cyclic AMP as an intracellular messenger for β-effects may not be confined to those affecting metabolism.

The increase in the force and rate of the heart beat produced by adrenaline is antagonised by propanolol. In toxic doses, adrenaline may produce a cardiac arrhythmia. Thus it is not normally given intravenously. Blood vessels are dilated by β-agonists. Adrenaline produces vasodilatation in skeletal muscle and increases blood flow through the myocardium and brain.

The stimulation of salivation, the secretion of tears and aqoeous humor in the eye and the release of renin from the kidney are β-effects of adrenaline. Relaxation of plain muscle is a very typical β-effect: adrenaline produces relaxation of the bronchioles, the fundus of the bladder, and the uterus in dioestrous.

α-effects of adrenaline include vasoconstriction. This is very marked in the skin, mucous membranes and viscera. Adrenaline produces both α- and β-effects, and normally it increases the arterial blood pressure due to a predominance of α-adrenoceptors in the vessels. A large dose of adrenaline produces a reflex bradycardia, the rise in blood pressure stimulating carotid and aortic baroreceptors. After blockade of α-adrenoceptors with phenoxybenzamine, adrenaline only combines with β-adrenoceptors, and produces vasodilatation and tachycardia.

In the eye, adrenaline produces dilatation of the pupil (contraction of the radial muscle of the iris), exophthalmos (contraction of the plain muscle at the back of the eye), contraction of the nictitating membrane and opening of the palpebral fissure. Other motor effects of adrenaline include contraction of the splenic capsule, oestrous uterus and sphincters of the alimentary tract and bladder. These effects are all blocked by phenoxybenzamine.

In the skin, adrenaline stimulates α-adrenoceptors in apocrine sweat glands and the errector pili muscles. The apocrine sweat glands are very numerous in horses and cattle. They seem to be without innervation and are stimulated by adrenaline in the circulation. The contraction of the errector pili causes the hair to bristle.

Effects mediated by both β- and α-adrenoceptors. Adrenaline inhibits the movements of the alimentary tract. Both propanolol and phenoxybenzamine inhibit this effect of the amine, which seems to be due to stimulation of β- and α-adrenoceptors. Electropharmacological evidence suggests that central effects of adrenaline are mediated by both β- and α-adrenoceptors. Adrenaline does not readily pass the blood–brain barrier, but if this structure is avoided by injection into the cerebral ventricles or cisterna magna, adrenaline produces drowsiness and, in most species, a reduction in body temperature. These central effects are not produced when the sympathetic nervous system is stimulated, and unlike the peripheral effects of adrenaline, do not prepare the animal for fight or flight.

Actions of noradrenaline

Noradrenaline is as potent as adrenaline in producing pharmacological effects mediated by α-adreoceptors. The efficacy of noradrenaline at β-adrenoceptors is variable.

Lands et al (1967) measured the potencies of a series of sympathomimetic amines in producing pharmacological effects mediated by β-adrenoceptors. For each pharmacological effect, the potencies of the amines was expressed relative to that of isoprenaline. The relative potencies of the amines was almost identical when increased contractility of a cardiac preparation, lipolysis and relaxation of the intestine were measured. Thus these effects seemed to be mediated by a common receptor, designated β1. In contrast, the amines exhibited another order of relative potencies common to pharmacological effects such as vasodilatation, bronchodilatation, relaxation of the uterus or glycogenolysis. These effects, which seemed to be mediated by a second type of adrenoceptor, were designated β2. Noradrenaline is about equi-active with adrenaline in producing β1 effects, and is a very weak agonist at β2-adrenoceptors.

In vitro, noradrenaline is about equipotent with adrenaline in increasing the force and rate of contraction of cardiac preparations. In vivo however, the effects of noradrenaline and adrenaline on the heart and circulation are dissimilar. Noradrenaline reduces the blood flow in skeletal muscle as well as that in the skin and viscera, bringing about a sharp increase in both diastolic and systolic blood pressure. The rise in blood pressure stimulates the carotid and aortic baroreceptors, producing a marked bradycardia which tends to reduce the oxygen consumption of the heart. In contrast, adrenaline produces vasodilatation in skeletal muscle and vasoconstriction in skin and viscera, thus redistributing the blood flow with comparatively little effect on the overall peripheral resistance. The diastolic blood pressure is not affected greatly by adrenaline, and the increase in mean arterial blood pressure is less than that after administration of noradrenaline. Thus adrenaline produces comparatively

less reflex bradycardia, and its direct action in stimulating contractility increases the oxygen consumption of the heart. The different
effects of noradrenaline and adrenaline on cardiac oxygen consumption, in vivo, may account for the less frequent incidence of
cardiac arrhythmias following substitution of noradrenaline for
adrenaline for intravenous administration.

Uses of adrenaline and noradrenaline

Solutions of catecholamines are susceptible to oxidation. Their activity is preserved by acidifcation to pH 5 or 6, and storage in air-
tight containers protected from light.

The acid tartrates of adrenaline or noradrenaline are used for
producing vasoconstriction. A swab dipped in adrenaline or noradrenaline (1:1000) will control the oozing of blood from capillaries
in mucous membranes or skin. Adrenaline or noradrenaline are
sometimes incorporated in preparations of local anaesthetics for in-
filtration anaesthesia. The vasoconstriction delays the absorption of
the local anaesthetic, prolonging its local action and reducing any
effect in the CNS.

In sudden cardiac arrest, an animal may be resuscitated by an
injection of adrenaline (1 : 1000) directly into the heart. Adrenaline
(subcut) can be used to relieve insulin hypoglycaemia.

In hypotensive states, noradrenaline acid tartrate (8 µg/ml) can
be infused intravenously to restore the arterial blood pressure to
normal. When given in conjunction with cyclopropane or a halogenated anaesthetic, the noradrenaline may produce a cardiac
arrhythmia.

Adrenoceptors

The β- and α-effects of the catecholamines are mediated by two
distinct groups of adrenoceptor, both heterogeneous. The me-
diation of β-effects by β1 and β2 adrenoceptors has been mentioned.
Most of the alpha agonists and antagonists combine with α-
adrenoceptors as a whole, and do not discriminate between receptor
subtypes. There are a few exceptions however, for example prazosin and phenylephrine combine selectively with one subtype of
alpha adrenoceptor (α1) and clonidine with another (α2). Some of
the postsynaptic alpha-adrenoceptors of the vasculature seem to differ from the α1- and α2-subtypes (Drew & Whiting, 1979).

Autonomic nerve endings are well endowed with receptors for

acetylcholine, adrenaline and other active substances. When an agonist combines with prejunctional receptors the nerve is stimulated antidromically, and this inhibits the release of transmitter from the nerve ending. The physiological significance of prejunctional receptors is unclear. When clonidine is administered, however, the ensuing effects are largely due to stimulation of prejunctional $\alpha2$-adrenoceptors.

Sympathomimetic amines

Phenylephrine (m-synephrine, neosynephrine) and *methoxamine* (Vasoxine) stimulate α-adrenoceptors, and are almost without cardiac or central effects. They produce vasoconstriction, and a reflex bradycardia which can be abolished with atropine. Both drugs may be used to increase the arterial blood pressure during spinal or general anaesthesia, and unlike adrenaline or noradrenaline, they are safe in conjunction with cyclopropane or one of the halogenated anaesthetics. Phenylephrine or methoxamine may also be used to produce local vasoconstriction, and decongestion of the mucous membranes of the nose. Phenylephrine is deaminated by MAO, and the effect of an intravenous injection lasts about 20 minutes. Methoxamine (Fig. 6.15) is neither a substrate of COMT, owing to the absence of free phenolic groups in the nucleus, nor of MAO, owing to a methyl substituent on the α-carbon atom of the ethylamine side chain. Injected methoxamine acts for 1–$1\frac{1}{2}$ hours.

Isoprenaline only stimulates β-adrenoceptors. It is more potent than adrenaline in stimulating the contractility of the heart and relaxing the bronchioles. It was used to produce bronchodilatation, but has been superceded by safer drugs which produce less cardiac stimulation.

Isoxsuprine (Duphaspasmin) acts on $\beta1$ and $\beta2$ adrenoceptors, and is given intramuscularly to relax uterine muscle. It may also produce tachycardia, palpitations and muscular shivers. An agonist acting selectively on the $\beta2$-adrenoceptors would relax uterine muscle while producing less cardiac stimulation.

Salbutamol (Ventolin), *terbutaline* (Bricanyl, Filair) and *clenbuterol* (Ventipulmin) stimulate $\beta2$-adreoceptors selectively. They relax bronchial and uterine muscle, and have little stimulant effect on the heart. These drugs are used for bronchodilatation, being given by inhalation, injection or by mouth. Their effects persist for 3 hours or more, and when they are given repeatedly tachyphylaxis may

Noradrenaline

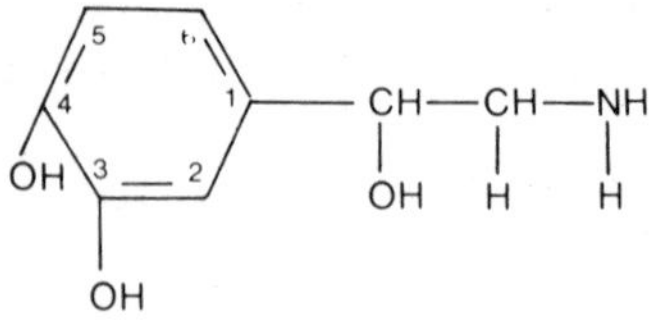

	4	3		OH	H	H
Adrenaline	OH	OH		OH	H	CH_3
Phenylephrine	H	OH		OH	H	CH_3
Methoxamine	H	H	$(2,5-OCH_3)$	OH	CH_3	H
Isoprenaline	OH	OH		OH	H	$CH(CH_3)_2$
Isoxsuprine	OH	H		OH	CH_3	$CH.CH_3.CH_2OC_6H_5$
Salbutamol	OH	CH_2OH		OH	H	$C.(CH_3)_3$
Terbutaline	H	OH	$(5,-OH)$	OH	H	$C.(CH_3)_3$
Clenbuterol	NH_2	Cl	$(5,-Cl)$	OH	H	$C.(CH_3)_3$
Dopamine	OH	OH		H	H	H
Tyramine	OH	H		H	H	H
Ephedrine	H	H		OH	CH_3	CH_3
Amphetamine	H	H		H	CH_3	H

Fig. 6.15 Chemical structures of sympathomimetic amines.

develop. In some human subjects salbutamol produces a fine tremor of the hands.

Dopamine (3-hydroxytyramine) is present in the brain, where it is stored in neurones that have cell bodies in the substantia nigra and axons passing to the basal ganglia. These dopaminergic nerves participate in the extrapyramidal control of skeletal muscle, a lesion in the nerves producing rigidity, tremor, and slowing and weakening of the voluntary movements.

In ruminants, dopamine is stored in cells resembling mast cells, which are present in the connective tissue of the viscera. Dopamine is rapidly metabolised by COMT and MAO. When given by intravenous infusion, dopamine (2–5 μg/kg/min) combines with specific dopamine receptors in the heart and vasculature, increasing the contractility of the heart, dilating the arterioles in the mesenteric and renal circulations and stimulating urine formation. These effects are antagonised by haloperidol. At higher infusion rates, dopamine acts on adrenoceptors and produces vasoconstriction.

Tyramine is a constituent of certain plants, and very large amounts may occur in silage. Tyramine is abstracted from extracellular fluid by Uptake 1, and subsequently releases noradrenaline from nerve endings. Thus tyramine produces sympathomimetic effects indirectly, without combining with adrenoceptors. The action of tyramine is terminated by MAO activity. Thus following inhibition of MAO, animals should not be given feeds containing tyramine.

Ephedrine occurs in the shrub *Ephedra sinica*. It acts indirectly by releasing noradrenaline from nerve endings. Ephedrine is not destroyed by COMT or MAO and so produces prolonged effects. It passes the blood–brain barrier, and produces wakefulness, alertness and anxiety. Although once use for nasal decongestion, mydriasis and bronchodilatation, ephedrine has been displaced by newer drugs.

Amphetamine (Benzedrine, Durophet) produces sympathomimetic effects indirectly. It is not metabolised by COMT or MAO, and is absorbed from the alimentary tract. Amphetamine passes the blood brain barrier and may be used for its central action, which is stronger than that of ephedrine. Amphetamine may be given to prevent attacks of sleep in narcoepilepsy or to reduce appetite in the treatment of obesity. *Dexamphetamine* (Dexedrine), the (+) isomer, is about twice as potent as racemic amphetamine. Large doses of these drugs produces tachycardia, palpitations, hypertension and central stimulation, which may be controlled with chlorpromazine. In some species, e.g. the horse, a large dose of amphetamine is liable to produce pulmonary oedema. Amphetamine and dexamphetamine are addictive, and as controlled drugs are subject to the provisions of the Misuse of Drugs Act. Moreover, because of their misuse for euphoric effects, the use of amphetamines is discouraged. Fenfluramine (Ponderax) is a derivative of amphetamine which produces anorexia and drowsiness. It is not a controlled drug.

Inhibitors of catecholamine inactivation

Cocaine inhibits Uptake 1, the mechanism which transports amines from extracellular fluid to adrenergic nerve endings. Thus cocaine potentiates the effects of catecholamines and abolishes those of tyramine and other amines acting indirectly (Fig. 6.16). In organs supplied with sympathetic nerve fibres cocaine produces sympathomimetic effects. Following sympathetic denervation and loss of the noradrenaline store, the sympathomimetic effect of cocaine is no longer demonstrable.

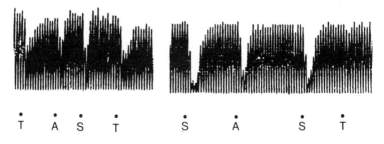

Fig. 6.16 Outflow from perfused rabbit ear, drop counter record returned to base line at 30 s intervals. Adrenaline 0.02 μg (A) and tyramine 15 μg (T) were injected into the arterial canula, and the sympathetic nerve stimulated for 20 s (S).
Left: control responses. Right: responses with cocaine (10^{-5}) in the perfusion fluid.
Cocaine potentiated effects of adrenaline or nerve stimulation and blocked tyramine.
(After Bartlet 1962 *British Journal of Pharmacology and Chemotherapy* 18: 480.)

MAO inhibitors are antidepressant. Sheep or guinea pigs become very aggressive when MAO activity has been inhibited by isocarboxazid. The behavioural excitation seems to be due to the increased amounts of noradrenaline, dopamine and 5-hydroxytryptamine in the brain.

Although inhibition of MAO activity in animals is not sought, it nevertheless occurs when furazolidone is given as an antibacterial or antiprotozoal agent. This is because the alimentary microflora transform the drug into an active metabolite which inhibits MAO activity in other organs.

Following inhibition of MAO, pethidine and narcotic analgesics must be withheld as they produce a severe febrile reaction which may be fatal. Feeds containing protein which has been subject to fermentation or spoilage are also dangerous, since they may contain large amounts of tyramine. The administration of an MAO inhibitor and an indirectly acting sympathomimetic amine produces a severe hypertensive reaction.

Adrenaline antagonists

Propanolol (Inderal) is structurally related to isoprenaline (Fig. 6.17), and is a competitive antagonist of $\beta 1$ and $\beta 2$-effects. In the heart, it inhibits the force and rate of contraction of the myocardial cells, and slows the passage of impulses through the conducting cells.

In non-ruminants, propanolol is well absorbed from the alimentary tract, a peak in the plasma concentration of the drug occurring 1–2 hours after administration by mouth. When given intravenously, propanolol may produce excessive bradycardia and hypotension, as it abolishes the influence of the cardiac sympathetic nerves but not that of the vagus. This effect may be avoided by giving atropine, then slowly injecting propanolol.

In veterinary medicine, propanolol may have a number of applications arising from its antiarrhythmic effect in the heart. The drug will prevent the onset or abolish cardiac arrhythmias produced by cardiac glycosides, general anaesthetics, exercise, emotion or hyperthyroidism. Although antagonism of the β-effects of catecholamines seems the prime mechanism of action of propanolol, the drug also has a potent local anaesthetic action which no doubt contributes to its antiarrhythmic effect.

Propanolol increases tolerance to exercise in subjects with angina, and in hypertension lowers blood pressure. It is not clear why the drug should lower blood pressure, but perhaps this is due to antagonism of an effect of the renal sympathetic nerves, which release renin from the kidney.

Unfortunately, propanlol sometimes produces bronchospasm, which is very undesirable in an animal with cardiac insufficiency or angina. A blockade of $\beta 2$-adrenoceptors in the lung causes the bronchoconstriction, which may be relieved with aminophylline (theophylline ethylene diamine). In patients with congestive heart failure, partial heart block or sinus bradycardia, the depressant effect of propanolol on the heart may prove fatal. The drug is also contra-indicated in patients with hypoglycaemia.

Atenolol (Tenormin) and *practolol* (Eraldin) are cardioselective antagonists of adrenaline, as they are more potent antagonists of the

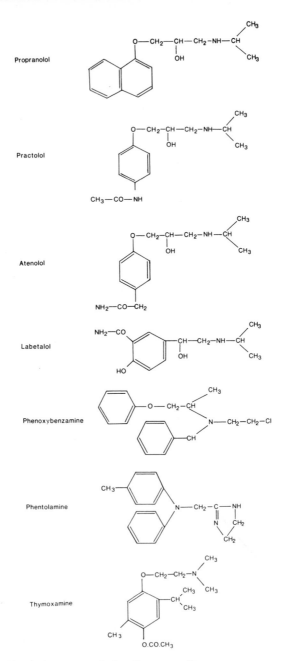

Fig. 6.17 Chemical structures of adrenaline antagonists.

β1- than the β2-effects, and are less likely to increase airway resistance than propanolol. Unfortunately, practolol can produce serious allergic effects in the eyes, skin and mucous membranes when given over several weeks.

Phenoxybenzamine (Dibenzyline) is transformed to an active metabolite which combines irreversibly with α-adrenoceptors, and antagonises the α-effects of catecholamines. The full effect of the drug takes up to an hour to develop after intravenous administration, and lasts for two days or more. The drug may be given by mouth, but it is irritant and not given by subcutaneous or intramuscular injection. Phenoxybenzamine produces vasodilatation, a decrease in arterial blood pressure, tachycardia, postural hypotension, drowsiness, nasal congestion, inhibition of ejaculation, miosis and dryness of the mouth. The tachycardia is very marked because the drug blocks the inactivation of catecholamines by Uptakes 1 and 2, and does not antagonise β-effects.

Phentolamine (Rogitine) is a competitive antagonist of the α-effects of catecholamines. The drug has been used in the diagnosis of phaeochromocytoma, a tumour of the of the adrenomedullary cells. When hypertension is due to this condition, an intravenous injection of phentolamine produces a fall in blood pressure lasting a few hours.

Prazosin blocks α1-adrenoceptors selectively, and antagonises the actions of phenylephrine more than those of noradrenaline. Prazosin antagonises the motor effect of noradrenaline in visceral but not digital arteries, whereas phentolamine blocks the effect of noradrenaline in both preparations. These observations suggest that prazosin and phenylephrine combine selectively with a sub-type of α-adrenoceptor, designated α1, whereas phentolamine and noradrenaline combine with all α-adrenoceptors. There are at least two types of α-adrenoceptor in the vasculature, which are prazosin-sensitive and prazosin-insensitive, respectively (Drew & Whiting, 1979).

Prazosin dilates arterioles and veins, thus reducing the peripheral resistance and venous return to the heart. It reduces the end-diastolic pressure in the left ventricle, and produces an increase in the efficiency of the heart. Small doses of the drug have been used together with frusemide for the management of congestive heart failure in the dog (Atwell, 1979). In a few patients, sudden collapse has followed the initial dose of the drug, which should therefore be small. The side-effects listed under phenoxybenzamine may occur, but their incidence and severity are not great, perhaps because prazosin does not block all the α-adrenoceptors in the vasculature.

Labetolol (Trandate) blocks both α- and β-adrenoceptors. It produces vasodilatation and a fall in arterial blood pressure, without compensatory tachycardia. Labetolol abolishes the reflex adjustment of vascular tone and produces postural hypotension. It has been given before the removal of a phaeochromocytoma, to block the effects of released catecholamines.

Reserpine

(Serpasil). This alkaloid produces a slow depletion of catecholamines and 5-hydroxytryptamine from the tissues of the body. This is because reserpine inhibits the storage of monoamines in the dense core vesicles present in adrenergic and tryptaminergic nerves, and choromaffin and enterochromaffin cells. The effects of reserpine develop over about 24 h, and include bradycardia, hypotension, nasal congestion, drowsiness, hypothermia, sedation, and an increase in gastrointestinal tone and motility. Reserpine has been used to prevent aortic rupture in turkeys and for the destruction of mice. In cases of poisoning, domesticated animals should be kept warm and the respiration stimulated with nikethamide as required.

Adrenoceptive mechanisms in the eye

The distribution of the sympathetic nerve to the ciliary body seems to be confined to the vessels and possibly the epithelial cells of the ciliary processes. Agonists which combine with adrenoceptors may influence the formation of aqueous humor by producing vasoconstriction (α-effect) or vasodilatation (β-effect) in the ciliary processes, and possibly by affecting its secretion by epithelial cells (β-effect). A change in the rate of formation of aqueous humor can be detected by measuring the rate of removal of fluorescein from the anterior chamber, an increase in rate of formation producing a more rapid washout of the marker. Adrenergic nerve fibres are present in the tissue of the trabeculum, and sympathomimetic amines and their antagonists affect the resistance to drainage of aqueous from the eye. This resistance can be assessed by measuring the fall in intraocular pressure (or loss of fluorescein) when fluid is forced from the eye by addition of a weight to a tonometer probe.

Adrenaline may be instilled into the eye in the treatment of simple (open-angle) glaucoma. It is contra-indicated in narrow-angle glaucoma however, as it is apt to dilate the pupil and produce a further increase in intraocular pressure. In human eyes, adrenaline may produce an increase (β-effect) or a decrease (α-effect) in the rate of formation of aqueous humor, together with a decrease in resistance to drainage of aqueous. Intraocular pressure is reduced by adrenaline, provided that pupillary dilatation does not block the drainage of aqueous.

Guanethidine (Ismelin) is an adrenergic neurone blocking agent, which blocks the release of noradrenaline caused by action potentials in sympathetic nerves. The amount of noradrenaline in adrenergic nerves is slowly reduced by the drug, and the effector cells become supersensitive to adrenaline and noradrenaline. Guanethidine reduces the resistance to drainage of the aqueous humor and lowers intraocular pressure. It is used either alone or together with adrenaline in the treatment of open-angle glaucoma.

Timolol (Timoptol) is about 5 times more potent than propanolol as an antagonist of the β-effects of the sympathomimetic amines. Its local anaesthetic activity is weaker than that of propanolol, however, so that timolol is preferred for application to the eye. Timolol blocks the increase in rate of formation of aqueous produced by adrenaline. The drug reduces the intraocular pressure without affecting resistance to drainage of aqueous humor from the eye. In the cat, timolol is less potent in the reduction of intraocular pressure than in man. In some individuals, the intraocular pressure increases slowly after several months of timolol administration. This may be due to a change in the nature of the adrenoceptors controlling formation of aqueous. Timolol inhibits tear production.

Thymoxamine is an α-antagonist, which blocks the effect of the sympathetic innervation to the dilator pupillae. This drug may be used to treat angle-closure glaucoma, or to reverse the mydriasis produced by a sympathomimetic amine. Thymoxamine has little effect on the cilliary muscles, and unlike parasympathomimetic drugs, does not produce discomfort or restrict accommodation.

Phenylephrine (α1-agonist) produces a biphasic change in intraocular pressure, a rise followed by a fall. In the rabbit, the rise in intraocular pressure is due to contraction of Müllers muscle in the orbit. Phenylephrine is not used in the treatment of glaucoma although it may be used to produce dilatation of the pupil.

Clonidine is a selective agonist at α2-adrenoceptors. The drug reduces intraocular pressure and seems to be very dependable for this purpose. α2-adrenoceptors are located mainly at prejunctional sites in adrenergic nerve endings. Stimulation of prejunctional α2-adrenoceptors reduces the influence of the adrenergic neurones on the effector cells. Other α2-adrenoceptors occur postjunctionally in effector cells, and agonists combining with them produce sympathomimetic effects. Following sympathectomy, clonidine is ineffective in the eye. This observation suggests that the ocular hypotensive action is due to a reduction in sympathetic tone, in consequence of the stimulation of prejunctional receptors. Unfortunately, the effect of clonidine is not confined to the eye. The drug is absorbed and produces central effects, including hypotension and fatigue.

SUGGESTIONS FOR FURTHER READING

Aldrige W N, Barnes J M, Johnson M K 1969 Studies on delayed neurotoxicity produced by organophosphorus compounds. Annals of the New York Academy of Sciences 140: 314–322

Ali B H, Bartlet A L 1982 Inhibition of monoamine oxidase in chickens and ducklings by a microbial metabolite of furazolidone. Quarterly Journal of Experimental Physiology 67: 69–79

Ambache N 1955 The use and limitations of atropine for pharmacological studies on autonomic effectors. Pharmacological Reviews 7: 467–494

Atwell R B 1979 Workload reduction as the basis for treatment of cardiac disease in the dog. Australian Veterinary Journal 55: 255–256

Axelrod J 1966 Methylation reactions in the formation and metabolism of catecholamines and other biogenic amines. Pharmacological Reviews 18: 95–113

Bowman W C, Rand M J 1980 Textbook of Pharmacology, 2nd edn. Blackwell, Oxford

Burn J H, Rand M J 1958 The action of sympathomimetic amines in animals treated with reserpine. Journal of Physiology 144: 314–346
animals treated with reserpine. Journal of Physiology 144: 314–346

Drew G M, Whiting S B 1979 Evidence for two distinct types of postsynaptic α-adrenoceptor in vascular smooth muscle in vivo. British Journal of Pharmacology 67: 207–216

Endo M 1977 Calcium release from the sarcoplasmic reticulum. Physiological Reviews 57: 71–108

Feldberg W (ed) 1957 Autonomic Nervous System. British Medical Bulletin 13: 153–226

Iversen L L 1971 Role of transmitter uptake mechanisms in synaptic neurotransmission. British Journal of Pharmacology 41: 571–591

Johns E J 1980 An investigation into the type of β-adrenoceptor mediating sympathetically activated renin release in the cat. British Journal of Pharmacology 73: 749–754

Koelle G B (ed) 1966 Cholinesterases and anticholinesterase agents. Handbook of experimental pharmacology, Vol 33. Springer-Verlag, Berlin

Kosterlitz H W 1967 Effects of choline esters on smooth muscle and secretions. Physiological Pharmacology 3: 97–161

Langer S Z 1977 Presynaptic receptors and their role in the regulation of transmitter release. British Journal of Pharmacology 60: 481–498

Nicholls J T 1976 Adverse effects of practolol. Annals of Clinical Research 8: 229–231

Potter D E 1981 Adrenergic pharmacology of aqueous humor dynamics. Pharmacological Reviews 33: 133–153

Trendelenburg U 1966a Transmission of preganglionic impulses through the muscarinic receptors of the superior cervical ganglion of the cat. Journal of Pharmacology and Experimental Therapeutics 154: 426–440

Trendelenburg U 1966b Mechanisms of supersensitivity and subsensitivity to sympathomimetic amines. Pharmacological Reviews 18: 629–640

Tu A T 1977 Venoms: Chemistry and Molecular Biology. John Wiley, New York

7

Depressants of the central nervous system

Narcotics are drugs which depress the central nervous system acting as either ataractics, sedatives, hypnotics, anticonvulsants or anaesthetic agents. However, the term narcotic is also used in a more restricted legal sense to denote drugs which often have addictive properties. It is necessary to appreciate the two different uses of the term narcotic. A hypnotic drug induces sleep. Pharmacologically, hypnosis is drug-induced sleep and this is distinct from neuro-hypnosis (of man). Ataractics are drugs which introduce an indifference to the surrounding animals and so produce calmness and make sleep easier. Sedatives have a similar but more pronounced effect. Drugs may have either ataractic or hypnotic effects depending on the dose of the drug and the animal species to which it is given.

The mechanism of anaesthetics

The mode of action of anaesthetics is uncertain, although there are a number of theories. One of the earliest explanations is the 'colloid theory' of Claude Bernard (1875). He suggested that a reversible aggregation of cell colloids causes or accompanies anaesthesia. It is now known, for example, that a number of anaesthetics including halothane reduce cytoplasmic mobility and will cause a reversible depolimerisation of labile microtubules. Microtubules are responsible for intracellular transport of organelles.

The 'lipid solubility theory' was proposed independently by Meyer (1899) and Overton (1901). They noted that certain substances with a high fat solubility and low water solubility were potent anaesthetics. The higher the fat/water partition coefficient the greater is the expected potency of the anaesthetic. Therefore they proposed that all chemically indifferent substances which are soluble in fats and fatty substances must exert a narcotic effect on living protoplasm in so far as they are distributed in it. This theory as a generalisation is well substantiated. However, it does not explain some observed differences in action between stereoisomers. There are other theories.

The 'cell permeability theory' proposes that anaesthetics cause a change in the membrane permeability of cells in the central nervous system. Biochemical theories have noted the reversible depressant effects of anaesthetics on oxygen consumption and ATP synthesis. Physical theories of Pauling (1961) & Miller (1961) involve water and the formation of gas hydrate microcrystals in the membrane or clathrates (an organised H_2O structure) over the membrane. Both hydrates and clathrates reduce membrane permeability. One of the more recent theories is the 'degenerate perterbation theory' of Metcalf et al (1974). This proposes that the functioning of membrane proteins which form ion channels activated by transmitters are selectively altered by changes in the fluidity of the membrane produced by the anaesthetic. In summary, there is not a single satisfactory theory of anaesthesia, so it is probable that narcotics are capable of producing anaesthesia by various molecular mechanisms.

CENTRAL NEUROTRANSMITTERS

Many central nervous system depressants, particularly the ataractics interact with central neurotransmitters to potentiate or depress their action. If a natural inhibitory transmitter is prevented from acting, it leads to a net excitatory effect on the central nervous system. Antagonism of a naturally excitatory transmitter leads to the opposite effect, i.e. central depression. Table 7.1 shows some of the neurotransmitters and their actions.

Acetylcholine depolarises Renshaw cells in the spinal cord by acting on both nicotinic (antagonised by hexamethonium) and muscarinic receptors (antagonised by atropine). In the brain acetylcholine causes excitation, mainly via a muscarinic action. The main pathway involved appears to be the ascending reticular activating system.

Glutamic acid and *aspartic acid* have been suggested to be excitatory transmitters in several sites in the central nervous system. Both depolarise and excite motor neurones. Ketamine antagonises NADA glutamate receptors.

GABA (γ-aminobutyric acid) hyperpolarises many central neurones. Purkinge cells in the cerebellum, for example, use GABA as a transmitter. It also produces pre-synaptic inhibition. GABA is synthesised by the enzyme glutaminic acid decarboxylase. GABA is antagonised by picrotoxin and by bicuculline and potentiated by the benzodiazepines and pentobarbitone.

Table 7.1 Putative neurotransmitters

	Acetylcholine	GABA	Glycine	Dopamine	Noradrenaline	5-HT	Substance P	Encephalin	Aspartate & Glutamic acid
Action	Excites arousal & motor function	Inhibits by a presynaptic action in spinal cord	Inhibits by a postsynaptic action in spinal cord	Inhibits extra-pyramidal	Inhibits mood regulation	Inhibits Involved in pain processing and behaviour	Excitatory from some primary afferents	Inhibits pain pathways	Excitatory on motor neurones
Antagonists	Nicotinic and muscurinic	Picrotoxin & bicuculline	Strychnine	Chlor-promazine haloperidol	propranolol	Methysergide			

Glycine has an inhibitory action hyperpolarising motor neurones. It is probably a post-synaptic inhibitory transmitter in the spinal cord. Its action is blocked by strychnine.

Noradrenaline terminals in the forebrain and spinal cord originate from cells in the pons and medulla. Others pass from the locus coerulus and pass to the cerebellar cortex and hippocampus. This was shown by fluorescent histochemistry. The central actions of noradrenaline are usually inhibitory and mediated by stimulation of adenyl cyclase, which increases cyclic AMP. Adrenergic α- and β-receptors are distinguished in the brain. β-blockers will antagonise the inhibitory actions of noradrenaline. Theophylline which inhibits phosphodiesterase and the breakdown of cyclic AMP potentiates the central actions of noradrenaline. It appears that noradrenaline is involved in the regulation of fear and mood. Stimulation of central α-receptors with clonidine and xylazine produces a fall in blood pressure.

Dopamine neurones project from the substantia nigra to the basal ganglia. Other dopamine pathways arise medially to the substantia nigra and project to the cerebral cortex. Dopamine receptors can be stimulated by apomorphine and ergot alkaloids. They are selectively antagonised by ataractic drugs like chlorpromazine and droperidol. Stimulation of dopamine receptors in the pituitary results in an inhibition of prolactin secretion. Stimulation of dopamine receptors in the chemoreceptor trigger zone produces vomiting in dogs and cats. Blocking of the dopamine pathway from the substantia nigra to the basal ganglia produces characteristic motor abnormalities in animals which is termed catalepsy.

Serotonin. (5-HT) neurones are localised in many areas of the brain including the raphé system of the brain stem. These nerves project from the medulla down the spinal cord. They are involved in the control of pain pathways which project from the spinal cord to the brain. This control can be blocked by L-p-chlorophenylalanine, which blocks the synthesis of 5-HT. It can be stimulated by tryptamine and α-methyl tryptamine, which prevents 5-HT uptake. Methysergide will antagonise the actions of 5-HT.

Substance P was first extracted by Euler & Gaddum in 1931 and is now known to be an undecapeptide. It is distributed throughout the nervous system particularly in areas like the dorsal horn of the spinal cord. It has an excitatory action on motor neurones and may be a transmitter of some primary afferents.

The encephalins and endorphins. In 1975 Hughes & Kostelitz described two naturally occuring pentapeptides, met-encephalin and

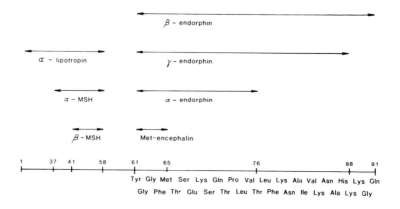

Fig. 7.1 Bovine β-lipotropin

leu-encephalin, which were recovered from brain extracts. They were shown to have morphine-like effects. Other peptides with similar actions were found and are now known as the endorphins. They are derived from a longer peptide β-lipotropin which was recovered from the pituitary. α--, β- and γ- endorphins, like the encephalins, have morphine-like properties. These compounds are believed to act as neurotransmitters on opiate receptors which are found in many areas of the brain including the substantia gelatinosa of the dorsal horn. They are believed to be active in the control of transmission of noxious stimulation as well as involved in the production of addiction. Many other peptides are now recognised as transmitters in the CNS.

CENTRAL NERVOUS SYSTEM DEPRESSANTS

Ethyl Alcohol (CH_3CH_2OH)

Alcohol is a narcotic, a disinfectant, a carbohydrate food and a useful solvent. It is rapidly absorbed from the gastro-intestinal tract and mostly metabolised in the body. Ethanol is metabolised by dehydrogenation ultimately to carbon dioxide and water, but forming on the way acetaldehyde and acetic acid. This oxidation is catalysed by an enzyme, ethanol dehydrogenase. It is interesting to note that one of the richest sources of this enzyme is horse liver. Ethyl alcohol has a disinfectant action by precipitating bacterial proteins. In veterinary practice its use is confined to disinfection of the skin.

Methyl alcohol resembles ethyl alcohol pharmacologically, the main distinction being due to the fact that in the body a large portion of the methyl alcohol is converted to formaldehyde. Although its immediate toxic effects are less than those of ethyl alcohol it is cumulative and will produce coma lasting days and is accompanied by a bilateral inflammation of the optic nerve and retina.

Chloral hydrate ($CCl_3CH(OH)_2$)

This white crystaline substance is used in veterinary medicine as a sedative and hypnotic for horses. It was the first synthetic hypnotic and was introduced by Liebreich in 1868. Liebreich knew that chloral hydrate in alkaline solutions liberated chloroform, and thought the same reaction would take place in the body. However, the narcotic effect is not produced by chloral hydrate or by chloroform but by trichorethanol.

Chloral hydrate is readily absorbed from the gastro-intestinal tract. It is irritant and is given to horses by stomach tube well diluted. It may be given to dogs well diluted with syrup. In the body it is reduced to trichlorethanol which is the active substance. This is conjugated in the liver with glucuronic acid to form urochloralic acid which is excreted in the urine. The urine is then capable of reducing Fehling's solution. Some of the trichlorethanol is oxidised

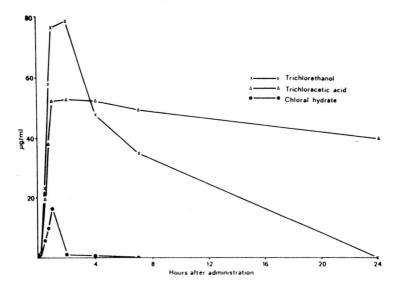

Fig. 7.2 The concentration of trichlorethanol, trichloracetic acid and chloral hydrate found in urine after i.v. administration of chloral hydrate.

to trichloracetic acid. This is a strong acid which binds firmly to plasma proteins and hence persists in the blood for some days after chloral hydrate has been given.

When given by mouth to the horse for colic, chloral hydrate produces its sedative effect after about 30 minutes. There is no initial excitement. It does not depress reflexes and is therefore of little use as an anticonvulsant. There is a slight fall in blood pressure due mainly to the peripheral vasodilatation. There is no good evidence of cardiac depression.

Since chloral hydrate is used occasionally in veterinary surgery as an intravenous narcotic and the margin between narcotic dose and toxic dose is not great, it is important to appreciate the drug's toxic properties. In acute poisoning the blood pressure is low, temperature falls and respiration is depressed. Delayed poisoning commonly occurs after prolonged narcosis and is characterised by fatty changes in the liver, heart and kidneys, causing death after two or three days.

BARBITURATES

This important group of narcotics dates from 1903 when Fisher & Von Mering introduced barbitone. Chemically they are dervied from the condensation of malonic acid and urea which forms barbituric acid. Although barbituric acid is not hypnotic it is modified by substitution to give the active barbiturates (Fig. 7.3).

A great number of barbiturates have been synthesised, mainly by substituting at position five in the ring (Fig. 7.3). The hypnotic activity of the barbiturate increases by substitution at position 5 until the number of carbon atoms at the two substituants totals seven. When the number of carbon atoms exceeds this the compound tends to be convulsive rather than hypnotic. It can be seen that pentobarbitone has a total of seven atoms in the two substituants and is approximately optimal. Methohexatone has more than seven carbons here and does show convulsant effects in dogs on recovery from the anaesthetic. It has been further shown that if the substituting groups in position five are branched the compound is a more potent narcotic than the straight chain isomeride. Pentobarbitone, methohexatone and thiopentone have branched side chains. Substitution at position one with methyl groups decreases duration of effect but this is often associated with excitation on induction and recovery (e.g. methohexatone). The addition of a phenyl group in position five gives specific anticonvulsant effects

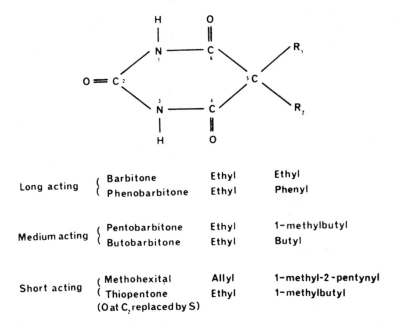

Long acting	{ Barbitone	Ethyl	Ethyl
	{ Phenobarbitone	Ethyl	Phenyl
Medium acting	{ Pentobarbitone	Ethyl	1-methylbutyl
	{ Butobarbitone	Ethyl	Butyl
Short acting	{ Methohexital	Allyl	1-methyl-2-pentynyl
	{ Thiopentone	Ethyl	1-methylbutyl
	(O at C₂ replaced by S)		

Fig. 7.3 The formulae of certain barbiturates found in common use.

(e.g. phenobarbitone). The replacement of the oxygen with sulphur at position 2 increases the speed of onset of the narcotic effect but decreases the duration (e.g. thiopentone). The speed of onset of a barbiturate depends on the lipid solubility of the compound as well as on the blood supply to the brain. These factors control the concentration which penetrate into the brain. Thiopentone is more lipid soluble than pentobarbitone, which in its turn is more lipid soluble than phenobarbitone. The speed of onset of the narcotic effect of thiopentone is faster than pentobarbitone, this in its turn is faster than phenobarbitone.

The duration of the narcotic effect is controlled by three factors. The first is redistribution, the second is metabolism and the third is renal excretion.

Redistribution is important for short acting barbiturates, particularly thiopentone. After intravenous injection thiopentone is carried to the brain and rapidly penetrates across the blood-brain barrier. This allows the rapid onset of narcosis. Redistribution from the brain to the other tissues particularly the fat depots then follows. Thiopentone is taken up by tissues with a lower blood perfusion rate and the plasma concentration falls. The concentration in the brain then falls allowing recovery. When thiopentone is released slowly from the fat it is metabolised by the liver. The fact that redistribution controls the duration of action of thiopentone accounts for the cumulative effects of thiopentone. On repeated injections the fat depots become saturated. In very lean animals like the greyhound, thiopentone is often not used because of the slow recovery. The duration of action is potentiated by intravenous administration of glucose or intermediates in its metabolism, such as lactate, pyruvate and glutamate. This should be remembered when using parenteral fluid replacement after barbiturate anaesthesia.

Table 7.2 Clearance of pentobarbitone

Species	Rate (per cent/hour)	Reference
Horse	46	Nicholson J D (1968) *Biochem. Pharmac.*, 17, I
Sheep	49	Rae J H (1962) *Res. vet Sci.* 3, 399
Dog	15	Taylor et al (1957) *Proc. Soc. exp. Biol. Med.* 95, 462

Metabolism is important for the medium acting barbiturates like pentobarbitone. The barbiturates are metabolised in liver by oxidation of the side-chains to form inactive compounds. This is accomplished by the P-450 oxidative enzymes in the liver microsomes. They require for their activity reduced triphosphopyridine nucleotide and oxygen. In addition to this, methohexatone is demethylated while thiopentone undergoes desulphuration to yield pentobarbitone. The metabolism of barbiturates is of some practical importance since liver damage can substantially prolong the duration of narcosis. The administration (to sheep) of carbon tetrachloride, which is a well-known liver poison, doubles the duration of action of pentobarbitone. There are some interesting and important species differences with respect to metabolism of barbiturates. Young calves appear to be deficient in oxidative enzymes and even short-acting barbiturates have a prolonged action in this species. Pentobarbitone given to a calf can produce anaesthesia of 20 hours duration and the animal may not recover. Sheep, on the other hand, appear to be well endowed with oxidative enzymes and the duration of action of pentobarbitone in sheep is not substantially longer than that of thiopentone. Presumably sheep can oxidise pentobarbitone as quickly as they can redistribute thiopentone. The horse appears to be similarly well-supplied with oxidative enzymes and the action of pentobarbitone in this species is little longer than thiopentone. In the dog pentobarbitone acts four or five times as long as thiopentone. Further evidence of the importance of oxidated enzymes in the liver in influencing the duration of activity of barbiturates comes from the use of an interesting compound SKF 525A. This compound is chemically diethylaminoethyl diphenyl propyl acetate. It has no apparent pharmacodynamic actions of its own but appears to inhibit oxidases and esterases in the liver microsomes. If this drug is given to an experimental animal and followed by a barbiturate such as hexobarbitone the duration of action of the barbiturate is substantially prolonged. Chloramphenicol has a similar effect on the liver microsomes and the duration of pentobarbitone narcosis. Pentobarbitone has an interesting property independent of its narcotic activity. It stimulates liver enzyme systems and can in the case of barbiturates cause tolerance to develop by increasing the activity of the oxidative enzymes of the liver. This type of activity is called 'enzyme induction'.

Renal excretion is important for the long-acting barbiturates like barbitone and phenobarbitone. Barbitone is excreted mainly in the urine. Phenobarbitone is partly excreted in the urine and partly metabolised. Barbiturates are weak acids and can exist as ionised and un-ionised moieties. Renal excretion can be increased by diuretics and by making the urine more alkaline with the administration of sodium bicarbonate. This prevents or reduces tubular reabsorption and shortens the duration of action of these barbiturates.

The short-acting barbiturates like thiopentone and methohexatone are used mainly for induction of anaesthesia. The longer-acting barbiturate pentobarbitone may be used for full anaesthesia. The longer-acting barbiturates like amylobarbitone, pentobarbitone and butobarbitone are used for sedation or as anticonvulsants.

All the barbiturates depress the central nervous system. They differ only in degree and are not analgesic unless consciousness is affected. They are particularly depressant to the motor areas of the cortex and are therefore useful in controlling convulsions of cortical origin. Depression of the sensory areas requires larger doses. There are several suggestions which attempt to explain the action of barbiturates. It is suggested that they act by depressing the utilisation of oxygen by the brain. Another suggestion is that they prevent synthesis of acetylcholine in the brain by blocking the conversion of pyruvate to acetate. It is also known that pentobarbitone potentiates the effect of GABA, an inhibitory transmitter. The mechanism of the anaesthetic action of the barbiturates, however, is still a matter for conjecture.

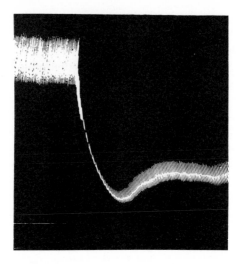

Fig. 7.4 The effect of pentobarbitone (10 mg/kg i.v.) on the respirations of a rabbit. The height of the tracing above the base line shows the volume of air breathed. Time interval 10 secs.

In veterinary surgery thiopentone and pentobarbitone are used to produce anaesthesia. They are given by intravenous injection as the soluble sodium salt of the barbiturate. The intravenous route is chosen because it allows the dose to be adjusted most readily to the animals requirements. These sodium salts form solutions which are markedly alkaline and therefore irritant. The intravenous route avoids this local irritation. However, perivascular injection will result in phlebitis or sloughing.

The barbiturates are particularly depressant on the respiratory centre and overdosage causes death from respiratory failure. Pulmonary oedema is occasionally produced. Two factors are involved in the respiratory depression: first, there is the direct depressant action of the brain stem respiratory centres, secondly there is the loss of sensitivity to CO_2 and hypoxia by the brain stem, carotid body and aortic body chemoreceptors. This means that using CO_2 to stimulate respiration which has been unduly inhibited by too much barbiturate is unlikely to succeed.

Therapeutic doses of barbiturates have only a small depressant effect on the cardiovascular system. Larger doses depress the vasomotor centre and may dilate and injure the capillaries, producing shock. Barbiturates have little effect on the digestive tract or on renal function. The barbiturates reduce the basal metabolic rate but do not damage the liver. The motor activity of the uterus is unaffected but the respiration is depressed in the newborn since the barbiturate passes across the placenta. This is an important factor in choosing an anesthetic for Caesarean section. The cerebro-spinal fluid is unaffected by the barbiturates. Overdose of barbiturates produce death either by direct paralysis of respiration or by causing prolonged coma which may lead to broncho-pneumonia. In treating barbiturate overdose during anaesthesia artificial respiration is invaluable.

ANTICONVULSANTS

Phenytoin sodium is an anticonvulsant drug chemically similar to diazepam. Phenytoin is well absorbed from the gut and destroyed in the body, less than 0.1 per cent appearing in the urine. A single dose of this compound may persist in the cat's body for several days because the cat is deficient in glucuronyl transferase. Hence, this drug in the cat is cumulative. Experimentally this compound was found to prevent convulsions produced in the cat by electrical stimulation of the brain. Clinically it will suppress epileptic convulsions and although it is not a general anticonvulsant like phenobarbitone, it has little hypnotic action. *Troxidone* is a drug which prevents convulsions induced by analeptic agents and is useful for controlling epileptic convulsions. It is readily absorbed from the gut and distributed throughout the body water. In dogs it is metabolised by demethylation. It has been found to damage the bone marrow. *Primidone* is an important anticonvulsant, said to be better than barbiturates and hydantoins and less hypnotic. It is used in dogs to control epileptiform convulsions and hysteria and to control convulsions in the foal. Prolonged treatment may cause incoordination. *Valproate* which inhibits the metabolism of GABA is also used as an anticonvulsant.

PHENOTHIAZINE ATARACTICS

An ataractic may be defined as a drug which produces in an animal a state of indifference to its surroundings. A number of derivatives of phenothiazine have been produced which possess this property. Several of these drugs have been very useful in veterinary practice, both to facilitate handling of difficult animals of all species and, in particular, to pre-medicate animals prior to general anaesthesia. When used in this way ataractics not only make the induction of anaesthesia easier but reduce the amounts of anaesthetic required and hence the liklihood of toxic sequelae.

Chlorpromazine inhibits a large number of enzymes and in consequence produces a wide range of pharmacological effects, the most conspicuous being due to depression of various functions of the central nervous system. Chlorpromazine inhibits the hypothalamus, the reticular formation and the chemoreceptor trigger zone. This latter property, due to its competitive dopamine antagonism, is utilised when the drug is given to prevent vomiting. It should be realised that chlorpromazine does not inhibit vomiting arising from stimuli from the gastro-intestinal tract or vestibular apparatus. Chlorpromazine has antihistamine, anticholinergic, antispasmodic and hypotensive actions. The hypotension may be due to its strong α-blocking activity and inhibition of centrally mediated pressor reflexes.

The animal given chlorpromazine remains conscious but is ataxic, refuses food, and shows some muscular relaxation, the head and tail drooping. Very occasionally muscle rigidity (catalepsy) is seen due to the interruption of the dopamine pathway between the substantia nigra and basal ganglia. The animal appears sedated but will react to stimuli. The effect of anaesthetics and hypnotics is enhanced. Body temperature falls and the production of hypothermia is facilitated. The uptake of oxygen by the tissues is reduced. Chlorpromazine is antagonistic to central stimulants and large doses may produce respiratory failure.

The phenothiazine ataractics have a complex metabolism and in the dog, less than 3% pf a single dose of chlorpromazine has been recovered from the urine unchanged. Many oxidation products are produced and in the dog tens of metabolites have been identified.

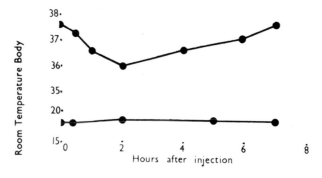

Fig. 7.5 The hypothermic action of chlorpromazine (1.5 mg/kg) in the horse.

Chlorpromazine is even more persistent in the cat than in the dog and it is important that this long persistence of the phenothiazines is appreciated. In veterinary practice, administration by the intramuscular route is usually preferred, the drug being used to render animals more tractable or as pre-anaesthetic medication.

Promazine has properties very similar to those of chlorpromazine but is much weaker. The hypotensive effects are particularly marked and it is claimed to be less toxic due to the absence of a Cl atom. It has proved popular in veterinary therapeutics.

Trimeprazine is similar to chlorpromazine in its activity but has stronger antihistaminic actions. It is used both as an ataractic and as an antipruritic. It is claimed that the ataractic action of trimeprazine is more reliable than that of chlorpromazine in the case of cats and horses.

Methotrimeprazine has marked hypotensive effects, but strong central analgesic actions, approaching morphine in potency. It is usually available in solutions with a pH of 4. Pain at the injection site may occur because of the pH and large volumes or repeated administration at the same site may cause necrosis of the muscle. Extrapyramidal effects have been reported with this compound.

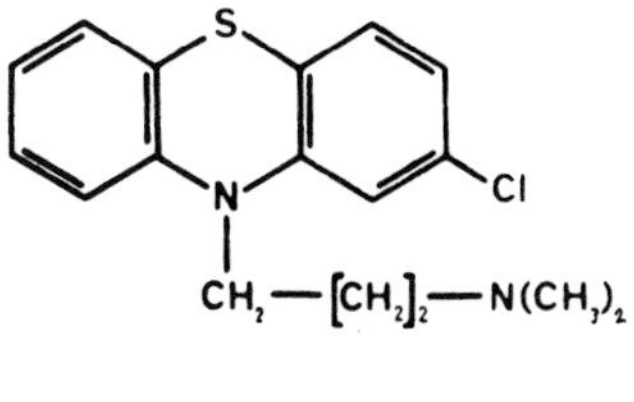

Chlorpromazine 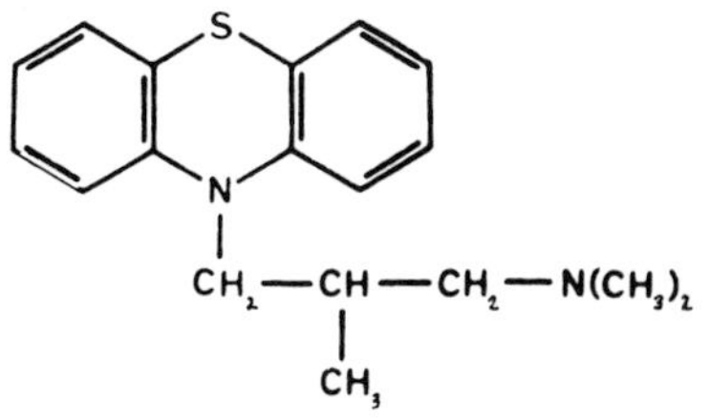   Trimeprazine

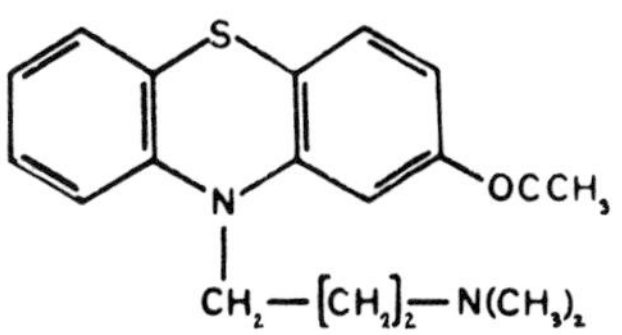

Acepromazine 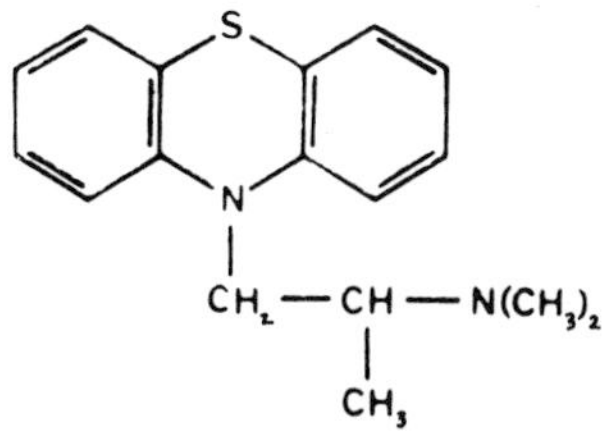   Promethazine

Fig. 7.6 Four phenothiazine derivatives.

Acepromazine has a potency similar to or even greater than chlorpromazine and it is alleged that acepromazine is less erratic in its ataractic activity, especially in the horse. It has been a popular drug for use in this species.

Promethazine is a phenothiazine used mainly as an antihistamine and is more effective than mepyramine. It has marked local anaesthetic properties and its central action is similar to chlorpromazine.

BUTYROPHENONES

These ataractic drugs inhibit purposeful movement so that the animal appears in a tranquil state dissociated from its surroundings. The butyrophenones have pharmacological similarities with the phenothiazines in that they have tranquillising, anti-emetic and slight α-blocking activities.

Azaperone is a butyrophenone with neuroleptic properties particularly suited for the sedation of pigs. It is given by intramuscular injection. The onset of sedation is produced within 10 minutes of injection, the effect is greatest at 15–20 minutes and may last as long as 2 hours. Although the hypothermic and α-blocking actions are less than with the phenothiazine ataractics, azaperone also produces a slight hypothermia and hypotension. Salivation and muscular termors occasionally occur.

Tritiated azaperone has been used to study the metabolism in rats. The drug was shown to be rapidly metabolised, 61% of the radioactivity appeared in the faeces within 24 hours. Azaperone has been used to prevent fighting amongst pigs immediately preceding slaughter. The problem of tissue residues demands special consideration in these circumstances as the drug is unevenly distributed in the body giving high levels in the liver. It would be inadvisable to slaughter within a few hours of administration.

Droperidol has ataractic actions and is a powerful anti-emetic. Large doses may produce extrapyramidol effects (catalepsy). Droperidol may be given in milk to primates to facilitate their handling.

Haloperidol has similar actions but its duration of action is longer. Fentanyl, a strong analgesic, is used with haloperidol to produce neuroleptanalgesia. It should not be used in horses.

BENZODIAZEPINES

The benzodiazepines are a group of drugs with ataractic and sedative effects. The site of action is the limbic system of the brain, particularly the hippocampus and amygdala. In addition to their sedative effects they also act as anticonvulsants. The mode of action is known to involve a potentiation of the inhibitory transmitter GABA. Their effect is therefore inhibitory in many areas of the central nervous system. There are many of these compounds. Their chief difference is potency. They have no anti-emetic or α-blocking actions like the phenothiazines and butyrophenones so they do not depress the blood pressure so readily.

Diazepam is a potent compound with tranquillising anticonvulsant, muscle relaxing effects acting on the ascending reticular formation. It is the only benzodiazepine that has been used to any extent in veterinary work. The marked anticonvulsant properties make it a useful agent in association with morphine in animal species where morphine drugs produce excitation. Because of its lack of α-blocking effect it is useful for tranquillisation in dogs suffering from shock.

Zolazepam is another benzodiazepine with similar actions, which has been suggested for use with tiletamine for exotic species.

HYPNOTICS

Hypnotic agents other than the barbiturates and opiates are discussed in this section. These drugs produce a hypnotic and analgesic effect which varies with dose, route of administration and the species.

Metomidate produces a hypnotic effect in fish, reptiles, birds and mammals. It has little analgesic effect but a strong central muscle relaxant effect. However, when used with azaperone or fentanyl it produces a condition which is like general anaesthesia. Azaperone followed by metomidate is particularly effective in pigs for many operations. It has also been used successfully in horses. It could be used for induction as an alternative to thiopentone but can cause intravascular haemolysis in this species. Etomidate is a derivative so far used only in human medicine.

Propanidid is a ugenol derivative, insoluble in water and dissolved in Cremophor El. It produces anaesthesia of very short duration because it is rapidly metabolised by liver and plasma esterases. It produces a fall in blood pressure which is particularly marked in dogs. This may result from a reaction to the Cremophor El. Its use is limited to rabbits and rats.

Alphaxalone-alphadolone acetate (Saffan). This is a steroid anaesthetic which can be used in cats, primates, rabbits, guinea-pigs,

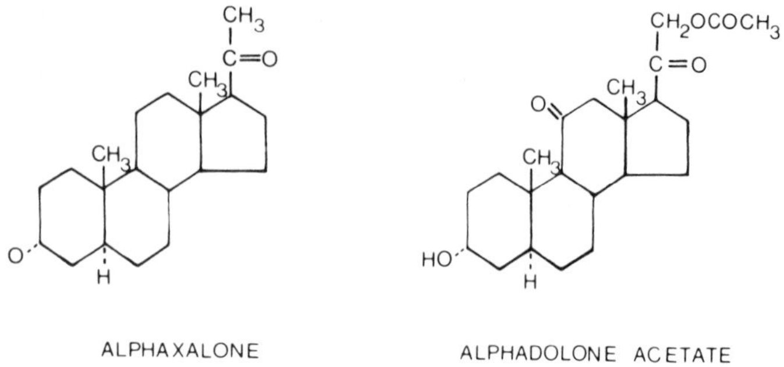

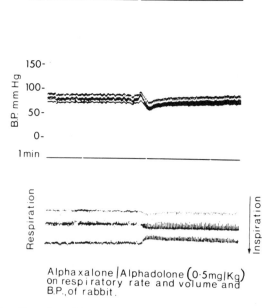

ALPHAXALONE ALPHADOLONE ACETATE

Fig. 7.7 The structural formulae of steroid anaesthetics.

birds, rats and mice. It was developed after the observations of Hans Selve (1941) who reported that steroids like progesterone and desoxycorticosterone have anaesthetic actions in rats. The advantage of steroid anaesthetics is that they have a greater therapeutic ratio and an action terminated by liver metabolism. However, steroid anaesthetics are insoluble in water and the compounds used to make them soluble are associated with undesirable effects. Saffan

sig

150-
100-
B.P. mm Hg 50-
0-
1 min

Respiration   Inspiration

Alphaxalone/Alphadolone (0·5mg/Kg) on respiratory rate and volume and B.P. of rabbit.

Fig. 7.8 The effect of steroid anaesthetics on respiration and blood pressure.

consists of three parts alphaxalone and one part alphadolone. Alphadolone has half the potency of alphaxalone and is included to improve solubility. Both are solubilised by the addition of Cremophor El (polyoxethylated castor oil).

After intravenous injection Saffan produces a rapid loss of consciousness lasting approximately 10 minutes. The muscle relaxation is good in most species. Recovery is rapid after a single injection although convulsive movements are seen on recovery in cats. This convulsive action seen on recovery may be due to a selective antagonism of the inhibitory transmitters GABA and glycine. Little or no tolerance or cumulative toxic effects are seen. It has a therapeutic index in rats four times that of thiopentone and has little oestrogenic effect. Intravenous injection causes a fall in blood pressure but cardiac output is maintained by an increase in heart rate. This returns to normal levels after two to three minutes. Respiration following induction may be depressed briefly.

The steroids are not bound exclusively to plasma proteins. Metabolism is rapid. Redistribution and metabolism are responsible for the fall in anaesthetic levels in the plasma. Metabolites are excreted in the bile with some enterohepatic recycling giving rise to some metabolites in the urine.

The drug is not irritant like thiopentone sodium and does not cause perivascular sloughs. Its main use is in the cat for intravenous induction. It may also be given by intramuscular injection into the quadriceps femoris muscle group. The action of the Cremophor El regularly causes oedema of the paw and ears of cats and sometimes pulmonary oedema. This action is due in part to histamine release and may produce hypotension and tachycardia. These side-effects due to the Cremophor El make the use of this drug unsafe in dogs.

Xylazine is a hypnotic with a selective α_2-agonist action and central muscle relaxant properties. It has some analgesic effects at higher doses in some species. The degree of central depression is also dose-dependent, varying from an ataractic effect to hypnosis in some species, particularly cows.

The heart rate and blood pressure shows an initial transient rise following intravenous injection. This is due to a peripheral α-agonist action and can be blocked with phentolamine. The blood pressure and heart rate and circulation time then falls. This fall in blood pressure is due to a central α-agonist action and a reduction in sympathetic output. At higher doses xylazine can cause partial A–V block and cardiac arrhythmias as reported in the horse and dog. The A–V block may be prevented by the administration of

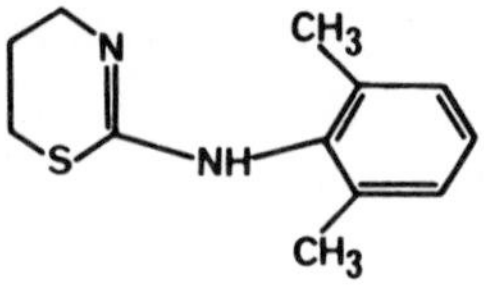

Fig. 7.9 The structural formula of xylazine and azaperone.

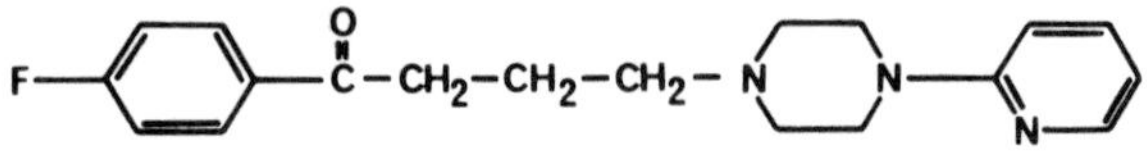

atropine. Respiration is depressed in horses, dogs and cats. There may also be a motor response to loud noises during sedation. This is seen in horses, dogs and cats. Cattle may also appear to struggle spontaneously. Vomiting is usually seen in cats and occasionally in dogs. Studies using xylazine labelled with radioactive sulphur or carbon showed that 90% is excreted as inorganic sulphur and CO_2 within 10–15 hours. Only 8% of the dose appears unchanged in the urine. 70% of the radioactivity appears in the urine and 30% arrives in the faeces via the bile.

Cows and goats are particularly sensitive to this drug and basal narcosis with some analgesia is produced with high doses. In horses it is an effective sedative but it does not produce recumbency in this species.

DISSOCIATIVE ANAESTHETICS

Three cyclohexylamines (phencyclidine, ketamine and tiletamine) have been used in animals to produce a state known as 'dissociative anaesthesia'. The site of action is thought to be the frontal cortex with little action on the reticular activating system. They produce a state of catalepsy, with loss of consciousness, analgesia but little muscle relaxation. The eyes remain open. Pharyngeal and laryngeal reflexes are only abolished if high doses of the drug are used. They may excite or depress respiratory and circulatory systems depending on dose and species. In man hallucinations and emergence delirium occur. It is not known if this occurs in animals. Salivation is produced in most species.

Phencyclidine is used mainly in the control of primates other than man. It has been used in a dart for the capture of wild animals but it is longer-acting than ketamine. In the horse this drug produces alarming excitement, unlike dogs, cats and birds, which are depressed. The profuse salivation produced can be countered with atropine.

Ketamine is similar in action to phencyclidine but has a short duration of action. It produces catalepsy and analgesia without muscle relaxation. Ketamine is metabolised by N-demethylation and hydroxylation to the cyclohexanone ring. It is then conjugated in the liver and excreted in the urine. Ketamine has a high therapeutic index, five times greater than pentobarbitone in dogs. It may be given by intravenous or intramuscular injection. Although it has been given to most small animals its use is recognised for the restraint of wild primates, birds and cats, following intramuscular injection. Ketamine is now used after premedication with xylazine to produce anaesthesia in cats and horses.

Tiletamine. This is similar in chemical structure and pharmacological activity to ketamine. Catalepsy is rapid in onset after intramuscular injection and lasts 30–50 minutes. It has been tested in clinical trials in association with zolazepam. A combination of these two drugs has been recommended for use in dogs, cats, sheep, primates and exotic species.

OPIATES

Opium is obtained from unripe seed capsules of the poppy plant, *Papaver somniferum*. It contains a number of alkaloids which are divided into two groups: the phenanthrenes, which contract smooth muscle, and include morphine, codeine and thebaine; the isoquinolenes, which relax smooth muscle, and include papaverine and narcotene.

The structure of morphine is illustrated in Figure 7.10 although morphine is difficult to synthesize it is easy to modify chemically. For example, methylation of morphine produces codeine; acetylation produces diacetyl morphine (heroin). Thebaine is easily modified to an antagonistic naloxone, or to a very potent agonist etorphine.

The main effects of morphine are on the central nervous system and bowel, producing analgesia sometimes hypnosis (dog), respiratory depression and decreased gastro-intestinal motility.

It is known that morphine acts on stereospecific opoid receptors which are found in the limbic system, amygdala, thalamus, hypothalamus, midbrain and the substantia gelatinosa of the spinal cord.

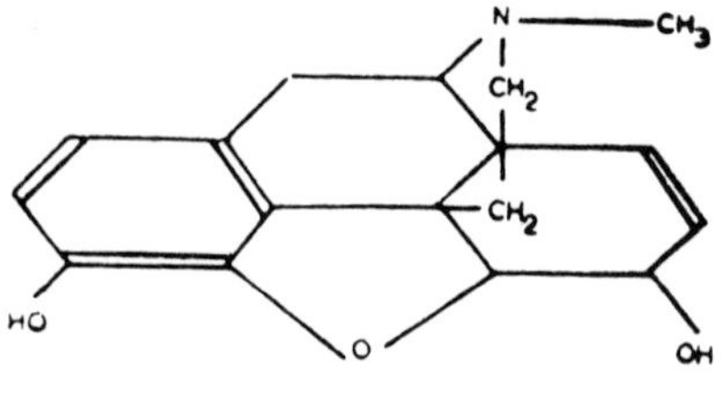

MORPHINE

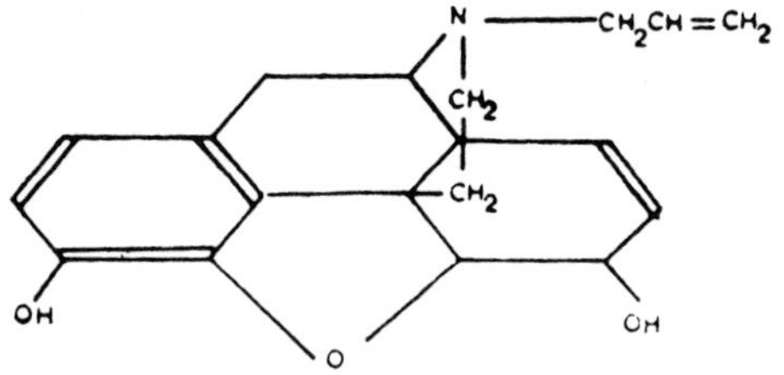

NALORPHINE

Fig. 7.10 The structural formulae of morphine and an antagonist nalorphine.

They are also present in the intestine and vas deferens. The opoid receptors appear to be the site of action of endogenous peptides known as leu-encephalin and met-encephalin as well as endorphines. There are at least three different types of opiate receptor (Gilbert & Martin 1977; Lord et al, 1979). These receptors are designated μ, κ and δ. The μ-receptor is stimulated selectively by normorphine to produce supraspinal analgesia, respiratory depression and physical dependence. The κ-receptor is selectively stimulated by pentazocine and ethylketocyclazocine to produce spinal analgesia, miosis and sedation. The mouse vas deferens contains δ-receptors which are selectively stimulated by leu-encephalin. The different opiates may act as agonists or antagonists at these different receptor sites. They may act as an agonist on one receptor site while acting as an antagonist at another receptor site.

Morphine is believed to act as a selective agonist at μ-receptor sites. In the dog, bird and rabbit, morphine produces analgesia, hypnosis and in large doses coma. In the cat it produces delirium in all but small doses. In the ox, horse and pig the effect is unreliable, sometimes producing narcosis and sometimes excitement.

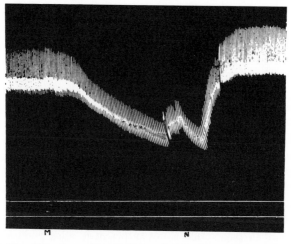

Fig. 7.11 The effect of morphine M (2.5 mg/kg) on the respirations of a rabbit and the antagonistic action of nalorphine N (2.5 mg/kg). The height of the tracing above the base line shows the volume of air breathed. Time interval 10 secs.

Morphine produces a pinpoint pupil in dogs due to stimulation of the oculo-motor nerve nucleus. In other species the pupil is dilated because of the excitement caused by this drug.

Morphine is a potent analgesic. The mechanism of this action involves an inhibition of the transmission of noxious stimuli from primary afferents to second order neurones which project towards the brain. This inhibition may be accomplished by the small cells in the substantia gelatinosa which are known to possess opiate receptors. A major descending inhibitory pathway consisting of 5-HT containing neurones is also stimulated by the opiates. Stimulation of these inhibitory nerves prevents the cranial transmission of noxious stimulation and contributes to the analgesia. Morphine also produces a slowing of the heart rate and initially increases gastro-intestinal activity, due to stimulation of the vagal centre. In species like the dog with a developed vomiting centre it stimulates vomiting and then inhibits it due to depression of the chemoreceptor trigger zone. In addition to vomiting, defaecation followed by constipation may occur. This is due to contraction of the plain muscle of the gut which subsequently impedes ingesta and leads to constipation. The constipation is accentuated by a reduction in the secretion of the intestinal glands and depression of the defaecation reflexes. Morphine also produces urinary retention by contracting the sphincter of the bladder.

Morphine is readily absorbed from the gut or after injection. Some undergoes glucuronide conjugation and excretion in the urine and bile. Thirty per cent of the dose is excreted in the faeces. However, most is destroyed in the liver and tolerances are quickly acquired to this drug.

The main use of morphine in veterinary practice is either as a pre-medication prior to anaesthesia or as an analgesic in the dog. It can be used to depress a troublesome cough but this is associated with the danger of respiratory depression. Morphine and crude preparations of opium are sometimes used to relieve diarrhoea.

Papaveretum is a preparation containing the water soluble alkaloids of opium (50% morphine plus 50% mixture of papaverine, codeine, narcotine and thebaine). It causes less vomiting in dogs than morphine. It has been suggested for the treatment of colic but the amount of papaverine is not sufficient to relax plain muscle.

Pethidine (also known as meperidine) has analgesic actions but is about ten times less potent than morphine. It has the added advantage of possessing spasmolytic properties like papaverine. It also has less hypnotic, and cough depressant effects. It relieves pain without interfering with muscular activity. It is rapidly metabolised in the liver, so that its effects are not long-lasting. Very occasionally it may cause serious histamine release in ruminants and dogs.

Methadone is a synthetic opiate with most of the properties of morphine, except that it is less hypnotic.

Diamorphine (heroin) is an acetylated analogue of morphine. It is more powerful than morphine and is very likely to produce addiction in man. It is not used in veterinary practice.

Pentozocine is a benzomorphan derivative with a selective agonist action on κ-receptors. It has, however, antagonistic actions at μ-receptors. It is a powerful analgesic and is approximately half as potent as morphine. It is only hypnotic in large doses. The lack of euphoric effects in man means that there is less liability to produce addiction. Although it is not subject to controlled drugs regulations it is still capable of producing misuse. It does produce some respiratory depression and stimulation of the vagal centre with slowing of the heart. However, vomiting, constipation or pupillary constriction are not likely to occur in the dog. It will antagonise the actions of morphine but is not itself antagonised by nalorphine or levallorphan. However, its effects can be antagonised by the antagonistic naloxone. An interesting technique of 'anaesthetie analgesique sequentielle', has been described. In this technique fentanyl is used throughout surgery and then its respiratory depression is terminated with pentazocine. This allows excellent post-operative analgesia.

Etorphine is a very potent opoid, such that sufficient of the drug may be loaded into a dart for immobilisation of wild game. It is approximately a thousand times as potent as morphine. Etorphine acts as an agonist on all the opiate receptor types. It produces central nervous system stimulation before depression, particularly in the horse. In an attempt to reduce the stimulation it is used with a phenothiazine ataractic (acepromazine or methotrimeprazine). However, despite this there are still pronounced cardiovascular effects. In the horse there is a dramatic rise in blood pressure and heart rate which can be reduced with propranolol. In the dog vagal stimulation produces a pronounced slowing of the heart rate. The combination of etorphine and a phenothiazine has a pronounced respiratory depressant action. A specific antagonist, diprenorphine is used to reverse the effects of etorphine. Excitement may occur after recovery in the horse, 6–8 hours after remobilisation. This is explained by the longer plasma half-life of etorphine compared to diprenorphine. Etorphine is excreted in the bile and undergoes entero-hepatic recycling. Other side-effects of etorphine associated with its use include hypothermia and priapism and sometimes paraphimosis as a sequel in horses. In dogs a sensitivity to metallic noises is seen during narcosis. Pigs are particularly sensitive to the respiratory depressant actions of etorphine and isolated cases of anaphalactic-type reactions have been recorded in pigs.

Etorphine has also very potent effects in man and is very dangerous, so that it is necessary to recognise its toxic effects. It can cause in man dizziness, nausea and pinpoint pupils followed by respiratory depression, cyanosis and eventually lower blood pressure, loss of consciousness and cardiac arrest. Treatment consists of prevention of absorption if possible, summoning of medical help and administration of naloxone (0.4 mg) i.m. or i.v. repeated at intervals of 2–3 minutes until the symptoms are reversed. If naloxone is not available diprenorphine should be given. It is vital to maintain adequate respiration and heart beat, if necessary by artificial respiration and external cardiac massage.

Fentanyl is a potent shorter acting synthetic opiate. Like morphine it produces analgesia in all animals as well as respiratory depression. In dogs, rabbits, rats and primates it produces narcosis but in horses and mice it produces excitement. Atropine can be used to reduce bradycardia seen in dogs. Fentanyl is used with do-peridol or haloanisone for neuroleptanalgesia in dogs, rabbits, guinea-pigs and primates.

Neuroleptanalgesia is a type of narcosis produced by the combination of a neuroleptic, for ataractic or sedative effects, and an opiate analgesic. Neuroleptanalgesia does not produce hypnosis. It is useful for minor surgery. However, the disadvantages include: a degree of respiratory depression and the two agents not having the same duration of action. The advantages are: the effects of opiate may be specifically antagonised; the mixture has minimal toxic effects on liver, kidney and myocardium.

OPIATE ANTAGONISTS

It is now known that there are several (μ, κ and δ) types of opiate receptor in the central nervous system and gut. Some morphine derivatives act as competitive antagonists at all of these receptor types but others may act at some sites as agonists and, at others, as competitive antagonists.

Naloxone, a morphine derivative, acts as a competitive antagonist at all the opiate receptors and is particularly effective at μ-receptor sites. Since it has no agonist action at the other receptor sites it is recommended that this compound, if available, should be used to reverse the effects of morphine-like compounds. Naloxone does not reverse the narcotic effects of barbiturates or other anaesthetic agents. Nalorphine acts as a competitive antagonist at μ-receptor sites but as an agonist at κ-receptor sites. It is an agonist–antagonist. This means that nalorphine will antagonise the respiratory depressant actions of morphine. However, when nalorphine is administered to normal animals without prior administration of morphine it has analgesic and respiratory depressant actions. It reduces the tone of plain muscle and increases intestinal muscle activity. The effects of nalorphine are less persistent than those of morphine. Levallorphan is a similar agonist–antagonist.

Diprenorphine is like nalorphine and is an agonist–antagonist. It is used in veterinary practice as a specific antagonist of etorphine and is prepared in a suitably high concentration.

Pentazocine will also antagonise μ-receptor actions of morphine but is itself an analgesic.

ANTITUSSIVES

Codeine resembles morphine in its activity but is less potent. It is mostly excreted unchanged in the urine and is used to relieve coughing, being given to dogs by mouth as codeine phosphate or syrup of codeine phosphate.

Dextromethorphan. This drug apparently has no analgesic or addictive properties, is devoid of narcotic activity and exerts no action on the gut. However, it raises the threshold for stimuli to coughing and has been used therapeutically to alleviate persistent or painful coughs.

SUGGESTIONS FOR FURTHER READING

Alexander F, Nicholson J D 1968 The blood and saliva clearances of phenobarbitone and pentobarbitone in the horse. Biochemical Pharmacology 17: 203

Boyes G R 1963–1964 Phenothiazine tranquilisers in veterinary practice, Vet. A. 5: 32

Bush M T, Sanders E (1967). Metabolic fate of drugs: barbiturates and closely related compounds. A. Rev. Pharmac., 7: 57

Franks N P, Lieb W R (1982) Molecular mechanisms of general anaesthesia. Nature 300: 487–493

Fraser H F, Harris L S (1967). Narcotic and narcotic antagonist analgesics. A. Rev. Pharmac., 7: 277

Gilbert P E, Martin W R (1975). The effect of morphine and nalorphine-like drugs in the non-dependent, morphine dependent and cyclazocine-dependent chronic spinal dog. Journal of Pharmacology and Experimental Therapeutics 192: 538–541

Hall L W (1971). Wright's veterinary anaesthesia, 7th ed Bailliere, London, Tindall & Cassell

Jaffe J H, Martin W R. Opoid analgesics and antagonists. In: Goodman & Gilman's The pharmacological basis of therapeutics, 6th ed. Macmillan, New York, p 494–534

Lord J A H, Waterfield A A, Hughes J, Kosterlitz H W (1977). Endogenous opoid peptides: multiple agonists and receptors. Nature 267, 495

Lumb W V, Winn Jones E (1973) Veterinary anaesthesia. Lea & Febiger, Philadelphia

Marsboom R (1971) The Development and Pharmacology of Butyrophenones in Human and Veterinary Medicine. Proc. Assoc. Vet. Anaesth., no 2, 81

Metcalfe J C, Hoult J R S, Colley C M (1974) The molecular implications of a unitary hypothesis of anaesthetic action. In: Molecular mechanisms in general anaesthesia. Halsey M J, Miller R A, Sutton J A Churchill Livingstone, Edinburgh

8

Depressants of the central nervous system: General anaesthetics

Alcohol and opium and substances containing hyóscine have been used from the earliest times to dull the pain of surgical procedures. Surgical anaesthesia was introduced very rapidly in the early years of the 19th century. Sir Humphrey Davey (1798) described the pharmacology of nitrous oxide (N_2O). Between 1842 and 1846 Morton and Long described and demonstrated the use of diethyl ether for surgical anaesthesia. In 1847 Simpson in Edinburgh demonstrated the use of chloroform anaesthesia. In animals ether was first used in 1846 at the Royal Veterinary College. Very soon after this the use of chloroform in the horse was a common practice all over the UK.

SIGNS AND STAGES OF ANAESTHESIA

General anaesthetics are used to produce a state of insensibility to avoid the pain of surgical procedures. Compounds like ether, chloroform and nitrous oxide have been used since the 1850s to produce general anaesthesia. It was Guedel who used ether to describe the signs and stages of anaesthesia in man. He described the transition from consciousness to complete surgical anaesthesia. Classically the signs were divided into four stages. They are more easily observed with slow acting compounds like ether but not so easily recognised with fast acting drugs like halothane or thiopentone. These separate stages can be recognised in domestic animals (Hall 1971). Stage 1 is called the stage of 'analgesia or induction or voluntary excitement'. Stage 2 is called the stage of 'delirium or involuntary excitement.' Stage 3 is called the stage of 'surgical anaesthesia' and can be divided into three planes. The first plane is called the plane of 'light anaesthesia', the second plane is called the plane of 'medium anaesthesia' and the third plane is called the plane of 'deep anaesthesia'. Stage 4 of anaesthesia is called the stage of 'medullary or 'respiratory paralysis'. It is also called the stage of overdose.

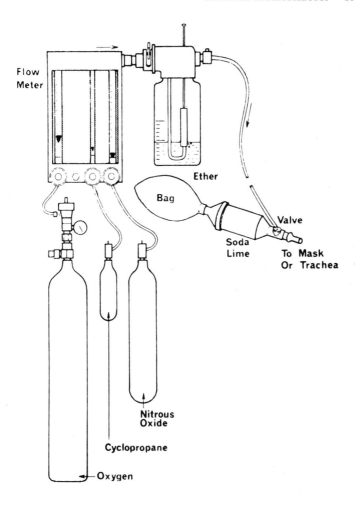

Fig. 8.1 Diagram of a simple anaesthetic machine for administration of gaseous and volatile liquid anaesthetics.

Stage 1: voluntary excitement

During this stage the animal is conscious and may resist the application of the anaesthetic agent. Breathing is under voluntary control and breath holding may occur. If the animal is frightened there may be an increase in the respiratory and pulse rates and dilatation of the pupils. If it is extremely frightened urine and faeces may be voided.

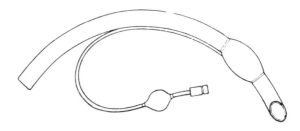

Fig. 8.2 A cuffed endotracheal tube.

Stage 2: involuntary excitement

The animal loses consciousness at the beginning of this stage. There may be exaggerated limb movements and response to sensory stimuli during this stage. Breathing may be very irregular and breath holding is associated with struggling. The swallowing and vomiting reflexes are present during this stage but become progressively depressed and disappear on entering stage 3. The cough reflex is also present during this stage and may produce difficulties on intubation.

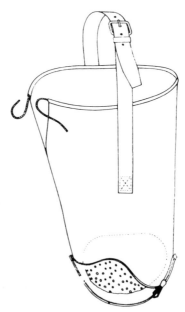

Fig. 8.3 Canvas mask for the administration of volatile liquid anaesthetics to the horse. The anaesthetic is applied to the sponge.

Stage 3: surgical anaesthesia

This stage was originally divided into four planes by Guedel but it is more usual to consider only three planes in this stage. This is because the fourth plane of Guedel indicates overdose and should be included in the next stage of anaesthesia. The three planes are:

The first plane (light) anaesthesia

This plane begins at the onset of regular and automatic breathing. There is no movement of the limbs. The eyeballs move from side to side and as anaesthesia deepens this movement becomes sluggish. Once the eye movement has finished and the eyeball becomes fixed the animal is then considered to have entered the next plane of anaesthesia. All the eye reflexes (palpebral, conjunctival, and corneal) disappear during this plane of surgical anaesthesia. They are no longer present in the second plane of surgical anaesthesia. However, in the dog and cat the pedal reflex is still present.

The second plane (medium) anaesthesia

There is little effect on respiration during this plane. Laryngeal reflexes remain until the middle of this plane. In dogs and cats the eyeball rotates downwards but in horses, cattle, sheep and pigs the eyeball is fixed and central. Muscle relaxation increases during this plane and is adequate for all except intra-abdominal surgery. In the dog and cat the pedal reflex becomes sluggish during this plane.

The third plane (deep) anaesthesia

During this stage the breathing is regular and automatic but has increased in rate, while the depth of respiration decreases. There is a pause between inspiration and expiration. The thoracic component of this inspiration gradually disappears during this stage leaving the abdominal component. If breathing becomes greatly depressed and is no longer regular and automatic the animal is said to have passed on to the fourth stage of anaesthesia. In both the dog and the cat the eyeballs, once again, become central and are no longer rotated downwards. This is due to the loss of tone of the eye muscles. The pedal reflex completely disappears.

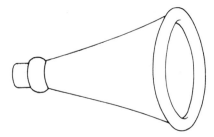

Fig. 8.4 Conical rubber mask for dogs and other small animals.

Stage 4: overdose

During this stage the thoracic muscles become completely paralysed and only diaphragmatic activity remains. Because of the paralysis of the thoracic muscles movement of the diaphragm causes the abdomen to bulge outwards and the chest to move inwards. Expiration causes a reverse of this. The movement of the diaphragm is often jerky during this stage. The pupils dilate while the pulse becomes rapid. There is also a cessation of lacrimal secretion which gives rise to a characteristic fish-eye appearance. If this stage continues cyanosis appears as respiration becomes progressively smaller in amplitude and rate. It will eventually cease. When cyanosis is replaced by an ashen grey colour of the mucous membranes of the eye it indicates heart failure.

THE EYE IN ANAESTHESIA

Eyeball movement is a reliable sign and indicates the presence of plane 1 (light) anaesthesia. The pupil size is an unreliable sign of the depth of anaesthesia, because it is inluenced by pre-medication with drugs like morphine and atropine and is also influenced by lighting. The exception is in stage 4, the stage of overdose where the pupil becomes widely dilated due to paralysis of the iris muscles. Conjunctival and corneal reflexes persist until the second (medium) plane of anaesthesia except in the horse where they persist until stage 4 (stage of overdose). The pupillary light reflex which can be tested by closing both the eyelids for 20 seconds and examining one eye uncovered in the presence of a strong light shone into it. If the light reflex is present the exposed pupil will constrict. This reflex disappears halfway through plane 3 (light anaesthesia). This reflex is not reliable if there has been pre-medication with atropine or morphine.

Minimum alveolar anaesthetic concentration

Merkel & Eger (1963) proposed the concept of minimum alveolar anaesthetic concentration (MAC). MAC is defined as the alveolar concentration of an anaesthetic that prevents muscular movement in response to painful stimulus in 50% of test subjects. Skin incision or tail clamping is used as the painful stimulus. Adequate time must be allowed for the alveolar and brain partial pressures to come to equilibrium (at least 15 minutes). The concept of MAC allows a comparison of the relative potencies of the gaseous and volatile anaesthetics. For example, halothane is more potent than ether. The MAC of halothane is 0.77% while the MAC of ether is 1.92%.

The EEG as an index of the depth of anaesthesia

Changes in the frequency and amplitude of the electrical activity of the brain recorded as the electroencephalogram (EEG) give characteristic patterns at different levels of anaesthesia but depend upon the anaesthetic agent used. However, a general picture can be described. A spontaneous rhythm, characteristic of a conscious patient is referred to as the α-rhythm. This consists of low amplitude high frequency waves. The frequency of the electroencephalogram becomes faster at the onset of anaesthesia and on further

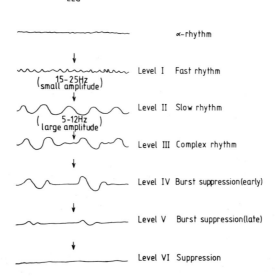

Fig. 8.5 A diagram of the effect of thiopentone on the EEG patterns

increase in the depth of anaesthesia the wave becomes larger in voltage but lower in frequency. The effect of a barbiturate on the EEG is illustrated in Figure 8.5. Six EEG levels are recognised in addition to the spontaneous α-rhythm of the conscious patient. Level I is referred to as the 'fast rhythm'; level II as the 'slow rhythm'; level III, 'the complex rhythm'; level IV, 'burst suppression (early)'; level V, 'burst suppression (late)'; and level VI, 'suppression'.

Gala et al (1958) have suggested that the various EEG levels can correspond to the different stages of anaesthesia. These workers found that the clinical signs and stages of anaesthesia lagged behind the EEG level of anaesthesia on induction. The electroencephalogram is unlikely to be used in routine veterinary practice because of the complicated interpretations of the patterns seen.

Pharmacokinetics

Gaseous and volatile anaesthetics are given by inhalation and must reach the brain to produce their effect. To do this the anaesthetic has to pass from the upper respiratory tract to the alveoli, be absorbed from the alveoli into the blood and carried by the circulation to the brain and other tissues. In the brain the level of anaesthesia is proportional to the partial pressure of the gaseous or volatile anaesthetic.

Transfer of anaesthetic from the upper respiratory tract to alveoli

The partial pressure of the anaesthetic in the alveoli will depend upon the partial pressure of the anaesthetic in the inspired gaseous mixture. Obviously the higher the partial pressure of the gaseous anaethetic in the inspired air the higher will be the partial pressure of the anaesthetic in the alveoli. Another factor which influences the partial pressure of the anaesthetic in the alveoli is the alveolar ventilation. An increase in alveolar ventilation increases the partial pressure of the gaseous anaesthetic reached in the alveoli. Alveolar ventilation in its turn is affected by the tidal volume, the dead space and respiration rate. For example, an increase in the dead space due to the addition of an endotracheal tube for anaesthesia decreases the tidal volume and hence alveolar ventilation. A reduction in the respiratory rate due to breath holding or a depression of the central respiratory centres will also reduce the alveolar ventilation. In addition to these factors there are two other factors which influence the partial pressure of the anaesthetic in the alveoli. These are the 'concentration effect' and the 'second-gas effect'. At higher concentrations of an anaesthetic gas, the alveolar partial pressure increases at a slightly greater rate than it would have done if a lesser concentration of the anaesthetic had been inhaled. This is because the volume of gas disappearing from the lung is replaced by fresh anaesthetic gas into the lung from the breathing circuit to replace the volume taken up. This means that the rate at which the inspired gas mixture is delivered to the lung is then greater than the minute ventilation would have provided without this effect. This effect is known as the 'concentration effect'. A closely related phenomenon, due to the simultaneous presence of two anaesthetic gases in the lung, is known as the 'second-gas effect'. This effect is seen for example with mixtures of N_2O (75%) oxygen (24%) and halothane (1%). The addition of N_2O to the O_2-halothane mixture speeds the rate of uptake of the halothane.

Transfer of anaesthetic gas from alveoli to blood

The speed with which the gaseous anaesthetic crosses from the alveoli of the lung into the capillary bed depends upon the partial pressure difference across this barrier and the diffusion constant of this barrier. The greater the partial pressure difference between the alveoli and the arterial blood the greater is the flow of the anaesthetic gas. The flow of the anaesthetic across the alveoli into the blood is also slowed in cases of pneumonia where there is an exudate present which increases the barrier to diffusion. Diffusion is also slowed when there is a reduction in the ventilation perfusion ratio of the alveoli. This may occur when there are pathological changes in the lung or during anaesthesia when an animal is positioned, as is usual, on its back. The solubility of an anaesthetic agent in the blood has a marked effect on the speed of which it crosses the alveolar endothelial barrier. The more soluble an anaesthetic agent in the blood the more that must cross the alveoli to raise the partial pressure of the anaesthetic in the blood. This means that the partial pressure of soluble anaesthetic agents rises more slowly than partial pressure of less soluble agents. The solubility of an anaesthetic agent is measured by the blood: gas partition coefficient (λ). Ether is very soluble and has a λ of 12. Halothane is less soluble and has a λ value of 2.4. N_2O is not very soluble and has

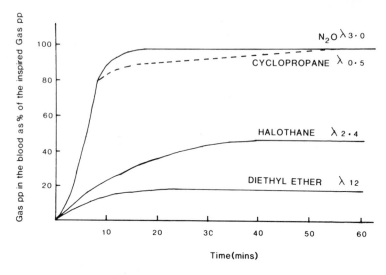

The % pp of the anaesthetic agents against time

Fig. 8.6 The % partial pressure in blood of different anaesthetic against time.

a λ of 0.5. It can be seen that because ether has the highest blood solubility it is slowest in reaching equilibrium. N_2O on the other hand is much less soluble and is much quicker at reaching equilibrium.

Circulation in the blood and diffusion into the tissues

Once the anaesthetic has reached the pulmonary blood circulation from the alveoli it is then distributed round the body in a manner

Table 8.1 The physical characteristics of some volatile and gaseous anaesthetics.

Anaesthetic	B.P. (°C.)	Saturated vapour pressure at 20 °C. (mm. Hg)	Maximum concentration obtainable at 20 °C.	Partition coefficient		
				Blood/ gas	Brain/ blood	Fat/ blood
Ether	35	442	58%	12	1.1	5
Halothane	50	243	32%	2.3	2.6	60
Chloroform	61	160	21%	10	1.2	26
Trichloroethylene	87	59	8%	9	—	106
Methoxyflurane	105	25	3%	13	—	63
Cyclopropane	− 33	—	100%	0.5	—	20
Nitrous oxide	− 88	—	100%	0.5	1.0	3

which depends on the tissue blood flow and the lipid or tissue solubilities. The higher the blood flow to a tissue the faster the partial pressure and concentration will rise in that tissue. Tissue solubility determines the final slope of the gas tension curve (Fig. 8.6). Those anaesthetics with a high tissue or lipid solubility like cyclopropane rise slowly in this area. Those compounds with a low tissue solubility rapidly achieve equilibrium like N_2O. A table of the physical properties of the anaesthetic agents is shown in Table 8.1

The elimination of gaseous anaesthetics

The major factors which influence the elemination of gaseous and voltaile anaesthetics are the same as those involved in uptake. They include tissue solubilities, blood flow rates, respiratory rates and tidal volumes. The whole process however is essentially behaving in reverse. Once the anaesthetic has been turned off and the animal is ventilated with no anaesthetic, the lung and blood partial pressures fall first; the brain partial pressure follows soon afterwards; the muscle and then the fat partial pressures follow more slowly.

A phenomena known as 'diffusion hypoxia' occurs in the early minutes following the end of N_2O administration, if the animal is breathing only air. This occurs because N_2O is removed rapidly from the body so that its appearance in the alveoli dilutes the available oxygen. Diffusion hypoxia only occurs to any significance level when N_2O has been used. It is easily overcome by ventilation on pure oxygen.

Other routes of elimination

Most of the anaesthetic gases are excreted through the lung. However, small amounts depending on the anaesthetic are retained in the body and metabolised. For example, 3% of ether may be oxidized in CO_2 and water while up to 4% of chloroform, 13% of halothane and 20% of methoxyfluorane can be retained and metabolised to various compounds. However, little of the insoluble agents like N_2O are metabolised. Induction of the liver enzymes can occur and be stimulated by the anaesthetic agents themselves as well as the preservatives included in them. This means that previous and prior exposure to an anaesthetic may result in an increase in the amounts of anaesthetic metabolised. This is important to recognise particularly if some of the metabolites are potentially toxic.

GASEOUS ANAESTHETICS

Nitrous oxide (N_2O)

Nitrous oxide is a colourless, odourless gas which is supplied in blue cylinders in a liquid form at a pressure of 46 atmospheres. It is not explosive or combustible. It is relatively insoluble in blood and body fluids so that induction and recovery are rapid. It has a weak narcotic action but only in concentrations above 80% will it produce light levels of anaesthesia. Concentrations above 75% N_2O (with 25% oxygen) should not be used because of the possibility of hypoxia. Despite the lack of potency of N_2O it is a useful vehicle for volatile anaesthetics. It will potentiate the effects of halothane and methoxyfluorane for example. Mixtures of N_2O oxygen and volatile anaesthetic are commonly used to produce a balanced anaesthetic.

N_2O is a weak narcotic only producing a moderate degree of depression (basal narcosis) at safe concentrations. Analgesia is weak at 50% of the inspired concentration. N_2O is not a marked respiratory depressant nor does it irritate the respiratory mucosa. Violent respiratory movements may indicate the presence of hypoxia. N_2O has little effect on cardiac contractility, venous return or arterial pressure. N_2O does not produce good muscle relaxation nor does it potentiate muscle relaxants. It can cross the placental barrier but without depressing the foetus.

Cyclopropane

This is a colourless gas with an odour like petroleum ether. It is stored in orange metal cylinders under pressure. It is explosive when mixed with air or oxygen. It is poorly soluble in blood (λ 0.47). This means that induction and recovery is rapid. It is more potent than N_2O and has a MAC of about 17% in rats. Anaesthesia may be induced with approximately 20% cyclopropane and oxygen and may be maintained with approximately 10% for light surgical anaesthesia.

Cyclopropane is a relatively potent anaesthetic and can produce any desired level of anaesthesia. Cyclopropane does not irritate the respiratory tract like ether but may produce respiratory depression. Cyclopropane has a complex effect on the cardiovascular system, apparently stimulating both sympathetic and parasympathetic outputs. Parasympathetic stimulation results in the bradycardia, laryngospasm and increase gut motility while if sympathomimetic responses predominate there is a tachycardia, an increase in myocardial contractility together with a raised peripheral resistance and decreased renal blood flow. There may also be metabolic changes such as raised glucose and lactate levels, indicating a metabolic acidosis. Because of the complex effect on the autonomic nervous system there is usually a hypertension during the early stages of anaesthesia but this can be followed by hypotension after long periods of anaesthesia. Cardiac arrhythmias are quite frequently encountered with this anaesthetic agent. They appear to be related to high concentrations of the anaesthetic and of carbon dioxide. Atropine should not be administered under these circumstances but artificial ventilation on pure oxygen should be applied to remove the cyclopropane.

Kidney function and urine output is depressed by the increase of ADH secretion together with the vasoconstriction in the kidney produced during cyclopropane anaesthesia. Muscle relaxation is good and adequate for most surgery. Cyclopropane crosses the placental barrier and may produce depression of the foetus.

VOLATILE ANAESTHETICS

Volatile anaesthetics have three properties in common. First, they are all liquids at room temperature; secondly, they are potent in low concentrations; and thirdly, they are more soluble in blood and fat than the gaseous anaesthetics. Their solubility retards equilibriation and hence slows induction. This means that tissue partial pressures will rise as anaesthesia continues, hence the depth of anaesthesia will continue to increase with time unless the partial pressure in the inspired air is reduced. As a consequence of this the levels of the anaesthetic required for induction are usually well above those required for maintenance. The higher tissue solubilities of the volatile anaesthetics also slows excretion via the lungs and the return to consciousness. A greater proportion of volatile anaesthetics are also retained and metabolised. Some of these difficulties can be reduced by using N_2O to produce basal narcosis and to supplement this by the addition of smaller amounts of volatile anaesthetic.

Ether — diethyl ether (C_2H_5O C_2H_5)

Ether was the first true anaesthetic employed for surgery. It is a clear liquid with a boiling point of 35°C. It is usually mixed with 3% ethanol and in the presence of copper used to retard oxidation preventing the formation of more irritant peroxides. The blood gas partition coefficient is 15. This means that ether is very soluble in the blood so that induction is very slow. Ether has a pungent odour and is irritant to the respiratory tract. This fact together with the high blood gas partition coefficient precludes its use for induction. Ether is explosive when mixed with oxygen.

The respiratory centre is paralysed before the vasomotor centre as anaesthesia is deepened to dangerous levels. Since ether is irritant to the respiratory tract it may induce laryngospasm in cats and rabbits. Salivary and bronchial secretions are seen in all species and may predispose to respiratory infections and can aggravate chronic respiratory problems. These secretions also increase the dead space of the respiratory tract.

One of the features of ether anaesthesia is the good muscle relaxation. This occurs because of the dual effect ether has on the neuromuscular junction, depressing it in a curare-like manner and a central depressant effect on the spinal cord motor neurones. Ether produces a greater degree of muscle relaxation than other volatile and gaseous anaesthetic agents.

During light levels of ether anaesthesia the sympathetic stimulation produced by ether increases the blood pressure slightly as well as the cardiac output and peripheral resistance. This is to some extent countered by the direct and strong myocardial depressant action ether exerts. During deeper surgical anaesthesia the cardiac depressant effects predominate. There may then be a fall in cardiac output and blood pressure. Ether does not sensitise the heart to the catecholamines and is not arrhythmogenic.

Approximately 90% of administered ether is recovered from the expired air. A small amount of ether is retained and metabolised to carbon dioxide and water. Small amounts of ether appear in urine, milk and sweat.

Chloroform (CH Cl₃)

Chloroform is a volatile anaesthetic which is readily oxidised by light to the poisonous gas phosgene. It is a very potent anaesthetic but induction is slowed by its high blood solubility. It is easier to administer than ether because it does not have the respiratory tract irritant effect. Chloroform is less safe than ether, because it predisposes to cardiac arrhythmias since it sensitises the heart to the effects of circulating catecholamines. Pre-medication with atropine may reduce the dangers of excessive vagal tone which has been shown experimentally to produce ventricular fibrillation. The incidence of arrhythmias may also be reduced by the use of β-blocking agents such as propanolol.

There are two other types of toxic affects seen following chloroform anaesthesia. The first type is due to a direct depressant effect of chloroform on the myocardium and occurs after prolonged anaesthesia. A second form occurs two to three days after the administration of the anaesthetic. This is called 'delayed chloroform poisoning' and is associated with liver damage and is more likely to occur when the liver glycogen levels are low and anoxia develops during anaesthesia. The symptoms of delayed toxicity in the dog consist of the signs of acidosis and vomiting. In the horse delayed toxicity is seen as a loss of appetite, jaundice, constipation, leading eventually to coma and death. The delayed toxicity is associated with fatty changes in the liver and kidney. In conclusion it may be said that chloroform is a potent anaesthetic agent occasionally useful in veterinary practice. However, it is important to be aware of the dangers of cardiac arrhythmias and the possibility of toxicity.

Trichlorethylene

This resembles chloroform but is less potent. It probably has the same cardiac effects as chloroform but may be less toxic to the liver. At deeper planes of anaesthesia trichloroethylene can produce tachypnoea rather than the more usual respiratory depressent action of anaesthetics. It is very important to remember that trichloroethylene is decomposed by alkalis and heat, to form a toxic and inflammable substance, dichloroacetylene. This means that this drug must not be used with a closed circuit apparatus containing soda lime to remove carbon dioxide.

Ethylchloride

Ethylchloride is a potent volatile anaesthetic. However, its main use now is in an aerosol form for skin application. This produces a transient local anaesthesia.

Halothane ($BrClCHCF_3$)

Halothane is a sweet smelling potent volatile anaesthetic sold in amber coloured bottles. Its stability is further enhanced by the addition of 0.01% thymol. Sodalime does not cause halothane to decompose but long exposure to light turns halothane brown due to the release of various bromides. These bromides are irritant. Mixtures of halothane with air or oxygen are not explosive. Most metals except nickel and titanium are corroded by halothane. Halothane interacts with rubber and some plastics and is highly soluble in rubber with a partition coefficient of 121. This can contribute to slowing of induction and recovery especially if low flow rates are used in the delivery circuit.

Halothane produces a dose-dependent depression of the central nervous system producing anaesthesia. Halothane is more potent than ether and is characterised by a marked dose dependent hypotensive effect. The classical signs of ether anaesthesia are difficult to recognise when using halothane. The best indicator of the depth of anaesthesia may in fact be the arterial blood pressure. The partial pressure of halothane increases progressively with time throughout anaesthesia when it is inspired at a constant concentration. This is because the blood gas partition coefficient (λ) is 2.3 so that halothane is relatively soluble in blood. Halothane is hypotensive at all levels of anaesthesia unlike ether. It is not a potent analgesic at subanaesthetic levels like ether. The MAC is 0.74%.

Respiration is depressed by all concentrations of halothane. The response to carbon dioxide is progressively lost as anaesthesia deepens. It is safe to use pure oxygen for ventilation provided spontaneous respiration is allowed. The brain partial pressure may rise too high however if forced ventilation is used. Halothane causes inhibition of laryngospasm, bronchospasm, and coughing but produces bronchial dilation because of a direct action on smooth muscle.

Halothane has a direct depressant effect on the myocardium and the vascular smooth muscle. It has a direct central depressant effect on the central vasomotor centre and has a sympathetic ganglionic blocking effect. All these effects combine to produce the characteristic hypotensive effect of halothane. Halothane depresses the arterial blood pressure, cardiac output, and peripheral resistance. This effect is dose dependent and increases as the level of anaesthesia is increased.

The sinoatrial node is depressed by halothane. Ventricular arrhythmias are rare during the administration of halothane but may occur in the presence of respiratory acidosis, hypoxia or other causes of sympathetic stimulation. It sensitises the bundles of His to the actions of circulating catecholamines. In this respect it resembles chloroform. Adrenaline should not be used for the control of bleeding when halothane is given.

Halothane causes a decrease in hepatic blood flow and also causes a reduction in glomerular filtration, decreasing sodium and water excretion. It has a minimal neuromuscular blocking action. Halothane relaxes uterine muscle and, unless carefully controlled, this relaxation may fail to respond to ergot derivatives and oxytocin. For this reason halothane is not recommended for obstetric anaesthesia except where uterine relaxation is required. Halothane readily crosses the placental barrier.

Halothane was introduced into clinical anaesthesia in 1956 but its metabolism was not reported until 1964. It is now known that between 10 and 20% of the total halothane absorbed is retained and metabolised and not excreted through the lung. The metabolites include trifluoroacetic acid, bromide, and inorganic fluorides. Recent studies have shown that halothane undergoes reductive defluorination by the cytochrome-P450 system in the presence of reduced oxygen tensions. Many halogenated hydrocarbons are known to be hepatotoxic and at least in certain individuals halothane is no exception. Liver damage may be seen three days to three weeks after exposure due to the production of hepatotoxic substances from the metabolism of halothane by the liver. Barbiturates and other substances which induce liver enzymes also increase the metabolism of halothane and its consequent toxicity. Halothane is toxic to the foetus and also has a teratogenic effect in rats when administered at anaesthetic concentrations. Electron microscope changes in the brain and other tissues and changes in behaviour have been reported in the offspring of mice exposed in utero to halothane.

Methoxyflurane ($CHCl_2CF_2$ O CH_3)

Methoxyflurane has analgesic and anaesthetic properties. The analgesia persists following the return of consciousness. It is very soluble in blood so that induction is much slower than with halothane. Methoxyflurane is also very soluble in fat but it has a high anaesthetic potency with a MAC of 0.3%. Like halothane, methoxyflurane decreases the cardiac output and peripheral resistance. However, methoxyflurane only produces a minimal sensitization of the heart to the circulating catecholamines. Methoxyflurane produces a dose-dependent depressant effect on respiration but it is not a respiratory irritant. Profound muscle relaxation is produced by methoxyflurane during deep anaesthesia.

Since methoxyflurane is highly soluble in fat a substantial proportion (approximately 20–30%) is retained and ultimately metabolised in the body. These metabolites include various halogenated organic and inorganic substances. One of the main disadvantages of methoxyflurane is the dose related renal toxicity which is caused by the release of large quantities of inorganic fluoride ion during the biotransformation of the drug. The signs of nephrotoxicity are a high output renal failure. Its slow recovery makes it unsuited for use in horses.

Enflurane ($CHFClCF_2$ O C F_2H)

Enflurane is relatively insoluble in blood with a blood gas partition coefficient of 1.9 and a MAC of 1.68%. Induction and recovery from anaesthesia are therefore rapid. Enflurane does not readily sensitise the heart to circulating catecholamines. Liver and kidney function tests suggest that enflurane is safer than methoxyflurane and halothane. The metabolites of enflurance resemble those of methoxyflurane but lower concentrations are found in the plasma and urine. Nevertheless several cases of nephrotoxicity due to this drug have been reported.

Isoflurane (CF_3CHCl O CF_2H)

Induction and recovery with isoflurane are more rapid than with halothane. The MAC is 1.3%. Isoflurane apparently produces a more profound respiratory depressant action than halothane. Less than 1% of an administered dose of isoflurane is metabolised in normal subjects. This suggests that isoflurane may be significantly less toxic. However, its full effects still remain to be evaluated clinically.

SUGGESTIONS FOR FURTHER READING

Campbell J R, Lawson D D 1958 Signs and stages of anaesthesia in domestic animals. Veterinary Record 70:545

Douglas T A, Jennings S, Lonstreath J, Weaver A D 1964 Methoxyflurane anaesthesia in horses and cattle. Veterinary Record 76:615

Evans F T, Gray T C 1965 General anaesthesia, 2nd Ed. Butterworth, London

Fisher E W 1961 Observations on the disturbance of respiration of cattle, horses, sheep and dogs caused by halothane anaesthesia and changes in plasma pH and plasma CO_2 content. American Journal of Veterinary Research 22:279

Featherstone R M, Muehlbaecher C A 1963 The current role of inert gases in the search for anaesthesia mechanisms. Pharmacological Reviews 15:97

Hall L W 1971 Wright's Veterinary anaesthesia, 7th Ed. Bailliere, Tindall & Cassell, London

Lumb W V, Jones E W 1973 Veterinary anaesthesia. Lea & Febiger, Philadelphia

Mitchell B 1966 Anaesthesia in small animal practice. Veterinary Record Clinical Supplement 3

Symposium on Inhalation Anaesthetics 1965 British Journal of Anaesthesia 37:644

Weaver A V 1966 Recent developments in anaesthesia of large animals. Veterinary Record Clinical Supplement

Westhus M, Fritsch R 1965 Animal anaesthesia, Vol 2. Oliver & Boyd, Edinburgh

Wood-Smith F G, Vicker M D, Stewart H C 1973 Drugs in anaesthetic practice, 5th ed Butterworths, London

Vandam L D 1966 Anaesthesia. Annual Review of Pharmacology 6:379

9

Stimulants of the central nervous system

The regulation of the body's vital functions is carried out by special nerve cells situated in the medulla. They are usually called the vital or medullary centres and include the respiratory centres, the vaso-motor centre, the vomiting and vagal centres. These centres are affected by a number of drugs, some of which cause stimulation, some depression and some a mixture of stimulation and depression. Drugs of the stimulating category are called **analeptics** or 'arousing' agents.

In veterinary therapeutics the medullary stimulants are of most value as stimulants of the respiratory centres. They are used mainly to stimulate respiration in animals which have stopped breathing during anaesthesia. It is usual nowadays to resuscitate such animals by means of artificial respiration and the medullary stimulants are a group of drugs which are of declining therapeutic importance. Two of the oldest stimulants of the central nervous system are caffeine and strychnine. They are no longer used to any great extent in therapy, but the latter is of toxicological importance.

Caffeine

This alkaloid occurs in tea and coffee and is derived from purine. Theobromine and theophylline are also purine derivatives with similar actions to caffeine. Chemically, caffeine, theophylline and theobromine are methylated xanthines. Caffeine is readily absorbed from the gut. In the body it is partly oxidised and partly demethy-lated. The purines are excreted in the urine as methyluric acids or methylxanthines, about 10% of the parent drug being excreted unchanged.

The central nervous system is stimulated from the cortex down-wards and there is no subsequent depression. Caffeine increases the motor effects of conditioned reflexes and, by acting on the motor area of the brain, decreases fatigue, thus increasing the work which a group of muscles can do. The respiratory, vasomotor and vagal centres are stimulated, and caffeine is sometimes used to stimulate respiration. Very large doses produce convulsions similar to strychnine convulsions.

Caffeine increases the blood flow through the brain and kidney, causing the latter organ to produce more urine. This increased blood flow is produced by the drug acting on the heart and blood vessels both directly and through the medullary centres. Its restriction to the brain and kidneys is due to these organs being poorly supplied with vasoconstrictor nerves. Caffeine acts directly on the heart muscle to increase the rate and force of contraction; at the same time the heart is slowed from stimulation of the vagal centre. Although the vasomotor centre is stimulated, the vasoconstrictor effect is counteracted by the drug dilating the vessels directly. The diuresis produced by caffeine is partly due to the effects on circulation and partly due to the drug decreasing tubular reabsorption of water.

The formation of prothrombin by the liver is increased by caffeine which by this action resembles vitamin K. The drug is used mainly as a diuretic, but occasionally to counteract centrally depressant drugs. It is usually given as the double salt caffeine and sodium benzoate because this is more soluble.

Theophylline and etamiphylline have similar actions to caffeine but are more powerful in their cardiac stimulant actions and diuretic actions. The methyl xanthines relax the smooth muscle of the bronchi, theophylline being the most effective. Theobromine has no action on the central nervous system and is used only for its diuretic properties.

An explanation for many of the pharmacological effects produced by the methyl xanthines has been provided by work on cyclic AMP. Cells respond to various hormones or drugs by acting on specific receptors on the membrane by showing an increase of intracellular cyclic AMP, this is thought to mediate increases in phosphorylase activity, lipolysis, gluconeogenesis or steroid production. Cyclic AMP has been called the 'second messenger'. Its activity is limited by a specific enzyme phosphodiesterase which converts cyclic 3′ 5′ AMP into 5-AMP which is inactive. This enzyme, phosphodiesterase, is inhibited by caffeine and other methyl xanthines with the consequent augmentation of cyclic 3′ 5′ AMP activity. The xanthines are also known to displace membrane bound calcium and increase muscle contractility. In addition cyclic AMP, calcium and inositol triphosphate are known to mediate the effects of some hormones.

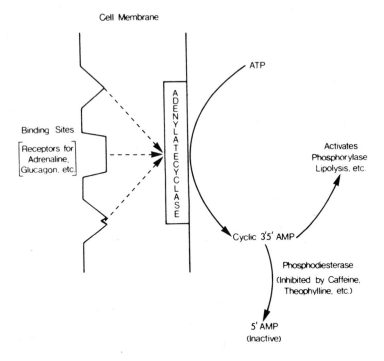

Fig. 9.1 A schematic representation of the role of cyclic AMP in the action of certain drugs.

Strychnine

This alkaloid occurs together with the chemically and pharmacologically similar Brucine in the Nux Vomica bean. Strychnine is more active and is absorbed quickly from the gut. It is rapidly fixed by the tissues and mostly destroyed in the liver by enzymes on the microsomes of hepatic cells.

About 20% is excreted unchanged in the urine; this takes about 12 hours and is therefore somewhat cumulative. Many proprietary 'tonics' contain small amounts of strychnine and their use by animal owners has given rise to cases of poisoning. Although strychnine is a particularly painful poison, it can still be legally employed to destroy moles and seals. It is surely time that a relatively painless poison was employed to kill these unfortunate creatures. An appreciation of the actions of strychnine is important to the veterinarian to enable him to take appropriate counter-action in cases of poisoning.

Strychnine has a bitter taste which in the mouth stimulates the taste buds, and in debilitated animals may cause a reflex stimulation of gastric secretion. However, the drug's most important action is on the central nervous system. Reflexes are first stimulated and then depressed; the motor effects of spinal reflex are increased and the latent period diminished. Nerve impulses in the spinal cord are restricted to their appropriate path by inhibitory neurones. Strychnine produces its characteristic pharmacological effects by a competitive antagonism of the inhibitory transmitter glycine. This produces an exaggeration of the reflex effects of sensory stimuli and a general enhancement of neuronal activity.

Although it antagonises the respiratory depression produced by morphine, the excitatory effects of morphine on the central nervous system are additive with those of strychnine. The blocking by strychnine of many post-synaptic inhibitory processes and consequent facilitation gives rise to increased irradiation, so that the nerve impulses are more widely spread within the spinal cord and the response to a nerve impulse involves more muscles than would normally be the case. Large doses exaggerate these effects, so that any small sensory disturbance sends all the voluntary muscles into violent convulsions which are extremely painful. These are followed by depression of the central nervous system and relaxation of the muscles. In a strychnine convulsion the limbs and trunk are extended, because in domestic animals the extensor muscles are usually stronger than the flexors, the position being termed opisthotonus.

The lethal properties of strychnine have led to its use for the destruction of dogs and cats. Such a procedure is quite unjustified because of the intense pain produced by the convulsions. Strychnine should never be employed for this purpose.

Strychnine exerts its main effect on the spinal cord, and, although the sensitivity to stimuli of the medullary centres is increased, drugs are available which exert a greater effect on the centres than the cord and are to be preferred. Strychnine is used as a bitter in the form of prepared Nux Vomica, which is the powdered bean standardised to contain 1.2% strychnine.

In strychnine poisoning the animal is restless; sensory stimuli, such as noise, cause jerking of the limbs and even convulsions. The convulsions are characteristic, the animal adopting a position of opisthotonus. Respiration usually fails after five or six convulsions. The treatment consists of controlling the convulsions by means of a barbiturate such as sodium pentobarbitone given intravenously, the animal being placed in a dark loose box or kennel and every effort made not to disturb the animal. Mephenesin, a drug acting on the inter-neurones of the spinal cord, has been suggested as a specific antidote to strychnine. Unfortunately, it is cleared relatively quickly and the dose has to be repeated almost hourly. In veterinary practice this is rarely possible. Ataractics are also useful in the treatment of strychnine poisoning.

Picrotoxin is a non-nitrogenous white crystalline substance prepared from seeds which come from an East Indian plant *Cocculus anamirta*. It is absorbed from all routes of administration, but since it is only used in emergency to stimulate respiration the intravenous route is the best. Since this drug leaves the circulation rapidly and is quickly destroyed, the dose can be repeated after a very short interval. It is a powerful stimulant of the central nervous system due to the non-competitive antagonism of the presynaptic inhibitory transmitter GABA. The effect on the mid brain and medulla being most marked. The cortex is also stimulated and may lead to convulsions. Stimulation of the central nervous eventually leads to depression.

Picrotoxin is an effective antagonist to the central depression produced by the barbiturates and this is its only therapeutic indication. It is too toxic to use in unanaesthetised animals and is of no value in morphine poisoning.

When using picrotoxin in barbiturate overdosage the solution should be injected slowly intravenously until tremors of the voluntary muscles are observed; to give more than is necessary to produce this effect is harmful. Two plants particularly poisonous to livestock contain active principles pharmacologically similar to picrotoxin. The plants are *Cicuta virosa* (cowbane; water hemlock) and *Oenanthe crocata* (water dropwort) which contain respectively cicutoxin and oenanthoxin. The best antidote to these poisons as to picrotoxin is a barbiturate given intravenously.

Leptazol (pentylenetetrazol) is a white crystalline substance, very soluble in water, and sterilisable by boiling. It is rapidly absorbed and quickly destroyed in the body so that half a convulsive dose can be repeated after an interval of two hours.

Leptazol is a powerful cerebral and medullary stimulant. It is probably the best analeptic or 'arousing' drug available, and counteracts the depression produced by hypnotics such as the barbiturates. The drug, however, has no value as a circulatory stimulant. Leptazol has been suggested to be a GABA antagonist.

Bemegride

This powerful stimulant of the central nervous system is used to antagonise the medullary depression produced by barbiturates. Because bemegride is chemically similar to the barbiturates, it was thought to be a specific competitive antagonist. However, its antagonism is probably due entirely to its analeptic properties. It will usually arouse dogs, sheep and rabbits from barbiturate-produced anaesthesia; cats are not awakened although the anaesthesia is lightened.

Bemegride is given in solution by intravenous injection. If this is not possible, the intraperitoneal route may be employed. The dose should be repeated at ten minute intervals until muscle tremors are seen. Bemegride's action lasts for only half an hour and cases treated should be kept under observation in case a relapse occurs.

Doxapram, nikethamide and ethamivan are now used as respiratory stimulants and have some selective action on the respiratory centre in sub-convulsant doses. They appear to act mostly by direct medullary stimulation but respiration is also stimulated via the peripheral chemoreceptors.

Procethamide is a mixture of *crotethamide and cropropamide* and is used for respiratory stimulation of newborn animals.

SUGGESTIONS FOR FURTHER READING

Hahn, F 1960 Analeptics. 12: 144–218 Pharmacological Reviews

10

Local analgesic agents

The effects of drugs on the various functions of the central and autonomous nervous systems have been considered. It remains to discuss substances which have direct action on nerve fibres and nerve endings, by far the most important being the local analgesics which are drugs with the property of reversibly impairing conduction in nerve fibres and paralysing nerve endings. Small diameter fibres are blocked more rapidly than the larger faster conducting A fibres because of the faster penetration of the local anaesthetic. This means that the sense of pain is lost first (carried by C fibres and small A_δ fibres) followed by the sense of heat then touch.

Local anaesthetics or analgesics act at the cell membrane where they interfere with a transient increase in the permeability of the membrane to sodium ions which is produced by depolarisation of the membrane and is an essential part of both the generation and conduction of the nerve impulse. Local analgesics block conduction without depolarising the nerve. The block in conduction is produced by the local anaesthetic plugging the sodium ion channels (ionophores). Although it is in the form of the free base that the tissues are penetrated and the local analgesia produced, the free base of the various local analgesic drugs is only slightly water soluble and is usually unstable. Local analgesics are usually used in the form of a water soluble salt which forms a slightly acid solution. However, these salts must be neutralised in the tissues, the free base liberated and the tissues penetrated before local analgesia is produced.

Local analgesics are used in a variety of ways to produce the effect desired. They may be applied directly to a mucous membrane to prevent pain arising from irritation or manipulation of the membrane. Most commonly they are injected subcutaneously or around nerve trunks; analgesia of a greater area of the body may be produced by injecting a local analgesic epidurally and paralysing a number of spinal nerve roots. A subarachnoid injection, or true spinal analgesic, has a similar effect but is less commonly used in veterinary surgery.

DESIRABLE PROPERTIES

A local analgesic must produce analgesia without damage to nervous structures and must be non-irritant. After absorption a local analgesic should have a low toxicity and should be effective in low concentrations. The analgesia produced should persist long enough for the surgical interference to take place, and should be produced quickly. The drug should act after injection and when applied locally to mucous membranes. However, few substances have all these properties, and amongst the defects which might be present in a local analgesic are the following: stimulation of sensory nerves may occur before analgesia; there may be local or general toxic effects; the drug may not penetrate mucosae and may be unstable in solution or insoluble in water.

The effect of local anaesthetics can be prolonged by the addition of a vasoconstrictor. This prolongation of effect is produced by delaying absorption into the circulation, and this in turn can reduce the systemic toxicity of the local anaesthetic. Adrenaline or noradrenaline in concentrations of from 1 : 80 000 to 1 : 250 000 are the vasoconstrictors commonly used. A vasoconstrictor should not be added when a local anaesthetic is used to block the nerves to an extremity because the intense vasoconstriction might cut off the whole blood supply thus damaging the organ. Moreover, when local anaesthetics are used in conjunction with a general anaesthetic attention should be paid to the fact that sufficient adrenaline or noradrenaline may be absorbed to produce dangerous cardiac arrhythmias. This is particularly probable when the general anaesthetic is a drug such as chloroform, halothane or cyclopropane which sensitises the heart to catecholamines.

Spinal anaesthesia may be produced by the injection of local analgesic solutions subdurally; on occasion, in small animals, the needle punctures between the lumbar vertebrae or the lumbar sacral space piercing the dura and arachnoid. In this case the injection is made into the cerebrospinal fluid and the specific gravity of the injected solution can influence its distribution and , hence, the zone of analgesia. In human surgery the extent to which the nerve roots are blocked can be varied by altering the specific gravity of the injection fluid; in veterinary surgery the volume of solution determines the extent of spread of the anaesthetic and hence the zone of anaesthesia produced. Spinal anaesthesia is not without risk, although epidural injections as commonly used in the cow are reasonably safe. There is a risk of paralysing the intercostal nerves or even the phrenic nerves if too large a volume is used. The blood pressure may fall partly because of blocking the splanchnic nerves and partly because the reduced respiratory movements may impede the return of the blood to the right heart.

Regional anaesthesia can be obtained by infiltrating the nerves supplying the region with local anaesthetic solution. This technique requires considerable knowledge of anatomy but is very popular, for example, in so-called 'paravertebral block' in cattle when the area of the flank can be anaesthetised to a sufficient extent to allow abdominal surgery to be carried out with the animal in a standing position.

GENERAL PROPERTIES OF LOCAL ANALGESICS

Local analgesics affect the central nervous system, autonomic ganglia, the myoneural junction and muscle fibres, in addition to their inhibitory effect on conduction in nerve axons. On the central nervous system they cause stimulation followed by depression and may give rise to death from respiratory failure. Medullary stimulants are ineffective in the treatment of this type of respiratory failure because the local analgesics themselves are central stimulants and the depression is characteristic of excessive stimulation, probably resulting from exhaustion of the mechanism.

Local anaesthetics also have quinidine-like actions on the heart. These are produced in a similar fashion to the effect on nerve cells namely by stabilising the membrane potential. They are occasionally used therapeutically for this purpose.

Cocaine is the oldest local analgesic and is obtained from the leaves of the South American plant *Erythroxylon coca*. It is destroyed by prolonged boiling. Absorption takes place from mucous membranes but not from intact skin, and after absorption it is partly destroyed by the liver and partly excreted in the urine. Cocaine is a very effective local analgesic paralysing sensory nerve trunks and endings without initial stimulation. It potentiates the action of adrenaline and therefore has a vasoconstrictor effect. Cocaine dilates the pupil but the light reflex remains, unlike the mydriasis by atropine. However, it has dangerous central actions which may be shown by doses lower than those required for local analgesia.

This drug produces a stimulation of the central nervous system which is followed by depression and starts at the highest centres. Large doses cause convulsions and small doses slow the heart by stimulating the vagal centre. Moderate doses increase the heart rate by central and peripheral sympathetic stimulation. It is subject to controlled drugs regulations. Cocaine is too toxic to use if a substitute can be found and neither cocaine nor butocaine should be injected.

In an attempt to find a less toxic substitute for cocaine, *procaine* was synthesised in 1905 and is still widely used. It has only one-quarter the toxicity of cocaine, forms a stable solution in water and dose not lead to addiction. However, it has poor powers of penetration and is therefore no good for the anaesthetisation of mucosae, being used mainly as an injection. Chemically most local analgesics are esters and are metabolised by hydrolysis. This takes place in both the liver and blood plasma, and it is probable that the enzyme responsible for the plasma hydrolysis is plasma cholinesterase. The fact that plasma cholinesterase may be responsible for much of the metabolism of certain local analgesics is of particular importance in the veterinary field when one considers the difference in the amount of plasma cholinesterase in different species.

There is considerable variation in the metabolism of the individual local anaesthetics in any one species and also of the same local anaesthetic by different species. Because of this variation the results of testing both anaesthetic potency and toxicity depends on the method of testing and the species used.

Local anaesthetics are often mixed with adrenaline, which limits absorption and acts as a local haemostatic, although this latter effect is not always advantageous as it may conceal haemorrhage which should have been dealt with by ligation of the bleeding points. The pH of concentrated solutions of drugs such as procaine may cause irritation by their acidity.

Many compounds have since been tested and several have come into general use. A more recent local anaesthetic popular in veterinary practise is *lidocaine* which gives anaesthesia both on injection and after local application. When used as a 1–2% solution it acts quickly and has about the same toxicity as procaine. It is also called lignocaine. Lidocaine is non-esteric and is metabolised in the liver and not by cholinesterase. This may explain in part the longer action of lidocaine. *Butocaine* is a good anaesthetic for mucous membranes but is too toxic to inject. *Amethocaine* is suitable for injection and anaesthetising mucous membranes. Orthocaine and benzocaine are insoluble local anaesthetic powders used only as dressings for painful superficial lesions. Cinchocaine is much more effective than procaine but is also more toxic. It is suitable for surface anaesthesia and produces a prolonged effect. However, cinchocaine may cause an inflammatory reaction at the site of injection and is no longer used for this purpose.

Prilocaine resembles lidocaine both chemically and pharmacologically. It is slower in acting but the effect lasts longer. It is used similarly. *Proxymetacaine* is used to anaesthetise the cornea if it is important not to dilate the pupil.

Butyl aminobenzoate is a surface acting local anaesthetic which is sometimes added to injections of drugs which would otherwise cause pain.

Sometimes local anaesthetic solutions have the enzyme hyaluronidase added to them. This enzyme splits the hyaluronides, which form an important part of connective tissue, and thus facilitates spread and penetration of the anaesthetic after injections.

SUGGESTIONS FOR FURTHER READING

Hall L W 1971 Wright's Veterinary anaesthesia, 7th Ed. Bailliere, Tindall & Cassell, London

Ritchie J M, Greengard P 1966 On the mode of action of local anaesthetics. Annual Review of Pharmacology 6:405

Westhues, M and Fritsch, R 1964 Animal anaesthesia Vol 1, Local anaesthesia. Oliver & Boyd, Edinburgh

11

Drugs acting on the alimentary system
Antacids, carminatives, emetics

The pharmacology of the digestive tract of the domestic animals is complicated by the diversity of form and by the fact that an important part of the digestive process is carried on by micro-organisms in the tract. These micro-organisms may be deliberately or inadvertently affected by drugs.

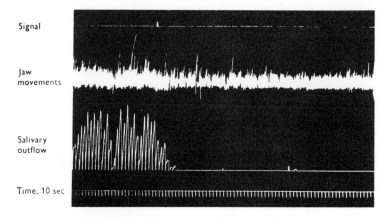

Signal

Jaw movements

Salivary outflow

Time, 10 sec

Fig. 11.1 The effect on parotid secretion of the horse of the administration of 250 mg of amethocaine in the feed. Amethocaine added at the signal. (Adapted from Alexander 1966 *Journal of Physiology* 184:646)

Salivary secretion in man and dogs can be stimulated by the sight or smell of food. This is called the psychic secretion and is not marked in the other domestic animals. Stimulation of the taste buds in the mouth causes an increase in secretion, and, in ruminants, eating and rumination has a similar effect. Salivation in the horse occurs as a consequence of mastication. A copious secretion is produced by pilocarpine, physostigmine and other parasympathomimetic drugs; inhibitors of the parasympathetics such as atropine also inhibit salivation. This fact is made use of in pre-medication

185

before a general anaesthetic, although in ruminants atropine only decreases the salivary flow and does not stop it completely.

The saliva of ruminants does not contain digestive enzymes but functions mainly as a buffer to neutralise the fatty acids formed during fermentative digestion in the rumen and is secreted continuously. Ruminant saliva also contains a substance which decreases the surface tension of the rumen liquor and this may be a factor in producing bloat. Horse saliva resembles that of the dog more closely than ruminant in composition, a point of difference being the relatively high calcium content of horse saliva.

Bitters

Reflexes from the taste buds when stimulated cause an increased secretion of saliva and gastric juice in the dog. The response to these reflexes is stimulated by bitter-tasting substances acting on the taste buds. These substances which are called *bitters* have no effect when given by stomach tube and work best in debilitated dogs. There seems little purpose in giving bitters to ruminants as these animals secrete an acid juice continuously from the abomasum. The continuance of this secretion depends on the passage of digesta through the abomasum and is independent of vagal innervation. The other parts of the ruminant stomach are non-secretory.

Bitters are classified into three groups, aromatic, simple and compound. Aromatic bitters include compound tincture of gentian, extract of orange peel, and gentian powder. Simple bitters, so called because they do not contain tannic acid and are therefore compatible with iron and alkaloids, include quassia; compound bitters such as compound tincture of gentian are incompatible. Many alkaloids have a bitter taste hence quinine and strychnine are used as bitters.

Antacids

There are few indications for the use of antacids in veterinary practice. In certain cases of disturbed ruminal function alkalies may be given to counteract excess acidity, and some inflammatory conditions of the dog's stomach may benefit from an antacid.

Sodium bicarbonate is the commonest antacid, acting quickly with the release of CO_2. When bicarbonates are given to ruminants, the CO_2 is removed by eructation after being formed in the rumen. The usual reason for giving bicarbonate to ruminants is when some indiscretion of diet has given rise to the production of large quantities of lactic acid in the rumen instead of the normal volatile fatty acids. This lactic acid can readily give rise to acidosis and a recognisable clinical syndrome. The sodium bicarbonate not only neutralises the lactic acid formed during fermentation in the rumen but may also be absorbed into the body where it assists to rectify the acidosis. The administration of sodium bicarbonate in excess to all species can give rise to an alkalosis.

Magnesium carbonate acts similarly to sodium bicarbonate; **magnesium oxide** does not release CO_2 but has the possible drawback of causing purgation. Frequent dosing with carbonates or bicarbonates may produce alkalosis causing vomiting and tetany in dogs. **Magnesium trisilicate** is an insoluble powder reacting slowly with acids to form magnesium chloride and colloidal silica. It acts as an absorbent and antacid and cannot cause alkalosis. Calcium carbonate is also an effective antacid but also has a constipating action which may sometimes be disadvantageous. Several salts of bismuth have been used as antacids. However, these compounds do not neutralise the gastric juice and are potentially toxic, hence there is no justification for their further employment.

DRUGS ACTING ON STOMACH MOVEMENTS AND SECRETIONS

Drugs can affect stomach movements by acting on the gastric muscles, reflexly by stimulating nerve endings in the gastric mucosa or through the autonomic nervous system. Parasympathomimetic drugs increase and sympathomimetic drugs inhibit stomach movements. Gastric activity is inhibited also by atropine, and stomach emptying is delayed by the spasm of the pylorus produced by morphine.

Gastric secretion is stimulated by excitation of the psychic reflex in some species, by drugs with muscarine actions and by drugs such as alcohol, histamine and insulin. In ruminants insulin reduces abomasal secretion. The secretion of gastric juice is inhibited by atropine, irritant drugs producing gastritis and by the direct action on the pylorus and duodenum of fats, cold and acids stronger than 0.2%.

As the structural differences might suggest, there are differences in the way in which the stomachs of the different species respond to drugs. Stomach movements in the horse stop when food is withheld for more than twenty-four hours. They are also inhibited by

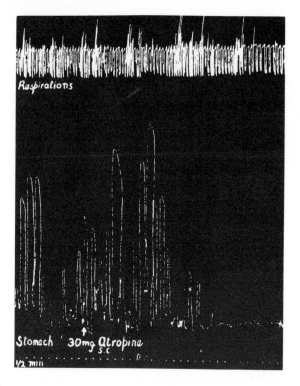

Fig. 11.2 The inhibition of stomach contractions in the horse by atropine. (Adapted from Alexander F 1951 *Quarterly Journal of Experimental Physiology* 36:139)

atropine and adrenaline but are not affected by carbachol or histamine. The reflex closure of the œsophageal groove in ruminants enables fluids to enter the omasum and abomasum directly. This reflex is stimulated by the presence in the mouth of a 1% solution of copper sulphate or a 10% solution of sodium bicarbonate. The reflex in sheep responds better to copper sulphate and in cows to sodium bicarbonate. The œsophageal groove reflex is inhibited by atropine and during general anaesthesia. The solutions which stimulate the reflex are useful adjuncts to give prior to the administration of other drugs which are required to act in the abomasum such as certain anthelmintics.

Carminatives are substances which facilitate the expulsion of gas from the stomach. They are of particular value in ruminants because these animals produce large quantities of gas in the rumen during the fermentation of carbohydrates. This gas is normally re-

moved by belching but if this mechanism is disordered, carminatives may assist the removal of the gas. The carminatives commonly
used in veterinary practice are the volatile oils such as oil of turpentine and volatile drugs such as ether, alcohol and preparations
of ammonia.

Antizymotics are drugs which kill or inhibit the rumen bacteria
thus stopping fermentation and consequently gas production. Formalin and the volatile oils are used for this purpose. Certain antibiotics such as the tetracyclines and streptomycin may be used as
antizymotics. This is a very undesirable use of antibiotics since they
readily give rise to resistant strains of bacteria. The protozoa which
are normally present in large numbers in the rumen and are probably an important factor in rumen digestion can be killed by very
low doses of copper sulphate.

BLOAT

Gases formed in the rumen during the process of fermentive digestion are normally removed by eructation. When, for any reason,
this mechanism fails the gas accumulates in the rumen and gives
rise to a condition known as bloat. In the clinical condition of
'frothy bloat' the gas formed cannot be removed by belching, the
gas accumulates and may give rise to fatal consequences unless appropriate remedies are applied.

A study of the foam in chronic or frothy bloat has shown that
the trapped gas exists in two forms: large bubbles and vast numbers
of small yellow bubbles, whereas under non-bloating conditions
very few yellow bubbles are present. The yellow layer enclosing
these small bubbles has a very high lipid and protein content and
it appears that these lipids constitute an important part of the
rumen's natural anti-foaming system.

The administration of a foam-dispersing drug into the rumen
disrupts the large bubbles and relieves the bloat as long as the drug
remains in the rumen. However, it does not affect the small yellow
bubbles, and after it has passed through the rumen, the animal may
bloat again. Drugs in this category include various vegetable oils,
mineral oils and fats, as well as synthetic compounds such as methyl
silicone polyricinate and an organo-polysiloxane which, together
with kaolin, has been used in the prophylactic treatment of bloat.

There is evidence that some detergents are more active preven-
tatives of bloat than foam-dispersing agents because they act on the

yellow bubbles to release the inactivated lipids in their walls. Certain low-foam detergents of the polyoxyethylene-polyoxypropylene series have been found to be very effective in the treatment and prevention of frothy bloat. One such drug, **poloxalene**, is given twice daily as a preventative in the concentrate or in the feed. Other drugs of this type include dioctyl sodium sulphosuccinate and nonyl phenyl-ethoxylate. An alcohol ethoxylate has been used prophylactically incorporated into a gel with ethyl cellulose; it is palatable and easily degradable. It has also been given in a slow-release capsule.

Various antibiotics have been used with some success but this is not a recommended treatment as although the drugs work for a short period resistance amongst the micro-organisms soon develops.

VOMITING

The vomiting reflex is controlled by a centre in the medulla which is situated near the cough and vagal centres. This centre is poorly developed in the horse and ruminant. These animals do not vomit in the true sense, although in certain pathological conditions stomach contents are ejected through the nasal passages. The vomiting centre can be stimulated directly or by peripheral stimuli. These stimuli include disturbances of the labyrinth, the stimulation of vagal nerve endings in the pharynx, stomach and duodenum and the stimulation of sensory nerves to the heart and viscera. Situated in the area postrema of the medulla is the chemoreceptor trigger zone (**CTZ**). This zone can be stimulated by certain drugs such as morphine and some of its derivatives such as apomorphine to produce vomiting. Destruction of the CTZ still allows the vomiting centre to respond to peripheral stimuli. Certain drugs which have anti-emetic properties such as the phenothiazine tranquilisers exert their effect on the CTZ and hence are more likely to be of value in preventing vomiting arising from the administration of drugs acting on the CTZ than vomiting brought about by stimuli from nerve endings in the alimentary tract or from the labyrinth.

Local or **reflex emetics** are drugs which stimulate sensory nerve endings in the stomach and duodenum. They include solutions of the salts of certain heavy metals and vegetable drugs such as Ipecacuanha.

Copper or **zinc sulphate** in 1% solution given by mouth to dogs produce emesis within a few minutes. This prompt action prevents damage to the gastric mucosa, and since these metals are absorbed very slowly there is little risk of poisoning. There is no nausea after the emesis or purgation; in fact small doses of these salts are astringent to the intestine. A crystal of washing soda given by mouth to a dog is also an effective means of inducing vomiting.

Ipecacuanha contains the alkaloids *emetine* and *cephaline* to which it owes its emetic properties. These alkaloids irritate all mucous membranes causing lachrymation, conjunctivitis and increased bronchial secretion. Emetine by mouth produces vomiting in thirty minutes. When this drug is given parenterally, much bigger doses are required. The slow action of ipecacuanha makes it a much less suitable emetic to use to empty the stomach in cases of poisoning. In subemetic doses it increases bronchial secretions and sweating and is used as an expectorant.

Tartar emetic produces vomiting but is too toxic to use for this purpose. However, it has been given by intravenous injection in certain protozoal diseases.

Central emetics are drugs which stimulate the vomiting centre through their action on the CTZ. They are effective in a smaller dose when given by injection than when the drug is given by mouth.

Apomorphine is the most important central emetic and acts selectively on the chemoreceptor trigger zone producing vomiting within ten minutes after a subcutaneous injection. When given by mouth, twice the dose is required and the effect is not produced for thirty minutes. Dogs whose CTZ has been destroyed no longer respond to the injection of apomorphine, although copper sulphate given by mouth still produces vomiting. This is part of the evidence for the existence of a CTZ separate from the actual vomiting centre. Therapeutic and large doses of apomorphine are depressant. Birds and pigs are said to be insusceptible to apomorphine emesis. Morphine also stimulates the CTZ in the dog as do the medullary stimulants. However, these drugs are never used for this purpose.

Motion Sickness

Travel sickness can be a problem in transporting dogs and cats and certain drugs are useful in the prevention of this condition. Motion sickness is a problem in human medicine and considerable effort has been applied to the study of drugs which are capable of preventing this condition. Dogs have been used as experimental animals for the study of motion sickness remedies, but unfortunately drugs which have been found effective in the dog have been less effective in man and vice versa.

In man the drugs of value in the prevention of motion sickness fall into two groups: the anti-acetylcholine drugs of which the most effective is the alkaloid hyoscine and a second group, the antihistamines, i.e., promethazine, diphenhydramine Trimeprazine and various piperazine antihistamines such as cyclizine and meclizine. The piperazine derivatives are equally effective as anti-motion sickness remedies as the other antihistamines and have fewer side actions and hence are the antihistamines of choice in this particular purpose, but in dogs and cats the central depression of the other antihistamines has advantages. Vomiting induced experimentally in dogs by putting them in a swing is not alleviated by the anti-acetylcholine type of drug but is, to some extent, prevented by the antihistamine type of agent. Barbiturates, whilst ineffective as anti-motion sickness agents in man, were shown to have an appreciable action when tested experimentally in the dog.

Vomiting arising from drugs acting on the CTZ or as a result of a disease process in which a so-called 'toxin' acts on the CTZ is best prevented by drugs of the phenothiazine type of antihistamine. Vomiting is often part of a clinical syndrome and occurs, for example, in intestinal obstruction and uraemia. Vomiting of this kind is treated by treating the cause. An undesirable feature of certain drugs is that they cause vomiting, and drugs such as sodium salicylate or digitalis given by mouth may have this disadvantage. Giving the drug in dilute solution may avoid this difficulty. Metoclopramide is occasionally used in small animal practice to prevent vomiting caused by the administration of drugs or anaesthesia. It has both a central and peripheral action; the latter facilitates gastric emptying. There is no evidence that it is effective against motion sickness.

SUGGESTIONS FOR FURTHER READING

Ayre-Smith R A 1971 Pasture bloat in cattle. Australian Veterinary Journal 47:162
Brand J J, Perry W L M 1966 Drugs used in motion sickness. Pharmacological Reviews 18:895
Clarke R T J, Reid C S W 1974 Foamy bloat of cattle. A review. Journal of Dairy Science 57:753
Howarth R E 1975 Review of bloat in cattle. Canadian Veterinary Journal 16:261
Wang S C 1965 Emetic and antiemetic drugs. Physiol. Pharmacol. 2:256

12

Drugs acting on the alimentary system

Reticulo-rumen, purges, astringents

THE EFFECT OF DRUGS ON RETICULO-RUMENAL MOVEMENTS

The reticulo-rumen shows a basic sequence of contractions which does not vary appreciably. The reticulum makes a double contraction at regular intervals of about one minute. This contraction forces the liquid digesta into the rumen and probably some digesta passes into the omasum with each reticular contraction. Digesta appears to pass continuously from reticulum to omasum and also to flow continuously from the abomasum. The movements of the reticulo-rumen depend upon the integrity of the vagi and there are various areas in the medulla which produce reticular contractions when stimulated. Rumination and the œsophageal groove reflex also depend on an intact vagal innervation.

Carbachol and similar parasympathomimetic agents usually increase the amplitude of the reticular contractions but not the frequency, and this increase is followed by inhibition. Acetylcholine and histamine inhibit the activity of both rumen and reticulum. It has been suggested that the inhibitory action of acetylcholine is due to the adrenaline which it releases from the adrenal gland. In support of this suggestion it has been shown that carbachol, in doses inhibitory to rumenal movement, also produced a rise in blood sugar. Carbachol is known to have strong nicotinic actions which would give rise to the release of adrenaline from the adrenal medulla, which in turn would produce the rise in blood sugar concentration. However, since both histamine and acetylcholine have marked effects on the cardiovascular system the inhibition of reticular rumenal movements by these drugs could be due to their interference with the flow of blood to these organs. Moreover, although adrenaline normally inhibits reticulo-rumenal movements, if the reticulum is quiescent, an injection of adrenaline or splanchnic stimulation produces a contraction. Atropine inhibits movement

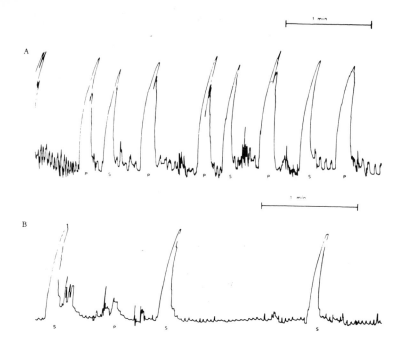

Fig. 12.1 The inhibition of rumen movements by carbachol (25 µg/kg) injected subcutaneously (A) before and (B) one hour after injection. (Adapted from Alexander & Moodie 1960 *Research in Veterinary Science* 1: 248.)

of the rumen and reticulum and etorphine has an even greater inhibitory effect which should be borne in mind when this drug is used in surgical procedures on the ruminant.

A mixture of alkaloids collectively known as **veratrine** are obtained from plants of the *veratrum* species. They have been used in man as hypotensive agents, and are of veterinary interest because when injected into ruminants they produce a phenomenon which is very similar to vomiting. It has been suggested that **veratrine** may be of use in the treatment of a certain type of bloat; at present the status of this agent is uncertain.

Very little absorption of drugs or products of digestion takes place in the stomach of simple-stomached animals. This is because most drugs are given as salts which ionise in the stomach and it is only the non-ionised moiety which passes through the gastric mucosa. Acidic drugs such as acetylsalicylic acid are readily absorbed through the gastric mucosa. However, in ruminants an appreciable absorption of both drugs and products of digestion takes place in the reticulo-rumen. Drugs such as pilocarpine, atropine, pheno-thiazine, cyanide and metabolites as, for example, ammonia and fatty acids, are absorbed through the rumen wall. The vital ions sodium and potassium pass through the rumen wall, the passage of potassium being passive but that of sodium is active, and can take place against a concentraion gradient. Water is absorbed along with sodium. Inorganic phosphate is both absorbed from the rumen and diffuses into the rumen.

Bile is continuously excreted by the liver and, in animals possessing a gall-bladder, is collected there and concentrated with the addition of mucin. Emptying of the gall-bladder is controlled in part by the vagal reflex and partly by humoral agents.

A number of drugs are excreted in the bile frequently in the form of a glucuronide. There are marked species differences in the proportion of glucuronide thus secreted and it is important to realise that the intestine in most species is rich in glucuronidases which hydrolyse the glucuronide freeing the drug in many cases for reabsorption.

Cholagogues are drugs which stimulate the liver to excrete bile. Bile acids increase the output of bile and such drugs are called 'choloretic agents'. The administration of bile salts has little effect on biliary flow. Vagal stimulation or drugs with muscarine actions contract the gall bladder and relax the sphincter of Oddi. Sympathetic stimulation and drugs which mimic it have opposite effects.

The hormone cholecystokinin which contracts the gall bladder is released by the presence of fat in the duodenum. This contraction throws bile salts into the duodenum causing the liberation of secretin, which in turn stimulates pancreatic secretion and the secretion of bile by the liver thus refilling the gall-bladder. Hypertonic solutions of magnesium sulphate in the duodenum cause contraction of the gall-bladder as does the injection of secretin. Bile acids themselves are used sometimes as cholagogues, being available as *Dehydrocholic acid.*

Certain iodine-containing drugs are radio-opaque and their excretion in the bile is utilised in the X-ray examination of the biliary system. Ipanoic acid and iodophthalein (a derivative of phenolphthalein) are given by mouth in dogs and outline the gall bladder in about ten hours. Iodipamide (as a methylglucamine) may be administered intravenously and is much quicker in its action.

Tablets containing pancreatic extracts known as **pancreatin** are used in the treatment of deficiency of pancreatic enzymes. This deficiency may arise from a number of causes and is not uncommon in dogs. These tablets are specially coated to resist digestion in the stomach and contain lipase, trypsin and amylase. Drugs such as the H_2 blocking agent cimetidine, which inhibit gastric secretion, may be used to increase the amount of enzymatic activity surviving passage through the stomach.

DRUGS ACTING ON THE MOVEMENTS OF THE INTESTINES

The intestines under normal conditions are constantly active, the purpose of their activity being to mix the digesta with the secretions of the intestines and associated glands and to expose this mixture to the intestinal mucous membrane. There are two basic types of activity: namely, mixing movements and propulsive movements, the latter moving the digesta along the tract from duodenum to anus. The division into these types of activity is not rigid. The mixing movements tends tends to move digesta aborally and the propulsive movements tend to mix the digesta. The aboral progression of digesta by mixing movements is brought about by the spontaneous activity of the plain muscle of the intestine which shows a gradient from duodenum to rectum. The rhythmic contractions decrease in rate from duodenum aborally. The propulsion of digesta is brought about mainly by the intrinsic nerve plexi and involves a co-ordinated contraction of the gut preceded by relaxation aborally.

Intestinal movements are influenced by the autonomic nervous system, vagal stimulation increasing and splanchnic stimulation decreasing the movements. Similarly, drugs with muscarine actions increase intestinal motility, and this effect is antagonised by atropine. Atropine also diminishes the propulsive movements of the intestine. Although in clinical cases of diarrhoea it often exacerbates the condition and even in healthy horses increases the faecal excretion of water and electrolytes. The intestines are also influenced by painful stimuli or irritation of the peritoneum which reflexly produce splanchnic inhibition. The response of the pyloric and ileocæcal sphincters to both nerve stimulation and adrenaline is opposite to that of the rest of the intestinal muscle.

The rate of passage of digesta along the alimentary tract varies in the different species and may affect the fate of drugs given by mouth. In carnivores a large part of digestion takes place in the stomach, and thereafter the food residue passes through the small intestine as a soup-like chyme, becoming firmer in consistency in the colon due to the re-absorption of water. The passage from mouth to anus takes less than 24 hours. Herbivores having a more complex gut take rather longer over this process, but in the horse not as long as might be expected. Food residues first appear in horse fæces about 22 hours after feeding and are not completely excreted until after 48 hours. In foals the over-all rate of passage is similar to that in the adult but the time spent in the stomach is much longer in the suckling foal than after weaning. The digesta in weaned foals passes quickly through the stomach but remain longer in the large colon. In ruminants the rate of passage is much slower; about 80% of food residue is excreted in from 70–90 hours after ingestion.

Drugs may influence intestinal movements by acting on the intrinsic or extrinsic nerves of the bowel or by direct action on the plain muscle. The sympathomimetic and parasympathomimetic drugs and their antagonists affect gut movement as discussed earlier. Histamine, barium, salts of lead, nitrates and the opium alkaloids act directly on the intestinal muscle.

Carbachol and physostigmine have been used clinically to stimulate bowel movements; specially in the horse this is a dangerous procedure. Atropine inhibits violent contractions of the gut and is useful in treating some types of colic. It is, of course, the antidote to carbachol and physostigmine and should be used if these drugs produce any untoward effects. Soluble salts of barium produce a violent contraction of intestinal muscle and profuse diarrhœa. Barium chloride was used in earlier times as a purge for the horse but this proved a dangerous practice as not only the muscle of the gut is affected but also that of the cardiovascular system, leading to heart failure.

PURGATIVES

It is sometimes therapeutically desirable to hasten the rate of passage of digesta along the tract and/or increase faecal water excretion. This is accomplished by the use of a purgative. Purgatives act either by increasing the bulk of non-absorbable contents in the bowel or by irritation or stimulation of the nerves or muscle of the gut.

Purgatives which increase bulk include *agar-agar*, a Japanese seaweed, liquid paraffin and the saline purges. **Agar-agar** in the presence of water swells to form a gel which is not absorbed. It is suitably for use in the dog and cat only as it is a carbohydrate and would be fermented in the alimentary tract of herbivores. **Liquid paraffin** is a mixture of aliphatic hydrocarbons. It is non-irritant and non-absorbable. It acts in part by softening the fæcal mass and lubricating the rectum and by virtue of its bulk. A practical objection, especially in household pets, is its tendency to leak through the anal sphincter. It also interferes with absorption of fat-soluble vitamins.

The **saline purges** all act in a similar fashion and depend on the fact that certain anions and cations are only slowly absorbed from the gut. These ions include magnesium, sulphate, phosphate, tartrate and citrate which, in the form of salts, remain in the gut, water passing through the intestinal wall until the cathartic salt is in isotonic solution with the tissues. This solution distends the gut and reflexly increases peristalsis, thus hastening the passage of contents along the small intestine, an increased volume of fluid enters the colon, which responds in a similar fashion to the small intestine, thus producing defæcation. If a saline purge is required to act quickly, it must be given in isotonic solution so that time is not taken for water to pass from the tissues into the gut or vice versa to make the saline solution isotonic.

Magnesium sulphate is a powerful saline purge typical of the class. It is not used for horses and if purgation is delayed there is a very slight risk of absorption of magnesium ions and consequent untoward effects. *Magnesium oxide* and *carbonate* are primarily antacids with slight cathartic properties. The latter salt is used sometimes as magnesium limestone to dress pastures on which hypomagnesæmia occurs.

Sodium sulphate is the saline purge of choice for horses and cattle. It is the cheapest and most effectibe saline cathartic which is best given by stomach tube because it has an unpleasant taste and the dose is rather copious. Sodium chloride is sometimes given to horses by stomach tube, in which species it acts to some extent as a saline purge.

Bile acids alter the fluid transport across the gut wall. This is probably mediated through cyclic AMP. They decrease sodium insorption and increase anion exorption. This effect resembles that of cholera toxin.

Contact cathartics

These drugs act on the mucous membrane of the gut affecting the net movement of electrolytes and motility. They include diphenylmethane, anthraquinones and castor oil. As well as affecting the permeability of the gut wall they released prostaglandins and increase cellular cyclic AMP. The effects of contact cathartics are inhibited by the application of local anaesthetics to the gut mucosa.

Castor oil is a bland non-irritant oil which is sometimes used externally as a protective dressing. It has no action on the stomach, but in the intestine it is hydrolysed by lipase to liberate ricinoleic acid. There is evidence that ricinoleic acid causes the exorption of water and sodium. It probably stimulates a cyclic AMP mediated secretory process. The catharsis produced may be due to the increase in water content of the intestinal contents and a decrease in circular muscle activity. The hydrolysis of castor oil depends on the presence of bile and lipase so the drug will not act in conditions where bile is absent. It is not used in adult horses or ruminants but is the purge of choice in foals and calves in which the large colon and rumen respectively have not fully developed.

The **anthracene purges** owe their activity to active principles derived from anthracene. Most of these drugs contain *emodin* (trihydroxymethylanthraquinone) and several contain *chrysophanic* acid (di-hydroxymethylanthraquinone). In such drugs such as aloes, senna, cascara sagrada and rhubarb these active principles are combined with sugars to form glycosides which require hydrolysis before the active principle is free to act.

The glycosides are absorbed from the small intestine, hydrolysed in the body to liberate emodin or chrysophanic acid which then act on the large intestine. This takes several hours whereas emodin given parenterally or placed in the jejunum of cats acts in about half an hour. Moreover, emodin or extracts of senna placed in the jejunum are effective even after the large and small intestines have been separated surgically. This evidence shows that the long latent period of the naturally occurring anthracene purges is due to the time taken for their hydrolysis in the body and not the time for them to pass down the gut to the colon.

These purgatives cause contraction of the colon and uterus and should never be given to pregnant animals because of the risk of producing abortion. There is some evidence that the anthracene purges interfere with the reabsorption of sodium from the gut. This may contribute to their purgative action. Emodin is converted in the body to chrysophanic acid which is excreted in the milk and urine. The chrysophanic acid acts as an indicator, turning red with alkalis.

Aloes, the traditional purge for horse, has been replaced by the synthetic compound **danthron** [*dihydroxyanthraquinone*] which has the advantage of being suitable to give mixed with the food. When given in this way *dihydroxyanthraquinone* takes about 24 hours to act; given as a suspension in water it acts more quickly. It is suitable for all the domestic animals when given in an appropriate dose. In horses it may cause abdominal discomfort and even colic.

Cascara sagrada is an anthracene purge used only in the dog and cat. It is the mildest anthracene purge and the gut does not become tolerant. It is given as either a dry or liquid extract.

Rhubarb, in addition to the anthracene active principles, contains a tannin and is therefore liable to produce constipation after purging because of the astringent action of the tannin on the bowel mucosa. To overcome this disadvantage it is combined with a saline purge. For example, Gregory's powder consists of powdered rhubarb and magnesium salts. Rhubarb as the powder or in the form of Gregory's powder (Pulv. Rhei Co.) is given to foals, calves and dogs to produce purgation.

Phenolphthalein is similar to the anthracene purges in the way it acts and in chemical structure. It may be given by mouth to dogs and cats, dissolves in the alkaline contents of the small intestine and is partly absorbed. The absorbed portion is partly excreted in the bile and partly in the urine. The excretion in the bile allows some of the dose to be re-absorbed repeatedly and thus prolongs the effect of the drug. Excessive prolongation of action may lead to irritation of the kidneys. Bisacodyl resembles phenolphthalein.

Mercurous chloride, calomel, is an insoluble compound which is slowly converted into a more soluble compound of mercury in the gut. It is usually a powerful purge, but should it not act, a saline purge must be given immediately to limit the absorption of mercury and consequent toxic effects. Calomel is rarely used now as safer means exist of producing a similar effect. It has been suggested that the mercurial purges act in a similar fashion to mercurial diuretics and by inhibiting enzymes with sulphydryl groups interfere with water absorption in the colon. The inhibition of water absorption distends the colon and so causes evacuation.

Dioctyl sodium sulphoscuccinate is an anionic-active agent which has a detergent-like effect on the contents of the intestine allowing the retention of more water. It causes the production of softer faeces and appears to have a laxative action. A 1% solution may be used as an enema in cases of faecal impaction. This anionic detergent is used occasionally to facilitate the disintegration of tablets.

Enemata are usually solutions of sodium chloride or soap injected into the rectum to stimulate defæcation. An enema of glycerine is sometimes used to treat constipation in dogs and cats. Enemata should be warmed before administration and injected by gravity not a pump. A suppository is occasionally inserted into the rectum of a dog or cat to stimulate defæcation.

The drastic purges colocynth, jalap and croton oil have no place in veterinary therapeutics.

Adsorbents are preparations used to remove undesirable substances, gases or poisons from the intestine. Substances are said to be adsorbed when they stick on the surface of a solid. Hence the greater the surface area of the solid the better adsorbent it is likely to be.

Kaolin, a naturally occurring aluminium silicate, is the commonest adsorbent used in veterinary medicine. It is practically insoluble, and when given by mouth forms a protective coating on the bowel wall. However, the main value lies in its absorption of toxins in certain entero-toxæmias. Magnesium trisilicate acts both as an antacid and adsorbent. *Prepared chalk* is used also in veterinary medicine as an adsorbent but is less effective than kaolin.

Preparations of belladonna are used to relieve spasm of the intestinal muscle and are termed '**Antispasmodics**'. Atropine, the active principal of belladonna may exacerbate diarrhoea by increasing the faecal water content.

Astringents are drugs which precipitate proteins and so form an insoluble layer of precipitated protein on the skin or mucous membrane. This layer protects the underlying tissue from further irritation and also inhibits exudation, secretion and small hæmorrhages. When given by mouth astringents tend to stop diarrhoea but are not as good as kaolin.

There are two classes of astringent, metallic astringents and vegetable astringents. The former includes salts of lead, zinc and aluminium which are used on the skin, and salts of iron and copper which are occasionally used as intestinal astringents. The vegetable astringents act by liberating tannic acid which precipitates protein. *Tannic acid* is not used as it irritates the stomach, damages the liver on absorption and precipitates food protein. The vegetable astringents liberate tannic acid slowly as they pass along the gut. *Catechu* is the main vegetable astringent used in veterinary medicine and by slowly releasing tannic acid as it passes along the bowel precipitates proteins on the inflamed mucosa thus forming a portective layer. Tannic acid should never be used to treat burn injuries because of the risk of damaging the liver with tannic acid absorbed from the burned surface.

Diarrhœa is a common symptom in all the domesticated species. It is interesting to note that intestinal motility is decreased during diarrhoea and increased in constipation. When it is produced by a specific agent the correct treatment is to eliminate the causal agent; various antibiotics have a useful function in this type of treatment where the cause is a specific organism. However diarrhœa may occur in which there is no obvious causal agent, and it has to be treated symptomatically. Astringents and adsorbents can be useful drugs in controlling this condition and it is important to remember that water and electrolytes can be lost in substantial amounts during diarrhœa and restorative treatment may be essential. Use may also be made in the treatment of diarrhœa of the spasmogenic action of morphine. This alkaloid increases the tone of the intestinal muscle and so delays the movement of digesta along the alimentary tract. It is usual in treating diarrhœa with morphine to use a preparation containing crude opium such as tincture of opium, or powdered opium.

Loperamide and **Diphenoxylate** are related chemically to pethidine and are used in the treatment of diarrhoea. They have opioid effects but are insoluble in water and almost unabsorbed from the gut. Diphenoxylate has been claimed to produce morphine-like effects in the cat. There is evidence that loperamide reduces the water content of equine faeces.

SUGGESTIONS FOR FURTHER READING

Alexander F 1963 Digestion in the horse. Contribution to the Rowett Research Institute collected papers for 50th anniversary. Oliver & Boyd, Edinburgh

Binder H J 1977 Pharmacology of laxatives. Annual Review of Pharmacology and Toxicology 17: 355

Dougherty R W, Allen R S, Burroughs W, Jacobson N L, McGilliard A D 1964 Physiology of digestion in the ruminant. Second International Symposium, Ames, Iowa

Farrar J T, Zfass A M 1967 Small intestinal motility. Gastroenterology 52: 1019

Menguy R 1964 Motorfunctions of the alimentary tract. Annual Review of Physiology 26: 227

Stewary J J, Gaginella T S, Olsen U A, Bass P 1975 Inhibitory action of laxatives. Journal of Pharmacology 192: 458

Texter E C 1964 The control of gastro-intestinal motor activity. American Journal of digestive Diseases 9: 585

Truelove S C 1966 Movements of the large intestine. Physiological Review 46: 457

13

Drugs acting on the heart

The heart is a vital organ used to pump blood around the body in the blood vessels. It has an intrinsic rhythmic contraction which is due to electrical activity in the sino-atrial (S-A) node. This spreads over the atria to the atrioventricular (A-V) node then through the bundle of His and Purkinje fibres into the ventricles. This electrical activity gives rise initially to the contraction of the auricles followed by the ventricles after a brief delay. This delay allows filling of the ventricles. The action of heart muscle, unlike skeletal muscle, has a long phase of contraction and a long refractory period. It is not capable of tetany. The heart rate is slowed by vagal activity involving stimulation of muscarinic receptors by acetylcholine. It is quickened by activity of the sympathetic nervous system involving stimulation of β_1-receptors. As the heart rate increases, the refractory period shortens so that the heart becomes more excitable with more rapid conduction of the electrical activity through the heart.

The heart may fail for a number of reasons including damage to the heart valves which impairs pumping efficiency. Heart muscle damage due to poison and ischaemia can also impair efficiency. Both can give rise to congestive heart failure. Pathological alterations in the refractory period, excitability and rate of propagation of the electrical activity can lead to ectopic beats of auricular or ventricular origin. The electrical activity may follow abnormal conduction pathways, giving rise to a reverberating circuit. In the atria this can give rise to atrial flutter or fibrillation. Some of these conditions can be alleviated by drugs which have inotropic or antidysrhythmic effects.

INOTROPIC DRUGS

Inotropic drugs alter the strength of the heartbeat. Sympathomimetic amines, acting on the β_1-receptors of the heart increase the force of contraction. However, their effect on blood pressure is

203

complicated by β_2-receptor stimulation giving vasodilatation. There is also the disadvantage that sympathomimetic drugs shorten the refractory period and increase excitability. This can give rise to irregularities of conduction, even fatal ventricular fibrillation.

Inotropic actions are produced by cardiac glycosides. Glycosides are most effective in left-sided heart failure due to muscle weakness, when uncomplicated by incompetent or stenotic valves. They are not usually effective in aortic valve disease.

The inotropic actions of the xanthines (e.g. caffeine) and Ca ions are dicussed elsewhere.

Cardiac glycosides

The purple foxglove, *Digitalis purpurea* is a the source of important cardiac glycosides and was introduced into orthodox medicine by William Withering in 1775. He was unaware of its cardiac action but used it as a cure for dropsy. The main active principle of the purple foxglove is digitoxin. Another important glycoside, digoxin comes from *Digitalis lanata* and is water soluble.

The basic structure of the glycosides consists of a steroid-like aglycone molecule joined to a sugar (glycone) such as digitoxose. This sugar molecule is important for the transport (of the glycoside) and fixation to the heart muscle. It exerts no action on its own. The aglycone by itself is less potent and shorter lasting than the glycoside.

The glycosides act on the heart directly and via the vagus nerve. They increase the force of contraction, the excitability of the heart muscle and increase the refractory period of the specialised conduction system. The inotropic effects of glycosides are best seen in congestive heart failure uncomplicated by valve defects. There is an increase in cardiac output despite a reduction in heart rate. The reduction in rate allows better filling and improved circulation. The improvement in circulation relieves oedema caused by venous congestion. There is a transient rise in arterial pressure and fall in venous pressure. Larger doses of glycosides can give rise to a conduction block between S-A and A-V nodes, partly due to vagal activity as well as depression of the A-V node and Purkinge fibres. The block can be partly relieved by administration of atropine. The effect of glycosides on muscle excitability will decrease the refractory period of the atrial muscle in flutter and can convert it further to fibrillation. However, electrical coupling between the fibrillating atrium and ventricles is reduced because of the longer refractory

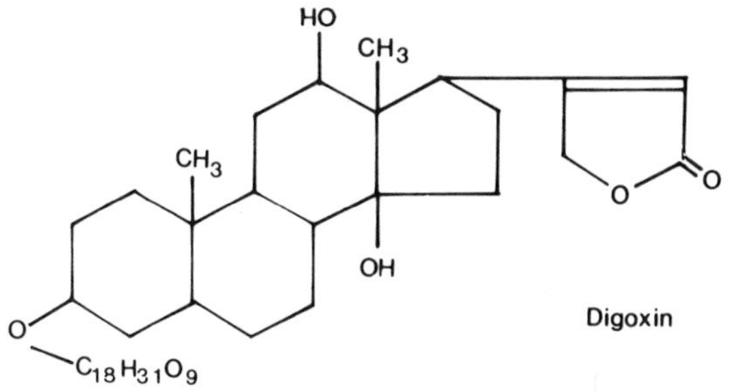

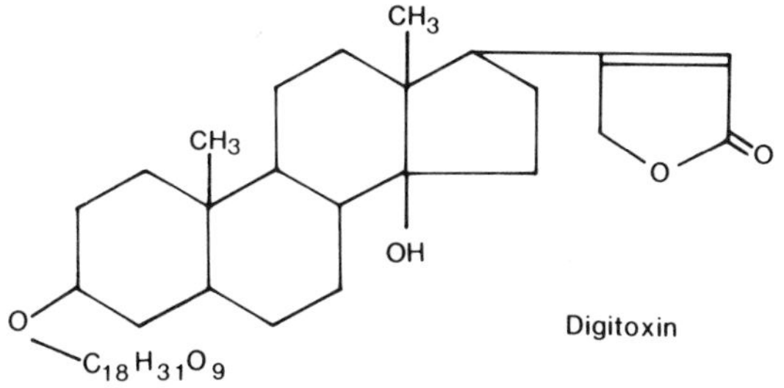

Fig. 13.1 The structure of two cardiac glycosides.

period of the A-V node. In cases of atrial fibrillation with a high ventricular rate there is a beneficial slowing of the ventricular rate allowing an increase in filling and consequently cardiac output. Glycosides effect the ECG. They prolong the P-R interval, due to depression of the conduction system. They shorten the Q-T interval and reduce or invert the T wave because of the direct excitatory action on cardiac muscle. In toxic overdose there may be a characteristic double beat or 'pulsus bigemini'.

The mode of action of the glycosides probably involves an increase in the labile calcium fraction of the sarcoplasmic reticulum. This calcium is released during depolarisation of the muscle fibre and activates the contractile proteins. The contractile response to depolarisation is then increased. It has been shown that the glycosides inhibit a muscle bound ATPase responsible for sodium and potassium transport. This could lead to an increase in the intracellular calcium because of a reduction in a sodium/calcium exchange mechanism. This normally extrudes calcium from the cell in exchange for sodium which enters under the electrochemical gradient. The increase in intracellular sodium may also directly increase the labile calcium fraction.

Glycosides and the effects of calcium on the heart are synergistic. Calcium should not be given during glycoside therapy because of the dangers of toxicity. Potassium depletion potentiates the effects of glycosides. This is important to remember if potassium-depleting diuretics are used for the treatment of oedema along with the glycosides. It may be better to avoid the thiazide diuretics.

The glycosides are absorbed from the small intestine after oral administration in monogastric animals but they are destroyed in the rumen of cows and sheep. The main factor which governs absorption is the degree of ionisation of the compound. The more non-polar or non-ionised compound is more lipid soluble and more readily taken up across the intestinal mucosa. Digitoxin, one of the most non-polar glycosides is well absorbed; digoxin, a slightly more polar glycoside is less well absorbed; ouabain, one of the most polar glycosides is poorly absorbed across the small intestine. In addition to these factors, however, the amount of absorption or the bioavailability varies with the preparation. Finely divided or micronised preparations of digoxin allow nearly 100% absorption. Glycosides are transported in the blood, bound to albumen and found free in the plasma. They are metabolised in the liver, the most non-polar glycosides undergoing the greatest degree of metabolism. They are then eliminated by the kidney in the urine or via the liver through the bile. The glycosides undergo entero-hepatic recycling. This recycling accounts in part for the differences in duration of action for a given glycoside in the different animal species. The half-life of digitoxin in the dog has been found to be about 21 hours. About 30% of an administered dose of digoxin is eliminated in 24 hours in dogs. Thus digoxin and digitoxin have a similar elimination rate in this species. In the cat the half-life of digitoxin is expected to be longer because of the lower level of conjugation in this species. In man the half-life of digitoxin is much longer than that of digoxin.

The powdered leaf preparation of digitalis is more irritant than digoxin. Dogs and particularly cats may vomit during treatment. This is likely in overdose. Anorexia may occur and it can be the first sign that digitalisation is nearly complete. Digoxin is sufficiently water soluble to be given by injection if it is necessary to avoid oral administration. Digitalis preparations are only given by mouth unlike the pure glycosides which may be injected. The slow onset of actions of the glycosides is mainly because they have to become fixed to the heart before they can act. The use of digitalis preparations appears to be confined to the horse, dog and cat. In general digoxin preparations are more controllable because of their

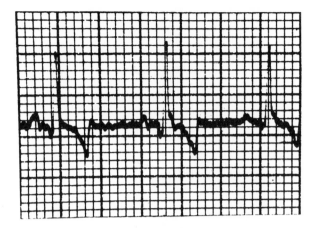

Fig. 13.2 An electrocardiograph showing atrial fibrillation in the dog (courtesy of G F Bodie).

shorter action. Often an initial loading dose is followed by a lower maintenance dose to achieve digitalisation.

Because there is a low therapeutic index it is important to recognise the signs of digitalis intoxication. These include anorexia, vomiting, diarrhoea, bradycardia, prolonged P-R interval and extrasystole. The presence of 'pulsus bigemini' and a big change in the ECG pattern are serious signs.

There are several reports of the successful treatment of atrial fibrillation in dogs and horse with glycosides. Sometimes digitalis has been used for the control of atrial fibrillation before treatment with quinidine and on occasion after withdrawal a normal sinus rhythm has resulted. The use of glycosides in the treatment of congestive heart failure without valve effects is recognised. However, in endocardiosis of dogs where there is a valve defect giving rise to oedema it may be more important to use diuretics. The use of α_2-blocking drugs like prazosin to reduce peripheral resistance and to reduce the load on the heart has also been suggested.

Strophanthin-K from *Strophanthus kombé* and strophanthin-G from *Strophanthus gratus* (ouabain) are chemically similar to the cardiac glycosides. Ouabain is destroyed by intestinal enzymes. It is therefore administered intravenously to produce a rapid effect. However, it is more rapidly destroyed in the body than digitalis. It has an advantage in cats where digitalis may cause vomiting. It has similar pharmacological actions to digitalis. Crystalline oubain or tincture of strophthanthus are available.

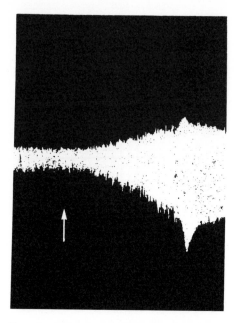

Fig. 13.3 The effect of ouabain on the contractions of the isolated guinea pig auricles.

The bulb of Squill contains the glycosides scillarin-A and B which resemble digitalis pharmacologically but are less effective. The tincture or syrup of squill is used as an expectorant. Red squill is a rat poison but this is not due to the cardiac glycosides.

ANTIDYSRHYTHMIC DRUGS

The S-A node cells and related conducting tissues depolarise spontaneously. The membrane potential follows the pattern illustrated in Figure 13.4. During phase 4 there is a slow depolarisation, which leads to 'firing' when it reaches the threshold potential. The cell then fires and depolarises rapidly during phase O. Until the cell repolarises below the threshold potential a second firing can not recur. The cell is then 'refractory'. The duration of the effective refractory period (ERP) includes phases 1, 2 & 3.

If extranodal tissue has a low membrane potential or if it deplorises more rapidly during phase 4 than the S-A node it leads to abnormal firing and extrasystole. There may be a regular ectopic rhythm. An abnormal circus movement of the electrical activity in the heart can develop under pathological conditions giving rise to

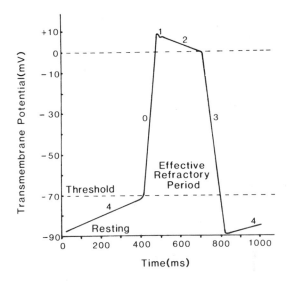

Fig. 13.4 The spontaneous depolarising potentials shown by pacemaker cells are divided into the five phases.

re-entry. This is believed to cause atrial flutter or fibrillation. In order to alleviate these conditions antidysrhythmic drugs are used.

Vaughan Williams (1970) has classified the drugs used for the treatment of dysrhythmias into four groups. *Class 1* drugs reduce spontaneous depolarisation (phase 4) and the maximum rate of depolarisation (phase 0); for example, lignocaine, phenytoin and mexiletine. *Class 2* drugs block sympathetic transmission; for example, the β-blockers. *Class 3* drugs prolong the effective refractory period; for example amidarone. *Class 4* drugs block the entry of calcium into the muscle cells; for example, verapamil. However, some drugs like quinidine, procainamide and disopyramide have both class 1 and class 3 effects. Although there are a large number of dysrhythmic agents available, only a few have been used in veterinary practice (mentioned below).

Quinidine, the dextro-rotatory isomer of quinine, can be used for the treatment of cardiac dysrhythmias such as atrial fibrillation and extra-systoles. It can cure atrial fibrillation where d.c. shock is not practicable. Its myocardial depressant action supresses ectopic pacemakers. Quinidine slows conduction in the bundle of His and depresses the excitability of the heart muscle. The frequency of atrial contraction is reduced and the ERP is increased. These actions assist the conversion of atrial flutter to normal sinus rhythm.

Quinidine is rapidly excreted, so high doses near the maximum are required. Sometimes quinidine causes sudden cardiovascular collapse. Other side-effects include skin rashes, anorexia, vomiting and diarrhoea. Quinidine has been used successfully in the treatment of atrial fibrillation in both dog and horse. It is usually desirable to use quinidine in this condition after prior digitalisation as this reduces the hazards of quinidine, due to the dislodging of thrombi from the auricular appendages.

Procainamide is a drug with a similar pharmacological action to the local anaesthetic procaine, but with more marked effects on the heart. The amide linkage renders it resistant to plasma esterase so that the majority of it is excreted unchanged in the urine.

Lignocaine has a cardiac depressant action and will suppress ventricular tachycardia. Phenytoin is more effective against supraventricular arrhythmias. The β-blocking drugs are also used in extra systoles and tachycardia of supra-ventricular and ventricular origin. However, they also depress cardiac contractility and are contraindicated in the presence of A-V block because of their further depressant action. *Propranolol*, a β-blocker, in addition to its other properties has a quinidine like action.

There are newer compounds like mexiletine, verapamil and amidarone which have yet to be evaluated in clinical veterinary practice.

SUGGESTIONS FOR FURTHER READING

Baggot J D, Davis L E 1973 Plasma protein binding of digitoxin and digoxin in several mammalian species. Research in Veterinary Science 15:81

Braunwald E, Pool P E 1968 Mechanism of action of digitalis glycosides (I and II). Modern Concepts of Cardiovascular Disease 37:129

Detweiler D K 1965 Cardiac glycosides in the treatment of congestive heart failure in dogs. Anim. Hosp. 1: 29

Detweiler D K, Knight D H 1977 Congestive heart failure in dogs: Therapeutic concepts. Journal of the American Veterinary Medical Association 171:106

Hamlin R L, Dutta S, Smith C R 1971 Effects of digoxin and digitoxin on ventricular function in normal dogs and dogs with heart failure. American Journal of Veterinary Research 32:1391

Harrison D C, Sprouse J M, Morrow A G 1963 The antiarrhythmic properties of lidocaine and procainamide. *Circulation* 28, 486

Jenkins W L, Clark D R 1977 A review of drugs affecting the heart. Journal of the American Veterinary Medical Association 171, 85

Pyle R L 1967 Conversion of atrial fibrillation with quinidine sulphate in a dog. Journal of the American Veterinary Medical Association 151, 582

Tilley L P, Weitz J 1977 Pharmacologic and other forms of medical therapy in feline cardiac disease. Veterinary Clinics of North America 7:2 415

Vaughan Williams E M 1970 Classification of anti-arrhythmic drugs. In: Sandoe
E, Fleusted-Jensen E, Oleson K H Eds Symposium on cardiac arrhythmias,
Elsmore 1970, p 449 Södertälje, A B Astra Sweden
Withering W 1785 An account of the foxglove and some of its medical uses.
Reprinted in part in: Willus F, Keys T E (eds) Classics of cardiology: A
collection of classic works on the heart and circulation, Vol 1. Dover, New
York

14

Drugs acting on the respiratory system

The respiratory centre is controlled in part by the CO_2 tension of the blood; an increase of as little as 0.2% of CO_2 in the alveolar air will double the volume of air respired. A large increase in CO_2 tension produces signs of asphyxia and a decrease causes apnoea. The respiratory centre is not directly stimulated by lack of oxygen, but such a lack makes the centre more sensitive to CO_2. Oxygen lack, therefore, does not cause hyperpnoea if the CO_2 tension is also lowered. In fact in these circumstances oxygen lack causes no very obvious effects excepting a marked cyanosis.

Carbon dioxide is the physiological stimulus to respiration and is often useful in treating respiratory failure in small animals. It is supplied in cylinders usually as a 5% mixture with oxygen and is given by intra-tracheal or intra-nasal tube or by means of a suitable mask. Such equipment is very useful in the operating theatre where a few minutes' treatment with an oxygen/CO_2 mixture can be invaluable in stimulating a failing respiration. However, in barbiturate poisoning the sensitivity of the respiratory centre to CO_2 is depressed; under these circumstances the administration of CO_2 is of no use.

The respiratory movements are partly controlled through the carotid sinus reflex. A rise in blood pressure in the sinus inhibits respiration and a fall in pressure causes stimulation. Respiratory stimulation is also produced by lack of oxygen or excess CO_2 in the sinus.

Carbon dioxide when inhaled for about one minute produces a brief cerebral depression. This has been used to make pigs unconscious prior to slaughter by bleeding; such animals bleed more thoroughly and bruising of tissues is avoided. Carbon dioxide is used also to render fowls and other small animals unconscious. Carbon dioxide decreases the force of contraction of the heart and by a direct action on the blood vessels causes vasodilatation. However, these effects are largely counteracted by the release of adrenaline and noradrenaline by CO_2.

The normal activities of all the tissues of the body depend upon an adequate supply of oxygen. The brain, however, is more susceptible to oxygen lack than any other tissue. Lack of oxygen is called hypoxia. Hypoxia gives rise to an increase in the respiratory rate. The extremities are cold and the mucous membranes cyanotic, and there is a depression of the central nervous system similar to that produced by alcohol.

Oxygen

Pure oxygen may be breathed for a few hours without harmful effects, but if this is continued for several days pneumonia and cerebral damage are produced. An atmosphere containing 60% oxygen can be breathed indefinitely without harm. Oxygen at a pressure of four atmospheres kills in a few minutes. This is due to certain enzymes in the brain being poisoned.

The main use of oxygen in veterinary practice is in general anaesthesia. It is best given by intranasal or intratracheal tube or suitable mask. Unless the anaesthetist is using a closed-circuit apparatus with a CO_2 absorber the oxygen should be given together with a 5% CO_2.

Oxygen, especially at high pressure (hyperbaric), is useful in overcoming the cellular hypoxia of cyanide poisoning.

Carbon monoxide is an odourless and colourless gas which on inhalation may produce a sudden loss of consciousness. The effects produced by this gas are entirely due to oxygen lack. Carbon monoxide combines with haemoglobin 200 times more readily than does oxygen; the combination is much firmer and excludes oxygen. The tissues are thus deprived of oxygen and tissue oxidation is inhibited because carbon monoxide also has a high affinity for the respiratory enzymes. The only treatment, which must be prompt, is to give oxygen to remove carbon monoxide from the blood. Under conditions of high oxygen tension, carbon monoxide is displaced from combination with haemoglobin and, in these circumstances, sufficient oxygen will dissolve in the plasma to maintain many functions. Carbon monoxide as produced by car exhausts or in coal gas is sometimes used to euthanise dogs and cats.

Cyanides may be absorbed from the lungs as hydrocyanic acid gas, or after ingestion or in ruminants following the ingestion of plants containing cyanogenetic glycosides. They act by interfering with the tissue oxidations inhibiting oxidative enzymes but not other enzymes. The cyanide ion reacts with trivalent iron, particularly the iron in cytochrome oxidase, and thus gives rise to histotoxic hypoxia. Very small doses of cyanides stimulate respiration by stimulating the carotid sinus. This stimulation is probably produced by cyanide blocking oxidative metabolism in the chemoreceptor cells of the carotid sinus and thus acting like a reduction in oxygen tension. This manner of stimulating respiration has long been discontinued because it is of no value when the medullary centres are depressed; moreover, cyanide has well-known and marked toxic effects. The treatment of cyanide poisoning must be very rapid if it is to be effective. The object is to form methaemoglobin which competes with cytochrome oxidase for the cyanide by forming a chelate cyanmethaemoglobin, thus freeing the cytochrome oxidase. Methaemoglobin is formed by giving sodium nitrite intravenously. Sodium thiosulphate should be given also by intravenous injection. Sulphur is transferred from the thiosulphate and replaced with cyanide to form thiocyanate in which form the cyanide is unable to combine with iron.

Cobalamin is a member of the group of B_{12} vitamins and is probably the treatment of choice in cyanide poisoning. It apparently combines with cyanide to form a chelate cyanocobalamin. Cobalt edetate has also been used as an antidote.

THE PHARMACOLOGY OF THE AIRWAYS

Mucociliary clearance is a critically important process in the lung defense mechanisms. Epithelial cilia are believed to function without nervous control. Their purpose is to transport the fluids and debris of the airways in a cephalad direction (the tracheal 'escalator') into the nasopharynx from where they may be either swallowed or expectorated. Ciliary activity may be impaired by chemical irritants, cold temperatures or infection. Fluids in the airways are, in part, under nervous control and are susceptible to the actions of drugs. Serous secretion is under autonomic nerve control and is stimulated by cholinergic agonists, inflammatory mediators (e.g. histamine) and expectorant drugs. Mucus, secreted by the goblet cells, is not considered to be so influenced. However, in many pulmonary diseases the mucus becomes very elastic and difficult to remove. It is sometimes useful to stimulate serous secretion therapeutically in order to lower fluid viscosity and assist its removal by cilia or by coughing. *Expectorants* are drugs which are used for this effect. They fall into several classes. (1) Reflex stimulants such as ipecacuanha, ammonia salts and squill. These drugs are emetics at high doses and expectorant at low doses. They probably act by stimulating sensory vagal nerve endings in the stomach and duodenum, causing a reflex increase in secretion of the bronchial tubulo-acinar glands. (2) Various volatile oils probably cause expectoration by direct irritation of the bronchial glands. These drugs include, turpentine, various 'balsams', pine oil and menthol. (3) Iodides, particularly potassium iodide are good expectorants. They are thought to act upon being excreted selectively by the tubulo-acinar glands (a diuresis-like effect). (4) Glyceryl guaiacolate is an expectorant with an unknown mode of action.

Occasionally it is considered therapeutically desirable to assist in the actual liquefaction of mucus. This is especially employed in chronic obstructive respiratory disease. Drugs with this 'liquefying' property are known as *mucolytics*. *Bromhexine*, when administered orally is said to be excreted into the airways and to depolymerise mucopolysaccharide-protein complexes and reduce mucus viscosity. *Acetylcysteine* liquefies mucus through its free sulphydryl groups which open up disulphide bonds in the mucoproteins, thus reducing the elastic properties of mucus.

The use of anticholinergic drugs, such as atropine, may seriously interfere with fluid secretions in the airways and may thus compromise mucociliary clearance very significantly.

Bronchodilators

Obstruction of the airways may be caused by many factors including spasm of the bronchial-bronchiolar smooth muscle. Other factors include vascular congestion and oedema, mucus 'plugging', foreign bodies and tumours. Differential diagnosis of airway obstruction may be difficult. However, some degree of obstruction is believed to accompany all forms of inflammatory lung disease. Several classes of drugs are employed to relieve bronchoconstriction:

 (i) *Anticholinergics*, e.g. atropine, block the muscarinic receptors in the smooth muscle, thus blocking reflex activity brought about by irritants which stimulate sensory vagal fibres in the sub-mucosa. (Refer to Chapter 6 for further details.)
 (ii) *Anti-inflammatory agents* have been described in Chapter 18.
 (iii) *Sympathomimetics*. These drugs are described in Chapter 6.

Most β-agonists exert bronchodilator actions. However drugs such as *adrenaline* or *noradrenaline* have mixed α-receptor and beta receptor activity. *Isoprenaline*, while generally devoid of α-agonist activity at normal doses, possesses mixed β-1 and β_2 properties — thus stimulating the heart and dilating certain blood vessels (β_1 effect) — properties which may not be desired. Drugs which selectively stimulate β_2-receptors in airway smooth muscle have little or no direct cardiovascular effect. Selective β_2-agonists include salbutamol, terbutaline and metaproterenol. These drugs have minimal effects on respiratory tract fluids. They do however have two further advantages: (a) they relax pulmonary venous smooth muscle and thereby may reduce pulmonary congestion and inflammatory pulmonary edema; (b) they inhibit the release of histamine from mast cells and lysosomal enzymes from leukocytes. A disadvantage to the use of systemic sympathetic bronchodilators in horses is the stimulation of the sweat mechanism.

The methylxanthine drug, *aminophylline*, is an effective bronchodilator which possesses β and α-adrenoceptor stimulating properties. The myocardial stimulation and vasoconstrictor action of aminophylline, while being potentially difficult side-effects, may be put to good advantage in the control of acute inflammatory pulmonary oedema because aminophylline dilates the bronchi, constricts the microvasculature, decreases vascular permeability (thereby reducing oedema) and improves cardiac performance. Specific 'decongestants' such as the α-adrenergic agonists *phenylephrine* and *methoxamine* have also been used. Additionally, a 'loop-acting' diuretic such as *furosemide* may be employed to decrease pulmonary capillary pressure and mobilise fluid.

RESPIRATORY STIMULANTS AND DEPRESSANTS

Stimulation of the respiratory centres is a valuable therapeutic measure in the treatment of respiratory failure, such as may occur during anaesthesia. The most important stimulants are CO_2 and the analeptic drugs which have already been described. The respiratory centre is more easily depressed than any other medullary centre and several drugs have this property. The centres are also made less sensitive to CO_2 stimulation by drugs. Morphine, diamorphine, and the barbiturates are powerful respiratory depressants, as are some of the morphine substitutes such as methadone. Morphine and diamorphine depress the cough centre, and, whilst this is sometimes therapeutically desirable, these drugs are usually avoided because of restrictions imposed by drug legislation under which they are scheduled in most countries.

Codeine is sometimes used in the relief of painful coughing, as it depresses the cough centre in doses which have little effect on respiration. This effect of codeine is not antagonised by nalorphine but is in fact augmented. Codeine phosphate and syrup of codeine phosphate are used as depressants of the cough centre in dogs.

Dextromethorphan is a newer anti-tussive (see p. 155) which does not have addictive properties.

SUGGESTIONS FOR FURTHER READING

Ran J L Jr 1984 Respiratory Therapy Pharmacology, Year Book Medical Publishers,

15

Drugs acting on the reproductive system

Hormones, ecbolics, relaxants

The principal drugs acting on this system are the gonadotrophins, the sex hormones and drugs which contract or relax the uterus.

Gonadotrophic hormones are present in the anterior lobe of the pituitary, the urine of pregnant women and the serum of pregnant mares. The pituitary gonadotrophins maintain the normal state of the testis and ovary and regulate the female sexual cycle. These effects are produced by the follicle stimulating hormone (FSH) and the luteinising hormone (LH).

FSH stimulates the development of Graafian follicles in the ovary and spermatogenesis is the testis. FSH increases the diameter of the seminiferous tubules, but probably both FSH and LH are essential for complete spermatogenesis. The effect of LH may be indirect, acting through the induction of androgen secretion and thus making complete spermatogenesis possible. LH stimulates the interstitial cells of the ovary and testis to produce their respective sex hormones, hence it is also termed the interstitial cell-stimulating hormone (ICSH). Provided maturing follicles are present in the ovary, LH causes ovulation and luteinisation of the granulosa cells.

Synthetic gonadotrophin releasing hormones (GnRH) have been produced which stimulate release of both FSH and LH. **Buserelin** for example, was developed by substitution of two amino acids in natural GnRH. This modification confers increased resistance to enzymatic degradation and therapeutic doses in mares and cows produce increased plasma concentrations of FSH and LH which persist for several hours. GnRH is used as an alternative to FSH and LH in mares and cows in the treatment of ovarian dysfunction and to improve the conception rate by inducing ovulation at the optimum tine for service or insemination.

Chorionic gonadotrophin is made in the human placenta and appears in the urine during pregnancy. The presence of this hormone provides the basis of various tests for pregnancy, such as the Ascheim-Zondek, Friedman and Xenopus tests. These methods have now been replaced almost entirely with immunologicol tests which are accurate, more convenient and much less expensive. Chorionic gonadotrophin is available for therapeutic purposes. Its effect is mainly luteinising. In female animals this hormone induces ovulation and reinforces the secretion of progesterone by the ovary. It is used to control the time of ovulation in mares because in these animals ovulation normally occurs towards the end of a long oestral period. This is also the case in the bitch and sow. Chorionic gonadotrophin is used also to induce ovulation in animals with recurrent anovulatory oestrus and for this purpose it is given by intravenous injection. However, the usual route of administering this substance is by intramuscular injection. It is widely used in the treatment of cystic ovarian disease especially where nymphomania is present and sometimes in the treatment of retained testicles (cryptorchidism). In male animals chorionic gonadotrophin is used to stimulate the secretion of testosterone by the testes.

Chorionic gonadotrophin has been used to treat persistent infertility in cows, but with such variable results that there seems little justification for its continued use.

Serum gonadotrophin

The pregnant mare does not excrete gonadotrophins in the urine, but the serum of such animals (PMS) provides a source of gonadotrophin in which FSH is the main hormone. Pregnancy tests in the mare are carried out on the blood serum during the 45th–90th day of pregnancy. Depending on the dose, the administration of serum gonadotrophin will cause one or more follicles in the ovary to develop and rupture, giving rise to a simultaneous oestrus. Ovulation takes place usually 2–5 days after a subcutaneous injection of serum gonadotrophin and it is recommended that mating should not take place at the oestrus induced by gonadotrophin because of the risk of multiple pregnancies. It is generally advisable that mating should follow the first spontaneous oestrus which follows the induced oestrus. The administration of serum gonadotrophin causes follicles to develop in the ovary and, if suitably timed, produces oestrus and ovulation. However, an ovarian response may occur without overt oestrus. The response appears to be quantitative but an excessive dose may inhibit ovulation. It is not certain, however, that normal cycles will be resumed; this is particularly the case when the treatment is given outwith the normal breeding season of the species.

Serum gonadotrophin has been used to increase the number of

developing follicles and ovulations at oestrus and thus increase the incidence of twins in cattle. It is administered during pro-oestrus, or following luteolysis induced with prostaglandin to stimulate pro-oestrus so that it reinforces the naturally produced FSH from the anterior pituitary gland. Serum gonadotrophin is used, in conjuction with progesterone or a synthetic progestagen, to induce oestrus in sheep — particularly for controlled breeding out of season. Administered at the end of the progestagen treatment serum gonadotrophin may improve the response of both the percentage of sheep showing oestrus and the number of ovulations induced.

In the male, gonadotrophins may be of some value in the treatment of infertility due to poor libido or low spermatozoa counts in ejaculated semen, but these defects are not commonly due to hormonal deficiency alone.

SEX HORMONES

The naturally occurring sex hormones are chemical substances with the basic structure of steroids. The hormones of the adrenal cortex,

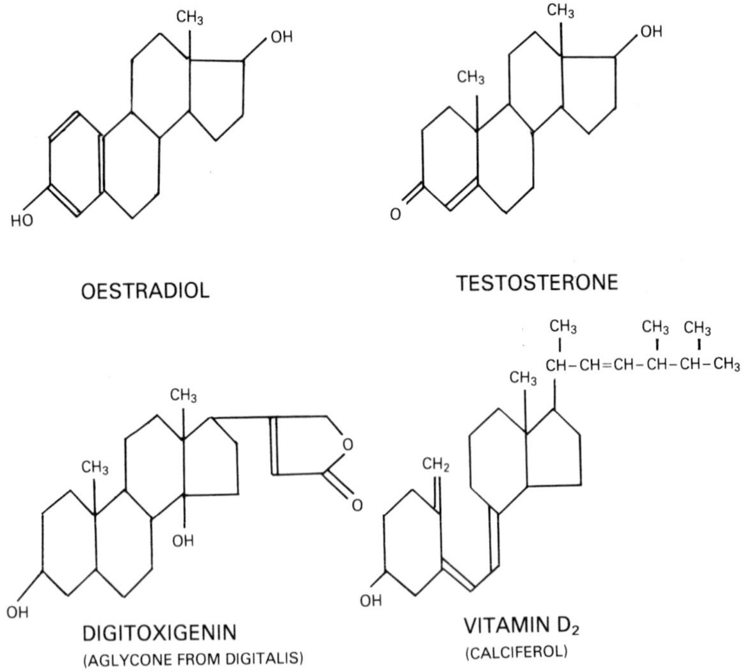
CH3
OH
HO
OESTRADIOL
CH3
OH
CH3
O
TESTOSTERONE
CH3
CH3
OH
O
O
OH
DIGITOXIGENIN
(AGLYCONE FROM DIGITALIS)
CH3 CH3 CH3
CH-CH=CH-CH-CH-CH3
CH3
CH2
OH
VITAMIN D2
(CALCIFEROL)

Fig. 15.1

cholesterol, vitamin D, the cardiac glycosides and some carcinogenic substances are also steroids. The pharmacological differences
between these compounds are due to small chemical groups attached to this basic structure (Fig. 15.1). They have, however,
some properties in common. For example, they dissolve only
slightly in water but are soluble in fats and fat solvents. This property is therapeutically valuable, because if they were water soluble
a single injection would flood the body and be quickly inactivated.
Since the effect of these hormones takes several days to develop,
such a water-soluble compound would be a very inefficient way of
administering the drug. These substances are most effective when
a low concentration is allowed to act for a long time, and these conditions are most readily obtained by injecting the drug subcutaneously or intramuscularly in a form from which absorption is very
slow. There are a variety of ways in which absorption may be delayed, mixing with a suitable oil, such as arachis oil, has this effect,
and by adding palmitic acid, which tends to solidify the fat, absorption is even further delayed. As the esters of some steroids are
less water soluble than the parent substance, absorption of the ester
proceeds more slowly. Absorption may be prolonged further by introducing the hormone in the form of a compressed tablet inserted
surgically into the subcutaneous tissue. Usually the administration
of steroid hormones by mouth is rather wasteful, as they are well
absorbed from the gut but rapidly metabolised in the liver. However, certain synthetic hormones such as ethinyloestradiol, megestrol and methyltestosterone are more slowly metabolised and are
thus suitable for oral administration.

Androgens and oestrogens are absorbed from the skin when applied in alcoholic solution. They are also effective when applied locally. After absorption the steroid hormones are partly combined
with glucuronic acid, the glucuronides so formed are inactive and
water soluble and are excreted in the urine. This glucuronide formation takes place mainly in the liver.

Androgens

Androgens are substances which stimulate the male accessory organs and produce the secondary sex characteristics.

Androgens reverse many of the effects of castration. Testosterone
is such a substance and is formed in the testis. Androsterone is
formed in the body from testosterone and is excreted in the urine.
There are many similar substances which come from the interstitial

cells of the testis and from the adrenal cortex. Synthetic androgens have been prepared. In addition to their effect on the male accessory organs, androgens possess powerful anabolic actions. These are shown by the increased retention of nitrogen and other elements essential for tissue formation, produced when androgens are administered.

The masculinising and anabolic actions of androgens are assayed in different ways. Masculinising activity, for example, can be assayed by measuring the increased growth of the comb of immature cockerels in response to the androgen. The increase in size of the prostate and seminal vesicles of the castrate rat in response to the administration of androgens can also be used as a measure of masculinising activity. Anabolic activity can be measured by determining the increase in nitrogen retention which takes place when a castrate rat is given androgen or the increase in size of the levator ani muscle produced in castrate rats in response to androgen.

Using the two different types of test, it has been possible to prepare compounds in which the virilising and anabolic activities are to a large extent separated. The compound nortestosterone (Nandrolone B.P.), for example, has a marked effect on increasing nitrogen retention and the growth and development of bone. It increases also the strength of healing wounds but has very slight masculinising activity and little progestonal activity.

The negative nitrogen balance and loss of weight produced by the administration of thyroxine can be reversed by testosterone. Testosterone also prevents the degeneration of muscles which occurs after the motor nerves to the muscle are injured. Laying hens can be protected against spontaneous osteoporosis by the administration of androgens. Another development has been the introduction of androgens with a long action. Some of these are fluorinated compounds, such as fluoxymesterone. This drug has about ten times the virilising activity and twenty times the anabolic activity of methyltestosterone. Androgens do not stimulate the testis of males but take its place, and, if the dose is big enough, actually depress the testis by depressing the anterior pituitary gonadotrophin secretion.

Although orally administered testosterone is well absorbed from the gut, when given by this route it does not produce its characteristic pharmacological effects because it is inactivated by the liver and does not reach the systemic circulation. Most of the synthetic androgens may be administered by mouth.

Testosterone is used to aid descent of the testicle but is not as effective as chorionic gonadotrophin. It has been used also to treat mammary tumours in the bitch with equivocal results.

Androgens administered as an aerosol spray can be useful in detecting oestrus in sows. The response of sows in oestrus to pressure on the back is more certainly elicited after such animals have been exposed to androgen in this way. The anabolic androgen trenbolone given as an implant has been used to increase carcase weight in heifers or steers being fattened for beef.

Anti-androgens. Although both oestrogens and progestagens are partial pharmacological antagonists to androgens, compunds have been sought which inhibit the action of androgens. One such compound delmadinone which is more active than progesterone as an androgen antagonist is used to treat prostatic hypertrophy in dogs.

Oestrogens

Oestrogens produce the female characteristics. Acting with other steroids, they produce the behavioural and physical effects known as oestrus when mating is permitted. The production of oestrogen in females is mainly cyclical; the periodic ripening of the Graafian follicles, the main source of oestrogen, being controlled by the gonadotrophins secreted by the pituitary gland. The main naturally occurring oestrogens are oestradiol, oestrone and oestriol. Oestradiol is converted in the body into the two other steroids.

Oestrogens stimulate and maintain the tissues of the reproductive tract, stimulating growth of both muscle and epithelium by a direct action. When oestrogens are administered to an ovariectomised rat or mouse and smears taken from the epithelium of the vagina, cornified cells are seen. These cells are characteristic of oestrus. This test has been used in the biological assay of oestrogenic activity for more than fifty years but bio-assays of various hormones have been virtually replaced by radio-immunoassay. A similar response is obtained when oestrogens are applied locally to the vagina and this response provides a very sensitive test of oestrogenic activity.

The increase in uterine growth which occurs when spayed rodents are given oestrogens is used as a test of oestrogenic activity. The sensitivity of the uterine muscle to pituitary oxytocin is increased by prior treatment of the animal with oestrogen, whereas prior treatment with progesterone diminishes the sensitivity of uterine muscle to oxytocin.

Growth of the mammary glands in both males and females is stimulated by oestrogens. The enlargement of the mammary gland is brought about by an increased growth of ducts and the deposition of fat. In ewes, goats and cows lactation is initiated and maintained. However, this effect in cows is too variable to be used commercially. Low levels of oestrogen activate the lactogenic function of the anterior pituitary but higher levels produce inhibition. Further, lactogenic doses of oestrogen are antagonised by progesterone. Oestrogens are concerned also in the distribution of female fat and sexual changes in the skeleton. They have metabolic actions not unlike those of the androgens, such as increasing the retention of salt, water and nitrogen, in addition to other elements involved in tissue formation. However, the anabolic effects of oestrogens are small compared to those of androgens.

The administration of low doses of oestrogens to anoestrus laboratory animals stimulates the release of gonadotrophins and may re-establish the normal oestrus cycle, but the evidence for this effect in domesticated animals is empirical, although oestrogens certainly induce a behavioural oestrus. Moreover, a single large dose, or repeated small doses, may produce cystic ovaries in the cow; alternatively, oestrogens may cause inhibition of FSH accompanied by a secondary degeneration of the gonads.

The naturally-occuring oestrogens are synthesised in the ovary and placenta. The natural oestrogens are inactivated for the most part in the liver; although some of the oestrogen reaching the liver is excreted in the bile and reabsorbed from the intestine. The endogenous oestrogens are inactivated by conjugation in the body with sulphate and with glucuronide, these conjugates are water soluble and readily excreted by the kidney.

The natural oestrogens are well absorbed from the gut and the reason why their effectiveness when given by this route is limited is probably due to their rapid metabolism in the liver. Certain derivatives of these natural oestrogens are more effective when given by mouth than others; this is because these compounds are more slowly inactivated.

Synthetic oestrogens

Certain simple synthetic substances have oestrogenic activity and these include stilboestrol, hexoestrol and dienoestrol. These stilbenes were previously the main oestrogens used in veterinary practice as they were inexpensive and effective by oral or parenteral administration. However, the demonstration of high residues of diethylstilboestrol in veal-based baby foods in Italy, following its illicit use in veal calves, was the cause of legislation which now prohibits the marketing of stilbenes intended for use in animals of all species throughout the EEC.

Certain esters of natural oestrogens, such as oestradio benzoate, are effective for parenteral therapy, but when oral administration is preferred, alternatives to stilboestrol must be used. Ethinyloestradiol is an example of a synthetic oestrogen which is active when given by mouth and in humans is about twenty times as potent as stilboestrol. It is used in veterinary medicine, in combination with methyltesterone, for suppressing lactation in bitches, but following the ban on the use of stilbenes, it may be used more widely in the future.

Oestrogens have various therapeutic applications. Very large doses may cause abortion by producing hypertrophy of the uterine mucosa and sensitisation of the uterine muscle to oxytocin. However, the results of this treatment for the induction of abortion are somewhat erratic, and prostaglandin or corticosteroid therapy is more reliable. Pregnancy following accidental mating of bitches is effectively prevented by the use of oestrogen within four days of the mating, when it may inhibit the rate of passage of the fertilised ova down the oviducts, in addition to its effect on the uterine mucosa.

Oestradiol is used for its effect on the uterine muscle and mucosa in the treatment of pyometritis and mummified foetus in the cow but as a corpus luteum is commonly present in these conditions, prostaglandins are more rational treatment. It is used, especially in cattle, to facilitate expulsion of the placenta. The effect is presumably produced by sensitising the uterine muscle to oxytocin. Oestrogens also help to increase the resistance of the uterus to infection. However, the use of such a drug in pyometritis in bitches increases the risk of toxaemia. Oestrogens are valuable in the treatment of urinary incontinence and vaginitis in spayed bitches. In the dog, they have been used in the treatment of prostatic hyperplasia and certain tumours, such as anal adenomata.

Sex hormones on growth

Both androgens and oestrogens affect growth and this is utilised in beef cattle by administering suitable preparations to increase the rate of live weight gain. Following the prohibition on the use of stilbenes however, the practice of using hormones for growth promotion in food producing animals is under review.

There is evidence that the growth promoting effect of oestrogens is associated with an increased plasma concentration of insulin and growth hormone, both of which increase tissue amino acid uptake and potentiate the initiation process of protein synthesis. Currently, two oestrogens, zeranol and oestradiol are used for growth promotion in cattle and are administered as solid implants injected subcutaneously at the base of the ear. The oestradiol is incorporated in a silicone rubber implant and provides a continuous low level release of hormone for at least a year. Offal containing those parts of the animal around the implant must be disposed of in a satisfactory manner.

The potent growth promoting properties of the androgens are well demonstrated by the accelerated growth of the musculoskeletal system at puberty. Various anabolic steroids have been synthesised which are derivatives of testosterone but in which the androgenic potency is markedly reduced. For example, trenbolone is used as an implant formulation in heifers or steers being fattened for beef and to improve carcase quality in cull cows. The use of anabolic steroids such as trenbolone, nandrolone and boldenone therapeutically, as opposed to meat production, is still in the stage of exploration. They are used for example, particularly in horses and small animals, to attempt accelerated tissue regeration during convalescence or when bone or tendon healing is delayed.

The androgenic anabolic steroids, unlike the oestrogens, do not appear to affect endogenous hormones, but their precise mode of action is unknown. There is a continuous turnover of amino acids between protein and the amino acid pool; growth and tissue regeneration depend on a positive balance between anabolism and catabolism. Androgens apparently act directly on muscle cells to decrease the rate of protein breakdown, thus increasing the net amount of protein. In addition, they promote the retention of calcium, phosphate, potassium and sodium ions; there is enhanced skeletal growth and increased retention of water.

Progesterone

Progesterone is the hormone released by the corpus luteum. It can be synthesised from a substance in soya beans. With the introduction of synthetic analogues of progesterone with a greatly increased potency and a potentially wide use in population control amongst human beings, the assay of progesterone activity has become increasingly important. Progesterone activity can be assayed in a variety of ways. An assay commonly used involves ovariectomised rats pretreated with oestrogen. The administration of progesterone to such animals causes proliferation of the endometrium which is proportional to the dose of progesterone and can be measured histologically. This test can be simplified by measuring, instead of histological proliferation, increased carbonic anhydrase activity in the endometrium. A test of a different nature involves the effectiveness of the substance under investigation in maintaining pregnancy in ovariectomised rabbits. Rabbits are used because in this species the corpus luteum is the sole source of progesterone. However, the use of these three different tests on the same compounds has given slightly different answers and so they may be testing different kinds of activity. Progesterone itself is assayed by radioimmunoassay and the technique is used, for example, in the differential diagnosis of ovarian cysts in cattle by assaying progesterone in serum or milk. The appropriate treatment for follicular cysts would be either chorionic gonadotrophin or GnRH, but animals with luteinised cysts, indicated by a higher milk progesterone concentration, require prostaglandin therapy.

Although progesterone is well absorbed from the gut it is not very effective when given by mouth, presumably because of its rapid metabolism. However, some of the new synthetic progestagens are very potent when given orally. In the body progesterone is converted into pregnandiol which is excreted in the urine as the inactive glucuronide. The tissues affected by progesterone only respond after having been acted on by oestrogens. Thus progesterone increases the thickness of the uterine mucosa and the complexity of the glands after the uterus has been sensitised by oestrogens. It is involved also in the proper development of the mammary glands, acting on them in conjunction with oestrogen. Progesterone depresses the response of the uterine muscle to oxytocin, and in this respect is antagonistic to oestrogen. The characteristic changes which occur in pseudopregnancy in the bitch are due largely to progesterone.

The chief function of progesterone is to prepare the uterus for the fertilised ovum. If pregnancy occurs the uterus becomes insensitive to oxytocin. This is not true of all animals. It does not happen, for example, in the cat. Progesterone has slight androgenic activity and some activity like that of the cortical hormones. Progesterone and its analogues suppress the formation of FSH and LH by the anterior pituitary. This effect is produced by a feed-back mechanism and has been used to suppress oestrus in the bitch and to synchronise oestrus in cattle, sheep and goats. In the mare, progesterone is produced mainly by the placenta and possibly myometrial activity is suppressed by the presence of a high local concentration of progesterone. This situation could not be imitated by injections, hence the use of progesterone in the treatment of deficiency in the mare does not appear to be very promising. It is interesting to note that, in women, myometrial contractions in threatened abortion can be suppressed by the injection of progesterone directly into the myometrium. That is a 'local' effect which cannot be imitated by intramuscular injections. The importance of progesterone from the corpus luteum in the maintenance of pregnancy in different animals is shown by whether or not the pregnancy is maintained after ovariectomy. In the mare ovariectomy does not cause abortion but is likely to do so in the sow. The corpus luteum appears to be essential throughout pregnancy in the pig and goat but not in ewe, dog and cat. The use of progesterone together with FSH to produce coincident pregnancies in sheep, cows and sows has been discussed (p. 220). The use of FSH is an insurance measure but doubles the cost of treatment. In ewes, a synthetic progestagen may be administered per vagina in the form of an impregnated tampon for this purpose.

Progesterone may be used to treat failure of nidation, for this it is given after ovulation and service. It may be used in the therapy of habitual abortion and to synchronise oestrus in cows. In male animals progesterone may produce an azoospermia which is reversible. The synthetic progestagens have been used to suppress heat in bitches but unfortunately this treatment was found to increase the incidence of cystic endometrial hyperplasia. *Megestrol, norethisterone* and *medroxyprogesterone* are all synthetic compounds with high progestonal acitivity. Medroxyprogesterone is used to impregnate tampons which are inserted into the vagina of sheep to control oestrus.

Prostaglandins

The prostaglandins as examples of autocoids and their role in inflammation are discussed in other sections. In relation to reproduction in domesticated animals, specific emphasis has been on $PGF_{2\alpha}$ and its analogues, although PGE_2 is used in human obstetrics in the induction of abortion and parturition.

There is strong evidence that $PGF_{2\alpha}$ is the physiological uterine luteolysin, released from the uterus at the end of dioestrus to cause luteolysis, possibly being transferred by a local counter-current mechanism from the utero–ovarian vein to the ovarian artery. Recent studies in sheep suggest that this luteolytic action is augmented by release of oxytocin from the ovary, but the physiological role of ovarian oxytocin remains to be determined. $PGF_{2\alpha}$ causes contraction of uterine muscle but also other smooth muscle, which may give rise to abdominal discomfort and respiratory embarrassment when it is used therapeutically. It may be involved in the initiation of parturition since there is an increased concentration of $PGF_{2\alpha}$ in uterine venous blood coincident with increased uterine motility and cervical dilatation. Oxytocin is measurable in plasma at this time and the two hormones appear to produce a cascade effect, each stimulating the release and ecbolic action of the other. Synthetic analogues of $PGF_{2\alpha}$ have been developed; for example, *fluprostenol,* *cloprostenol* and *tiaprost.* The luteolytic activity of these drugs is much greater than that of $PGF_{2\alpha}$ but without a corresponding increase in spasmogenic potency. This is utilised for example in the treatment of anoestrus in cattle and mares, to synchronise oestrus in cattle and sheep, and in the treatment of pyometra and mummified foetus in cattle. In those species dependent on luteal tissue for the maintenance of pregnancy, the drugs are particularly effective in inducing parturition or terminating unwanted pregnancies at certain stages.

FERTILITY CONTROL

In veterinary practice the usual problem in fertility control is to ensure conception and normal pregnancy. The use, for example, of progesterone analogues and gonadotrophins in the timing of pregnancy in ewes has been discussed.

In man, as is well known, one of the major problems of the world is the regulation of pregnancy so as to prevent the population exceeding the food supply. A considerable amount of work in this field has been carried out and is proceeding with the object of providing cheap and satisfactory methods of controlling pregnancy in man. The chemicals used as contraceptives in man are sometimes of interest in veterinary medicine because the same substances may be of value in the control of malignancy and may also provide a possible alternative to some of the poisons and other objectionable methods at present used to control certain species which may become pests. Seals, for example, are controlled at present either by shooting, or by giving strychnine. These procedures are unsatisfactory and not devoid of cruelty and it seems possible that antifertility drugs could control the seal population in a more humane fashion.

Fertility control in the male

The chemical control of spermatogenisis can be exercised either by drugs which inhibit spermatogenesis, and are without effect on the endocrine functions of the testis, or by drugs which, by suppressing pituitary gonadotrophin secretion, inhibit both spermatogenesis and the endocrine function of the testis.

Four types of compound have been found to have activity of the first kind, namely nitrofurans, thiophenes, bis (dichloroacetyl) diamines and dinitropyrrole compounds. The nitrofurans are primarily bacteriostatic drugs, and are also used in the treatment of coccidiosis. When given orally or parenterally in appropriate doses these drugs cause a degeneration of the seminiferous epithelium resulting in arrest of spermatogenesis: this is reversible. The thiophenes have similar activity but both thiophenes and nitrofurans are regarded as too toxic to use in man for their effect on spermatogenesis. However, a series of bis (dichloroacetyl) diamines have been synthesised which inhibit spermatogenesis reversibly without having any effect on the spermatagonal, Leydig or Sertoli cells. In man these drugs have caused gastric upsets and an increase in the sedimentation rate.

The dinitropyrrole compounds arrest spermatogenesis at the primary spermatocyte stage. A single dose of these drugs will inhibit spermatogenesis for as long as four weeks. It appears that the gonadotrophins are essential for activity of the dinitropyrrole drugs. Salts of cadmium have a specific effect on the elements of the testis, causing degeneration which is usually permanent.

Clomiphene (p. 232) is an anti-oestrogen, which acts by inhibiting the secretion of gonadotrophin by the pituitary gland, and thus interferes with spermatogenesis. It also prevents the development of the very young embryo. Methallibure is a hydrazine compound with similar activity which has been withdrawn from the market because of possible hazards due to teratogenicity.

Fertility Control in the Female

Since ovulation does not occur during pregnancy, it appeared highly probable that progesterone was involved in the supression of ovulation. When this probability was investigated, it was found that although progesterone would suppress ovulation, a very large dose was required. However, the introduction of the synthetic progestogens with greatly increased potency has provided a method for controlling pregnancy in man and certain of the domesticated animals.

The use of medroxyprogesterone impregnated tampons for oestrus synchronisation in sheep has been mentioned earlier (p. 228). The suppression of oestrus in cattle has been attempted with a number of synthetic progestogens such as chlormadione, megestrol and melengestrol but with only limited success. Similarly, attempts to synchronise oestrus in goats using medroxyprogesterone have not been entirely satisfactory.

Progestogens are used in the bitch and queen to suppress oestrus. In the bitch, the use of such preparations is either by oral administration, the use of a long-acting injection, or short-term administration. Several untoward sequelae have resulted from the use of these preparations for example, various endometrial disorders have occurred such as cystic glandular hyperplasia. This conditions is more likely to occur after the use of a high dose and/or treatment during pro-oestrus, oestrus or met-oestrus before the endometrial restoration is complete. *Hydroxymethylprogesterone* is used to suppress oestrus in dogs, cats and mares, *norethisterone* is used for this purpose in queens and bitches, *megestrol* in bitches, and *medroxyprogesterone* in bitches and queens.

Delmadinone is a synthetic progestogen which has also anti-oestrogen and anti-androgen properties. It is used in male dogs and cats in the treatment of hypersexuality and in dogs to treat circumanal adenomata and prostatic hypertrophy. Delmadinone has a thymolytic action like cortisol but is devoid of anti-inflammatory action. It is not anabolic but has anticonvulsant properties.

Other methods used for the chemical control of pregnancy have involved drugs which act by inhibiting the implantation of the embryo, or by destruction of the blastocysts. It has also been found that several anti-progestins interfere with nidation; although these compounds were effective in rats and mice they did not act in rabbits. The non-steroid anti-oestrogen compounds have an antifertility action due to their anti-oestrogenic activity.

Anti-oestrogens

This term could include androgens and progestins, excepting the latter compounds act with oestrogen to produce the typical pregnancy changes in the vaginal mucosa. There are, however, many compounds which show anti-oestrogenic activity. Their administration to mice prevents the vagina responding to an oestrogen given subsequently. One compound with high activity of this type is clomiphene. This drug inhibits the gonadotrophic function of the pituitary gland. Small doses stop the oestral cycle of rats and large doses inhibit spermatogenesis. The compound does not appear to have progestational or androgenic activity. It will prevent the action of oestradiol on the mouse uterus but does not interfere with pituitary–adrenal or pituitary–thyroid function and may be useful in regulating pregnancy.

Fertility Control in Insects

Certain insects have been eradicated by releasing sterilised members of the particular species into the infested area. The eradication is effected because the sterile insect on mating with its fertile counterpart produces no progeny. This technique has been applied with success in the control of the screw-worm Fly (*Cochliomyia hominivorax*). The larva of the screw-worm fly live on the flesh of mammals and cause a great deal of harm to livestock. The males of this species mate frequently but the females only once, hence, by releasing a number of sterile males, the fly population can be substantially reduced. In the early experiments of this nature the insects were sterilised by irradiation, but now chemicals are used to produce sterility; one of the best of these is 5-flurouracil.

ECBOLICS (OXYTOCICS)

Drugs which cause contraction of the uterus are called ecbolics or oxytocics. A very important drug with this property is ergometrine, an alkaloid obtained from a fungus or ergot which grows on rye. The fungus is called *Claviceps purpurea*. It contains several other alkaloids and pharmacologically active substances.

The alkaloids of ergot are derived from lysergic acid and include (in addition to ergometrine) ergotoxine, ergotamine, ergosine, ergocristine and ergotycryptine. Pharmacologically they fall into two groups, one group including only ergometrine and the second group the remainder, of which ergotamine is a typical member. This last group is of very little therapeutic value but has an importance in toxicology. Some forage plants become infected with ergots and when eaten by grazing animals produce toxic effects similar to the effects produced by ergotamine.

Characteristic of ergot poisoning are coldness of the extremities and tips of the ears and in pregnant animals foetal death and abortion. Interference with the blood supply to the extremities and ears may lead to necrosis and gangrene.

Ergotamine stimulates contraction in all plain muscle by direct action after a delay of 15–30 minutes. The blood pressure is raised by the contraction of the arteriolar muscle, and if this action is prolonged gangrene of the extremities will be produced. The sphincter pupillae muscle contracts, giving a very small pupil. The sympathetic nervous system is stimulated by the action of ergotamine on the central nervous system. This effect is of limited duration because the effects of adrenergic nerve stimulation are antagonised by ergotamine.

Ergometrine differs from all the other ergot alkaloids in several respects. It is readily soluble in water and rapidly absorbed even when given orally to non-ruminants. Ergometrine produces uterine contractions within five minutes and is the most important constituent of crude preparations of ergot. Plain muscles other than the uterus are little affected by this substance, hence it does not cause gangrene. It stimulates the sympathetic system by direct action but does not paralyse adrenergic nerves. The alkaloid is available as the maleate but is usually considered too expensive to use except in the dog or cat. Because of its prolonged affect, ergometrine should not be used to facilitate parturition. It may cause foetal entrapment leading to hypoxia and death, or in other cases uterine rupture may result. However, the drug is valuable for all control of post-partum haemorrhage and may be used for this purpose after Caesarian operation.

Extracts of the posterior pituitary gland contain an oxytocic principle, *oxytocin*. This active substance is a polypeptide which can be prepared synthetically. The synthetic hormone is available commercially and has the advantage over extracts of the natural gland in being free of antidiuretic hormone. Although a number of synthetic oxytocins have been prepared they have no therapeutic advantage over the original. The main action of oxytocin is on uterine muscle and the myoepithelial cells of the mammary gland. Oxytocin contracts the uterus by direct action on the muscle. As pregnancy progresses the uterus becomes increasingly sensitive to oxytocin. The uterine cervix can contract independently of the body or cornua. The sensitivity of the body of the uterus to oxytocin increases throughout the second half of pregnancy, the increase accelerating just before parturition, whereas the response of the cervix to oxytocin is high in the oestrogenic phase and low in the luteal phase of the reproductive cycle. Oxytocin increases the rate at which spermatozoa ascend the female reproductive tract and is released during coitus in both male and female. Oxytocin causes vascular plain muscle to relax. This action is particularly marked with avian muscle in which species hypotension is produced and is antagonised by the antidiuretic hormone.

The oxytocic principle stimulates the myoepithelial cells of the mammary gland and so produces the 'let down' of milk. The effect on the myoepithelial cells of the guinea-pig mammary gland is used in the assay of oxytocin because it is a very specific response. In conducting parallel quantitative assays, other tests include the response of the uterine muscle of guinea-pigs, or rabbits after the muscle has been sensitised by pre-treatment of the animal with an oestrogen. Specific radio-immunoassays for oxytocin have been developed and are widely used in experimental studies to measure concentrations of the hormone in plasma.

Oxytocin, being a polypeptide must be administered parenterally, it is quickly destroyed in the body by a specific enzyme, and half an administered amount is destroyed within 2–3 minutes in the human, rat, sheep and rabbit. The kidneys and splanchnic organs appear to play an important part in the removal of oxytocin from blood and, in lactating animals, the mammary gland may also be implicated. The specific enzyme, oxytocinase, has so far only been found in the pregnancy plasma of primates and is formed in the placenta. Evidence for the same enzyme being present in the domesticated animals is lacking. The injection of oxytocin given intravenously is the drug of choice to produce the 'let down' of milk as it avoids the complications for which the pressor principle is responsible. These complications include cardiovascular collapse rising from the risk of constriction of the coronary arteries. For the effect on the uterus, oxytocin is given intramuscularly, this route may also have to be used to produce the 'let down' effect in sows.

Oxytocin may be used to induce parturition but this procedure is not devoid of risks. In species in which multiple pregnancies are usual, it sometimes happens that a foetus is prevented from being delivered by a band of contracted uterine muscle induced by the administration of oxytocin causing the foetus to be trapped in a uterine horn. Used with caution, oxytocin is of value in the treatment of dystokia associated with uterine inertia providing always that there is no mechanical obstruction to birth. Oxytocin has been used with advantage in retention of the foetal membranes in cows. For this purpose it is given by intramuscular injection, repeated if necessary at intervals of 20–30 minutes for up to four or five injections. It has been used also in the treatment of bovine mastitis to aid debridement drainage utilising the 'let down' effect and to reduce the size of the uterus in prolapse.

THE INDUCTION OF PARTURITION

The cross-breeding of certain cattle can give rise to dystokia arising from the calf being too big to traverse the genital passage. This can be avoided by inducing labour at an earlier date than the natural parturition. Moreover, there are economic reasons for inducing parturition within a specified period so as to facilitate the deployment of labour. The induction of parturition is also an important method of synchronising deliveries so as to breed at the most desirable time. Elective Caesarian hysterotomy remains the best technique in dogs and cats, but in farm animals, various drugs are used to mimic the hormonal changes associated with parturition.

The induction of parturition by glucocorticoids is possibly accounted for by the high concentration of corticoid in the blood which mimics the signal normally produced from the foetus. This causes the placenta to produce increasing amounts of oestrogen at the expense of progesterone and sensitises the uterus to oxytocin. Glucocorticoids are most effective in cattle and sheep, but only when there is a living foetus, and in cattle, the technique is associated with a high incidence of retained placenta.

In the mare at full-term, the most effective inducing agent appears to be oxytocin, administered intramuscularly in cautiously increased doses. When the cervix is not softened, it may be preceded with oestradiol, injected about 18 hours before the oxytocin. $PGF_{2\alpha}$ has been used as an alternative and as there is no corpus luteum at that stage, the effect is presumably on the cervix and/or the myometrium.

Prostaglandins may be used as alternatives to glucocorticoids to induce parturition in cattle and indeed, where there is a dead foetus, the latter would not be indicated. In the goat and pig, where the corpus luteum is necessary throughout pregnancy, prostaglandins, by virtue of their luteolytic action, are the drugs of choice to induce parturition.

The luteolytic effect of prostaglandins is utilised in all species except dogs and cats to terminate early pregnancy, for example following inadvertent mating or the diagnosis of twin pregnancy in mares. A safe prostaglandin analogue has not yet been introduced for small animals.

UTERINE RELAXANTS

Drugs which cause relaxation of the uterus may have either an anticholinergic or a β-mimetic action. The former appear to be of more value in reducing intestinal tone than in reducing uterine contractions and the group includes hyoscine and methindizate, usually combined with an analgesic.

There is little documentary evidence on the use of β-mimetics such as isoxuprine and clenbuterol (which is also a bronchodilator) in obstetrical work. Preliminary clinical reports suggest that such drugs may be useful before caesarian section, particularly when xylazine has been used, to permit better perfusion of the placenta and improved oxygenation of the neonate, presumably because of uterine relaxation. Relaxation of the uterus is desirable before correcting a foetal malpresentation. In first calf heifers, β-mimetics will delay parturition for up to 14 hours, which permits soft tissues to stretch to facilitate delivery. There is evidence that these drugs will prevent abortion following the stress of laparotomy in mares and cows and they may prove useful, as in human medicine, in the prevention of threatened premature parturition due to other factors.

SUGGESTIONS FOR FURTHER READING

Jones D E, Knifton A 1982 Oestrogen therapy without stilbenes. Veterinary Record 110: 441–443
Laing J A (ed) 1979 Fertility and infertility in domestic animals. Baillière Tindall, London
Lamming G E, Foster J P, Bulman D C 1979 Pharmacological control of reproductive cycles. Veterinary Record 104: 156–160
Proceedings Prostaglandins Symposium 1980 Upjohn Ltd
Short R V (ed) 1979 Reproduction. British Medical Bulletin 35: Number 2
Stabenfeldt G H 1980 Reproductive cycles in domestic animals. In: Phillipson A T, Hall L W, Pritchard W R (eds) Scientific foundations of veterinary medicine. Heinemann, London
Woods A J, Jones J B, Mantle P G 1966 Gangrenous ergotism in cattle. Veterinary Record 78:742

16

Drugs acting on the skin

The chief effects which can be produced on the skin by pharmacological means are, cleansing, antisepsis, stimulation, relief of irritation, inflammation and destruction of parasites. The preparations used for these purposes include lotions, powders, ointments, pastes, dips and sprays. Inflammatory conditions of the skin not caused by a pathogenic organism or parasite are of frequent occurrence, especially in dogs, and are sometimes very difficult to treat. Objective evidence of the efficacy of treatment in such conditions is sparse. A method of testing a remedy for this type of condition is to apply the treatment to one side of the animal only, that is where the disease effects both sides, and, using the other side as a control, the local treatment can be assessed.

Cleansing is usually achieved by the use of soap and water; carbolic soap should not be used on dogs as they are often sensitive to it. The synthetic detergents are useful for both cleansing and disinfecting the skin. They should not be used regularly because they remove natural fats and penetrate the epithelium, making the skin liable to infection. Antisepsis is achieved by using an appropriate disinfectant, stimulation by counter-irritation. The relief of irritation sometimes requires a local anaesthetic and inflammation can be relieved by using a corticosteroid. Corticosteroids used locally must be in the active form because they cannot undergo biotransformation until they are absorbed; for example, preparations containing cortisol and not cortisone should be used. Certain skin diseases in dogs and cats are associated with disturbances of the metabolism of the sex hormones and are treated by the administration of oestrogens, anabolic steroids, or progestagens.

The destruction of ectoparasites involves the use of specific parasiticides. It is sometimes possible to treat parasitic conditions of the skin by giving drugs systemically, for example, ringworm, a disease caused by a fungus, may be treated with griseofulvin given systemically. Certain organophosphorus compounds can be given orally to treat warble fly infestation.

When irritation and itching of the skin occurs, animals usually make matters worse by adding mechanical damage by scratching, biting or rubbing the part. It is known from experiments on man that histamine, histamine liberators, certain proteolytic enzymes and bradykinin when applied locally cause itching or irritation. This observation led to the use of antihistamines as local applications to alleviate pruritis. Unfortunately such local applications were found to be ineffective.

The absorption of most drugs through the skin takes place very slowly. However, some substances are well absorbed such as lipid soluble substances and their absorption can be accelerated by being applied in a fat solvent.

Dimethylsulphoxide is a widely used industrial solvent. Pure preparations of this water-miscible organic solvent have potential therapeutic uses. It is rapidly absorbed through the skin or gut an appreciable amount passing through the skin within 30 minutes. After topical application about 70% appears in the urine partly unchanged, partly conjugated with sulphuric acid and partly as other metabolites such as dimethyl sulphone. This latter metabolite has been found in blood and milk after the use of the compound in cattle. Dimethylsulphoxide has mild antiseptic properties. When applied locally it produces analgesia around the affected area. As single or repeated doses its toxicity is low. It has some solvent action on collagen and has been used as an anti-inflammatory agent. However, its main potential use is to transport steroids and large molecules across biological membranes — especially skin.

Occasionally the passage of drugs through the skin has been promoted by electrophoresis. In this technique the drug is driven by an electrical current through the ducts of the sweat glands. It has little practical applicability in veterinary medicine.

The skin of mice is frequently used as the test organ for carcinogenic activity. Many chemicals with carcinogenic activity will show this property when applied to the skin of the mouse over a period of weeks or months.

Powders are used as antiseptics and to relieve irritation. Boric acid is a common antiseptic powder but has a very feeble action. Magnesium trisilicate (talc) is an insoluble inert powder mainly used to allay friction. Talc should not be used to powder rubber gloves or any appliance likely to be introduced into the abdomen as the talc particles act as foreign bodies and cause a tissue reaction.

A suitable powder for dusting gloves and instruments is sterile starch powder which is absorbed.

Lotions are preparations containing medicinal substances either in suspension or solution. They are of various kinds, such as antiseptic, irritant, protective and astringent lotions. Protective lotions are probably the most important, the commonest being calamine lotion which acts by depositing calamine, zinc carbonate, on the skin. The drying effect of watery lotions on the skin is reduced by adding 3% glycerin.

Astringent lotions precipitate the proteins of the surface epithelium and thus harden the epidermis. An example of such a lotion is a dilute solution of lead acetate. This lotion is popular in equine circles for application to horses' legs. Alcohol is also a good astringent.

Ointments consist of one or more active ingredients mixed with a fatty base and are intended for application to the skin. The main difference between ointment bases is that some are absorbed through the skin. These include lanoline, lard and emulsifying bases. Soft paraffin and bees-wax are not absorbed. The latter substance is used to stiffen an ointment. Emulsifying bases are of two kinds, those making an oil-in-water emulsion such as 'lanette wax' and the water-in-oil emulsion 'cold cream' in which the oil forms the continuous phase. Applying an ointment with vigorous rubbing increases the absorption. Sometimes it is necessary to stiffen an ointment. This is done by adding inert powders such as zinc oxide or starch. If the powder represents more than 10% of the preparation it is called a *paste*. Pastes are often preferred to ointments because they are cleaner to apply and less is required.

The water soluble emulsifying ointments are mixtures of macrogels and polyethylene glycols. They are readily removed and used as lubricants and as vehicles to allow the passage of active drugs such as hydrocortisone into the skin.

The application of an ointment or paste is the most popular method of treating a skin disease, excepting where the cause is a parasite for which a specific treatment exists. Sulphur ointment is sometimes used to treat infections of the hair follicles and in some amounts of hydrogen sulphide. An ointment for treating eye infections is made with yellow oxide of mercury which exerts a mild antiseptic action. It may cause inflammation. Although ointments containing antibiotics and chemotherapeutic agents are very popular, they are not necessarily always better than the older, simpler preparations because they may cause sensitivity reactions and are usually more expensive. The conjuctiva can be protected from irritation, such as may occur when certain volatile anaesthetics are given by mask, by introducing into the eye a few drops of castor oil.

Preparations containing hydrocortisone or other glucocorticoid are popular in the treatment of a variety of skin diseases. They are effective in certain allergic conditions and may reduce the response of the skin to injury. There are, however, hazards associated with even their local application, this is especially the case with the very potent fluorinated steroids. With these latter compounds sufficient quantities can be absorbed from local applications to produce systemic effects including adrenocortical depression. They may also be teratogenic. They reduce the normal defence mechanisms of the skin and thus may aggravate an existing infection or allow infection to supervene. To overcome this hazard they are sometimes combined with an antibiotic, this in turn introduces new factors. Cortisone and prednisone are ineffective as local applications because they require conversion to the active forms hydrocortisone and prednisolone which should be used in their place. The most potent compounds for use on the skin are the fluorinated compounds such as betamethasone and triamcinolone.

Potassium hydroxyquinoline sulphate is a drug with antibacterial, antifungal, deodorant and keratolytic properties. It may be used in the treatment by local application of fungal and bacterial infections. **Chlorquinaldol** is a drug with properties similar to those of potassium hydroxyquinoline sulphate and is used for similar purposes. **Polynoxylin** has antibacterial and anti-fungal actions. It acts by releasing formaldehyde and has been used as a cream or powder for the treatment of skin infections particularly those due to gram negative organisms. **Miconazole** nitrate has a wide range of antifungal activity. It also has some antibacterial actions. There is evidence that betamethasone used as the valerate is particularly effective against inflammatory conditions of the skin. It may be necessary to combine this glucocorticoid with a suitable antibacterial agent.

Depilatories are substances which remove hair from the skin. Barium sulphide produces this effect by dissolving the hair shaft and in this way resembles shaving. Exposure to an adequate dose of X-rays produces a slight erythema and loss of hair on the part exposed. Larger doses of X-rays cause permanent damage with ulceration and scarring. Such burns may result from a single large dose or from repeated small doses. The hair does not fall off until about three weeks after exposure, and regeneration takes up to three months. Exposures to X-rays have been used to treat ring-worm and some skin tumours.

The elimination of shearing by using drugs to allow sheep to be plucked is now a possibility.

Cyclophosphamide given orally or intravenously produces a thinning of the wool fibre which enables the fleece to be plucked 7 days after administration. It is preferable, however, to wait for 3 weeks before plucking, thus allowing a short growth of new fleece. The drug probably acts by interfering with mitosis and doses which produce de-fleecing do not appear to cause any obvious toxic effects.

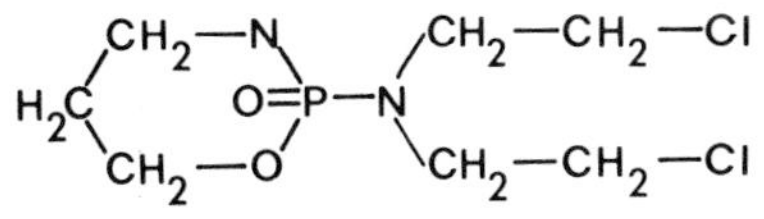

Fig. 16.1 Cyclophosphamide

Cyclophosphamide when given in gelatine capsules to sheep is completely absorbed within three hours of administration. Within 24 hours of administration between 60–80% of the dose is excreted in the urine, however, the drug can still be detected in the liver, kidney, lungs, heart and spleen up to 14 days of the treatment. When given together with streptomycin and penicillin it is more than 90% efficacious in the treatment of mycotic dermatitis in sheep.

Cyclophosphomide is an alkylating agent developed from the mustard war gases and used in tumour chemotherapy.

Several drugs are used to destroy unwanted living tissue such as warts, horn buds and excess granulation tissue. The mildest of these agents are called *keratolytics*, e.g. salicylic acid, and the strongest *caustics*. Some caustics, such as caustic soda, tend to spread and thus destroy more tissue than intended. Other caustics penetrate too deeply because the compound formed between the caustic and skin protein dissolves in a solution of sodium chloride; mercuric chloride behaves in this fashion. The best caustic is silver nitrate because it is self limiting, being precipitated by sodium chloride. However, it causes a good deal of pain when applied to exposed tissues. Copper sulphate is also used as a caustic but is more painful than silver nitrate.

Styptics are substances used to control small superficial haemorrhages. They act by precipitating protein. The commonest styptics are alum, tannic acid, ferric chloride and Friar's balsam.

Counter-irritants are agents which cause local vasodilation and increase the blood flow to an affected part. This increased blood flow is presumed to facilitate healing. Counter-irritants stimulate sensory nerve-endings, thus producing vasodilation by reflexes acting through the posterior roots. This stimulation of sensory nerve-endings can also stimulate medullary reflexes concerned with respiration and circulation.

Rubefacients are substances causing redness of the skin which is accompanied by heat and swelling. These signs are those of early inflammatory change and are produced in a variety of ways. The simplest method is the application of hot water as in hot fomentation; a longer-lasting heat may be applied by a heated poultice. Kaolin poultice (cataplasm of Kaolin) is one of the most convenient. A similar effect is produced by rubbing the affected part with a liniment. *Liniments* are made by incorporating an active substance with an oil. Examples of such preparations are liniments of camphor, ammonia and turpentine. A rubefacient effect can be produced by repeatedly painting the skin with iodine, by applying a mustard plaster, by radiant heat, diathermy short wave and infrared therapy.

Methyl salicylate in an ointment or liniment combines counter-irritation with the anti-inflammatory and analgesic properties of the salicylates as an appreciable amount of this drug can be absorbed through the skin.

Vesicants or epispastics are agents which cause blisters to form in the skin. They produce first a rubefacient effect which is followed by the exudation of lymph beneath the stratum corneum, raising it to form a blister. The local anodyne effect is followed by pain which subsides when blisters form. The vesicants used in veterinary practice are 'green blister' made from cantharides and 'red blister' from biniodide of mercury. 'Blisters' are used in horse practice to treat chronic inflammatory conditions of the limb joints and tendons. Whether their use is justified other than by custom is open to question.

A more powerful counter-irritant than a vesicant is a *pustulant*. This is a drug which when applied to the skin causes blisters which involve the deeper layers. This blister is accompanied by the migration of leucocytes, suppuration and scarring. These effects are produced by croton oil and tartar emetic, substances which should have no place in veterinary therapeutics. The use of the actual cautery or 'firing' is also used to produce counter irritation in horses. There is no evidence of 'firing' being of any value and the practice should cease.

SUGGESTIONS FOR FURTHER READING

Barr M 1962 Percutaneous absorption. Journal of Pharmacological Science 51:395
David N A 1972 The pharmacology of dimethylsulphoxide. Annual Review of Pharmacology 12:353
Keele C A, Armstrong D 1964 Substances producing pain and itch. Arnold, London

17

Autocoids, inflammation and hypersensitivity

Inflammation is a highly dynamic reaction of living tissue to injury. The purposes of the inflammatory process are presumably to counteract the injurious agents and facilitate the repair of damaged tissue. Inflammation, as a normal part of homeostasis, is essential to the survival of the organism. However, in certain circumstances, it may become even more harmful than the original injuring agent. The inflammatory mechanism comprises a very complex series of events, the fundamental characteristics of which are similar, irrespective of the anatomical location and the nature of the offending cause. The inducers of inflammation include physical and chemical injury, antigen-antibody interactions and the products of tissue lysis.

ACUTE INFLAMMATION

The so-called 'cardinal' signs of inflammation have classically been considered to be pain, heat, redness, swelling and impairment of function. Pain is probably caused by chemical mediators, coupled with pressure of extravascular fluid, acting on sensory nerves. Local heat and redness arise from dilatation of the microvasculature, particularly the venules. Swelling is produced by increased permeability of the venules with consequent loss of fluid, electrolytes and proteins from the plasma into the tissue spaces. This process may be referred to as transudation or exudation, depending on circumstances. The nature of impaired organ function is obscure and may simply be an avoidance of activity in a painful swollen organ or there may be unknown biochemical alterations underlying it.

The acute inflammatory mechanism may be classified arbitrarily into three broad phases: (a) the *haemodynamic* phase; (b) the phase of *increased permeability*; (c) the *cellular* phase. The haemodynamic changes comprise arteriolar dilation followed by venous congestion. opening of capillary beds, concentration of red cells and stasis of flow. These events are accompanied by, or followed by, oedema formation caused by extravasation of plasma constituents through the junctions between adjacent endothelial cells and the basement membrane of the blood vessel. The third phase of acute inflammation involves the appearance of leucocytes in the extravascular spaces at a site of inflammation. The sequence of events is: (a) margination and 'pavementing' of circulating leucocytes (i.e. layering of leucocytes on the endothelial cells); (b) emigration (escape) of leucocytes into extravascular sites; (c) chemotaxis or migration of leucocytes towards foci of attractive chemicals; (d) aggregation of leucocytes followed by phagocytosis and release of lysosomal enzymes from the leucocytes.

CHRONIC INFLAMMATION AND REPAIR

In the late phase of acute inflammation it is postulated that neutrophils release chemical substances which are attractive to mononuclear cells, including macrophages and lymphocytes. These, in turn, are apparently responsible for stimulating fibroblasts and causing capillary regeneration, necessary for proper wound healing. In circumstances where an irritant persists, mononuclear cells and capillaries proliferate excessively and create a chronic inflammatory lesion persisting for weeks or even years. This may even give rise to discrete growths or granulomata. Generally speaking, removal of the irritant is accompanied by disappearance of the reaction.

Hypersensitivity (allergy) refers to a complex group of immunological reactions which are characterised by heightened responsiveness to antigen, to which an animal previously has been exposed (sensitized). Hypersensitivity may often be an important cause of acute and chronic inflammation. Four types or classes of hypersensitivity have been proposed. *Type I*, or immediate, hypersensitivity occurs when antigen combines with mast cell or basophil-bound antibodies, usually IgE. The cells degranulate and liberate a variety of chemical substances including histamine (see below). Examples of this reaction include allergies to certain drugs, vaccines and parasites, and systemic anaphylactic shock. *Type II* hypersensitivity involves the antigens of cell membranes, e.g. the blood-group antigens of erythrocytes. Transfusion of blood into an imcompatible host results in an interaction between donor red cells and the recipient's plasma antibodies, leading to haemolysis and complement fixation. Some drugs bind to cell membranes and create a 'foreign' surface which thus becomes antigenic and may lead to a similar cytolytic effect. *Type III* allergic reactions are induced by non-cytotropic antibodies which fix complement and form complexes with antigen. Such immune complexes may be phagocytosed by neutrophils and macrophages and lead to the release of lysosomal enzymes which cause tissue destruction characterized by vasculitis, thrombosis and haemorrhage. Localized type III reactions (tissue antigen encounters circulating antibody) are called *Arthus* reactions. Generalised type III reactions are exemplified by systemic vasculitis or *'serum sickness'*. *Type IV* hypersensitivity, commonly known as *delayed hypersensitivity*, occurs in the absence of demonstrable antibody and is the result of previously sensitized lymphocytes (T-cells) encountering the sensitizing antigen. Activated T-lymphocytes release a series of chemicals known as lymphokins or cytokins which further recruit other mononuclear cells and neutrophils to the site. Classical type IV responses include the tuberculin reaction and 'contact'dermatitis.

CHEMICAL MEDIATORS OF INFLAMMATION

Injury, irrespective of the cause or location, always induces inflammation by liberating a mixture of chemical (pharmacological) mediators. The exact mixture and relative importance of each chemical constituent depends on the animal species, the organ-system affected and the nature of the injury.

These agents are sometimes referred to as autacoids, a term derived from two Greek words meaning 'self' and 'remedy'. There are many autacoids in the body with widely different chemical structures and mechanisms of action but sharing many pathophysiological properties. Smooth muscle and sensory nerve stimulation, promotion of vascular permeability, and recruitment of leucocytes are properties generally shared among most of the chemical mediators. Anti-inflammatory and anti-allergic drugs generally act by preventing the synthesis or liberation of chemical mediators or by acting as physiological or pharmacological antagonists to the mediators.

THE BIOGENIC AMINES

Histamine is formed by decarboxylation of the dietary amino acid histidine (Fig. 17.1). The enzyme histidine decarboxylase is present in most tissues which, consequently, are capable of synthesising

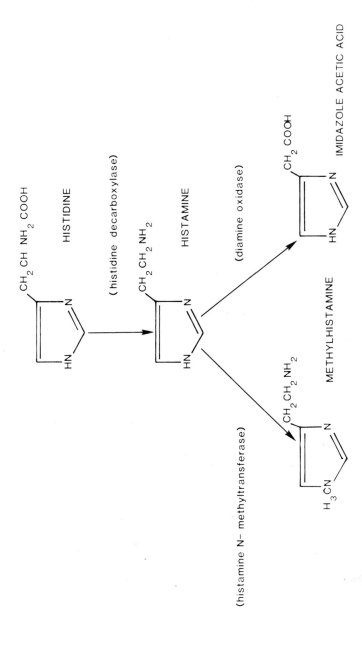

Fig. 17.1 Synthesis and catabolism of histamine

histamine. Although histamine is present in central nervous system neurones and in epithelial cells, the amine in these locations probably does not participate in inflammatory processes. The histamine pool which responds to inflammation and hypersensitivity is stored mainly in tissue mast cells, circulating basophils and, in some species, platelets. In these cells histamine is stored in granules bound to heparin and protein. Tissue injury by physical, chemical or immunological means causes mast cells and basophils to degranulate and to release histamine. Injury may also enhance histidine decarboxylase activity and thus increase the quantity of histamine formed. This may account in part for delayed vasodilatation and chemotaxis, characteristic of some forms of inflammation. Many common drugs release histamine and heparin from mast cells and basophils. These include curare, morphine, the diamidines, organic arsenicals, polymyxin and succinylcholine. In addition, lysosomal proteases, bacterial toxins, complement components, insect, reptile and fish venoms may liberate histamine from mast cells and basophils. A powerful and selective histamine releaser known as Compound 48/80 is a mixture of polymers of N-methylmethoxyethylamine and formaldehyde. This drug has been extensively used experimentally as it has been shown to mimic 'allergic' histamine release in some laboratory animal species.

Histamine is well absorbed from all parenteral sites of administration, but only a little is absorbed after oral administration because histamine, given by mouth or produced in the gut by the activity of bacterial decarboxylating enzymes, is rapidly metabolised by intestinal bacteria and by enzymes in the intestinal mucous membrane. Histamine is metabolised partly by methylation to produce methylhistamine and partly by oxidation to imidazole acetic acid. In herbivores the major route of inactivation of histamine appears to be by oxidative deamination and no inactivation by methylation occurs in this species, whereas in the dog and cat methylation predominates. The oxidation of histamine is catalysed by an enzyme histaminase (diamine oxidase). Herbivorous animals excrete in the urine a substantial quantity of acetyl histamine which is pharmacologically inactive. It arises mainly as a result of the acetylation of histamine by intestinal bacteria.

The original assays of histamine were conducted on the isolated guinea-pig ileum, the cat's blood pressure and the guinea-pig uterus. More recent developments in chemical assay of biologically active substances have yielded more sensitive and more accurate methods. These include spectrophotofluorimetry and radioimmunoassay. For further information the reader should consult the literature.

Pharmacological actions

Histamine possesses very marked biological activity which has been the subject of intensive medical research interest since the beginning of the 20th century. Among the more important actions of histamine are dilatation and increased permeability of the microvasculature. Although it is common to speak of increased capillary permeability, it is probably the very small venules which show this phenomenon. The effect of histamine on the arterioles varies with the species; in rodents the arterioles contract, in cats the contraction is only slight and in the dog there is dilation of the arterioles. Big doses of histamine generally cause blood to collect in the capillaries and the plasma to be filtered off; this results in haemoconcentration and produces a clinical condition which is called shock.

Histamine causes contraction of nearly all smooth muscle. However, different species vary in their response to histamine; the guinea-pig is very sensitive and histamine causes death in this animal by producing a marked broncho-constriction and asphyxia. In the dog death is said to be produced by constriction of the hepatic veins and a fall in venous return. In ruminants and swine, histamine produces systemic hypotension and pulmonary hypertension, the latter due principally to histamine constricting the pulmonary veins. This not only decreases venous return to the heart, reducing cardiac output and blood pressure; it also increases pulmonary vascular hydrostatic pressures which, coupled with increased vascular permeability, is thought to be a major cause of inflammatory pulmonary oedema in these species.

Histamine antagonists (antihistamines)

Specific inhibitors of the actions of histamine were first described in the 1930s as potential anti-allergic agents. Antagonists of histamine are now classified in several ways. *Physiological* antagonists are substances such as adrenaline, isoprenaline and many other sympathomimetics (see Ch. 6). Such drugs have many actions opposite to those of histamine and therefore are antagonistic to it. *Competitive* antagonists are said to act by competing for occupancy of the same receptors in the tissues. Competitive antagonists generally have a molecular structure similar to the agonist and are evaluated by measuring their ability to protect against the actions of histamine in living animals or isolated tissues.

Competitive histamine antagonists are now further classified according to which of the two known histamine receptors is inhibited. The two classes are H_1-*receptor* or H_2-*receptor*-blocking agents. All compounds which antagonise histamine in inflammation are H_1-receptor blockers, inhibiting the actions of histamine on smooth muscle, vasculature and exocrine glands.

Many H_1-*antagonists* have been synthesized and introduced into clinical practice. They include *mepyramine* (pyrilamine), *tripelennamine, promethazine, trimeprazine, diphenhydramine, dimenhydrinate, chlorcyclizine* and *chlorpheniramine* (Fig. 17.2).

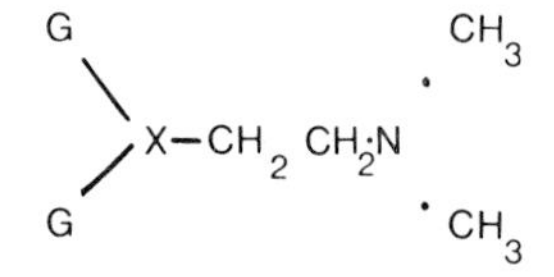

Fig. 17.2a Structural formula of a typical Histamine H. antagonist

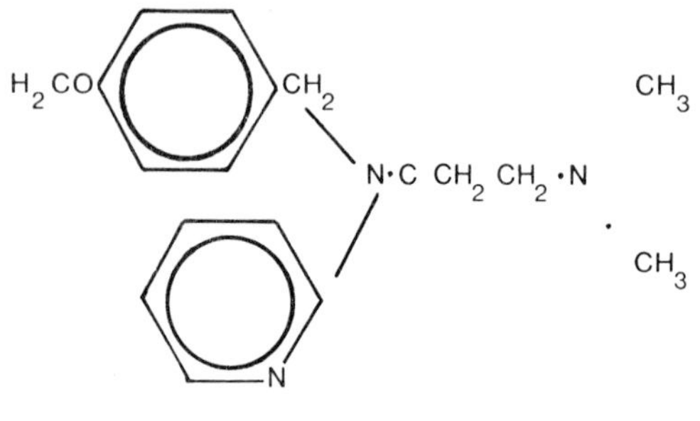

Fig. 17.2b Formula of mepyramine (pyrilamine)

Mepyramine (pyrilamine) is a typical antihistamine and may serve as a general model. It is specific and very active; protecting guinea-pigs against 80 times a lethal dose of histamine. Mepyramine antagonises the actions of histamine on the blood vessels, bronchi and intestines, but not on gastric secretion. The drug has a powerful local anaesthetic effect and a quinidine-like action on the heart. It has some atropine-like effect, however the other antihistamines have greater atropine-like actions; are generally less specific and more depressant to the CNS. The antihistamines protect against the effects of histamine released either in anaphylaxis or by drugs, however they do not prevent the release of histamine in these circumstances. The degree of protection against inflammation by antihistamines varies with the species, for example, they give essentially no protection in rats and mice, a little in ruminants, an appreciable amount in man and dog and almost complete protection in the guinea-pig. Whether or not an antihistamine protects against anaphylaxis depends in part on the sensitivity of the particular species to histamine. The rat and mouse, for example, being relatively insensitive are not protected. Moreover anaphylaxis, in the species which are not well protected by antihistamines, involves active substances other than histamine (see below).

Mepyramine is absorbed from the intestine, producing a maximum effect in one to two hours which lasts three to four hours. Promethazine reaches a maximum effect after oral administration in four to five hours and persists for 24 hours. Antihistamines are partly destroyed in the body and partly excreted in the urine. In the large animals they are given by injection. If these drugs are given by rapid intravenous injection, a fall in blood pressure is produced. This may be due to depression of the heart and it does not generally occur when they are injected slowly. The antihistamines are used therapeutically to counteract various allergic conditions, and to antagonise the effects of histamine released by drugs.

Antihistamine drugs are also of value in the prevention of motion sickness (p. 191), although not all compounds are equally suitable. Diphenhydramine, chlorcyclizine and promethazine are valuable for this purpose. They do not appear to act on the CTZ because apomorphine-induced vomiting is unaffected by pre-treatment with these antihistamines. Similarly their effect does not seem to be simple depression of the vomiting centre. Promethazine and trimeprazine are used as tranquilisers. Diphenhydramine is an antihistamine with marked depressant actions on the central nervous system. Certain antihistamines, e.g. tripelennamine, may stimulate the central nervous system. This effect is utilised for the stimulation of the recumbent cow. Destructive antagonists of histamine include the enzyme histaminase and are not of therapeutic importance.

Antihistamines possess several clinical limitations. Unlike the sympathomimetics, antihistamines lack any direct ability to reverse (repair) the inflammatory process or to inhibit mediator release. As their actions are relatively slow in onset (compared with adrenaline), antihistamines are generally useless in treating peracute reactions such as anaphylactic shock. Apart from allergic dermatoses and nasolachrymal hypersensitivities, H_1-receptor blocking agents have not been particularly rewarding drugs in clinical veterinary medicine.

H_2-receptor antagonists were first announced in 1972 with the discovery of the drug *burimamide*. These drugs now number five or six. However the only one currently licensed for human and veterinary use is **cimetidine**. This agent is principally used to block the stimulating action of histamine on gastric acid production; an H_2-receptor-mediated mechanism. Curiously, H_2-blockers antagonise the gastric acid secretagogue effects of histamine, vagal activity (acetylcholine) and gastrin/pentagastrin. Cimetidine is highly effective in controlling gastric hyperacidity and peptic ulceration. Because H_2-receptors may also be important constituents of mast cells and leucocytes; mediating negative feedback mechanisms which inhibit chemical mediator release, H_2-blockers may enhance inflammation rather than inhibit it. As T-type lymphocytes possess modulatory H_2-receptors, their blockade with H_2-antagonists may cause lymphocyte stimulation. Thus, cimetidine is under investigation as a potential immunostimulant (Fig. 17.3).

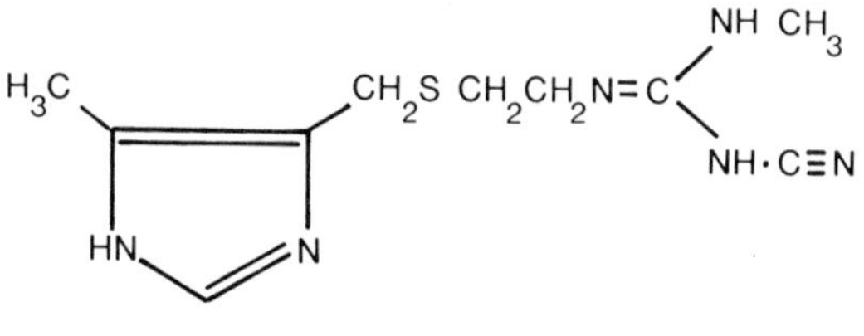

Fig. 17.3 Formula of cimetidine

5-hydroxytryptamine (*5-HT; serotonin*) is an amine which shares many of the biological properties of histamine. It is present in the tissues and causes contraction of smooth muscle in very low concentrations. Most of the 5-HT in the body is synthesised by the hydroxylation and decarboxylation of tryptophan and stored in in the chromaffin cells of the intestine, and in the brain. When 5-HT is liberated in the body or added to blood in vitro it is rapidly taken up by the platelets. When the platelets aggregate 5-HT is liberated. It is also released by drugs such as reserpine and in allergic reactions. 5-HT is destroyed by mono-amine oxidase and excreted in the urine as 5-hydroxyindoleacetic acid (5-HIAA), some of which is conjugated with glucuronic and sulphuric acids. 5-HT is quickly absorbed after parenteral administration but is ineffective when given by mouth.

5-HT stimulates the smooth muscle of the arteries, veins, bronchi, uterus and intestine to contract. The sensitivity of smooth muscle to 5-HT varies with the species. Avian and rat smooth muscle appears very sensitive whilst that from guinea-pigs is relatively insensitive. Sensory nerves are stimulated as are chemoreceptors in the large vessels and lungs, causing a slow pulse and apnoea. The sensory receptors in the intestinal mucosae are also stimulated, promoting peristalsis. It has been suggested that a function of 5-HT in the gastrointestinal tract is to regulate peristalsis. Ganglionic transmission is enhanced by small doses and blocked by large doses of 5-HT. the response to 5-HT varies not only among species but among individual members of a species.

5-HT antagonists. There are a number of drugs which antagonise the effects of 5-HT: some of these act as physiological antagonists, e.g. catecholamines which have pharmacological actions which are directly opposed to the actions of 5-HT. Other drugs antagonise 5-HT by acting on the nervous pathway through which the 5-HT is acting. An example of this type of drug is shown when the slowing of the heart, which is produced by 5-HT, is prevented by the prior administration of either atropine or a ganglion-blocking agent. Atropine or the ganglion-blocking drug prevent the effect of 5-HT by blocking the efferent limb of the reflex on which the cardiac slowing depends.

A third group of 5-HT antagonists selectively inhibit the combination of 5-HT with its receptors on either smooth muscle or nerve cells. These antagonists are various ergot alkaloids or derivatives of these alkaloids containing *lysergic acid*. An important member of the latter group is lysergic acid diethylamide (LSD). In man this drug has interesting central actions in that it gives rise to hallucinations. Reserpine, which is a potent tranquiliser, depletes the brain of its 5-HT. It has been shown that 5-HT is a neurotransmitter in the central nervous system. A potent antagonist of 5-HT is the lysergic acid derivative *methysergide*. However, no single antagonist of 5-HT completely blocks all its pharmacological activity. Recently it has been possible to classify 5-HT or tryptamine receptors into two types: 5-HT_1-receptors in the nervous system and 5-HT_2-receptors predominantly in smooth muscle. A newly announced 5-HT_2-receptor antagonist, *Ketanserin*, is currently being evaluated as an inhibitor of the inflammatory effects of 5-HT.

5-HT is a component of the venoms of certain animals and

plants. It is involved also in some of the responses to inflammation shown in rodents and ruminants. In these species 5-HT is synthesised and stored in mast cells from which it is released by injury together with histamine. 5-HT does not appear to be present in the mast cells of other species.

Dopamine has been located in the mast cells of ruminants, from where it is released following mast-cell-dependent inflammatory reactions, e.g. type I hypersensitivity. Dopamine possesses few if any, inflammatory properties in its own right. However, this catecholamine stimulates a specific dopamine-receptor-mediated positive feedback mechanism on the mast cells of ruminants, leading to enhanced release of histamine and SRS-A. *Dopamine antagonists* such as *spiperone* and *haloperidol* possess anti-hypersensitivity activity in ruminants. This observation awaits full clinical investigation.

CHEMICAL MEDIATORS OF PROTEIN ORIGIN

Kinins constitute an important group of related polypeptides derived from precursors in the plasma α_2-globulin fraction, collectively known as *kininogen* (Fig. 17.4). The proteolytic enzymes responsible for protein cleavage are called *kallikreins*. These enzymes are to be found as precursors in plasma in a pre-enzyme form

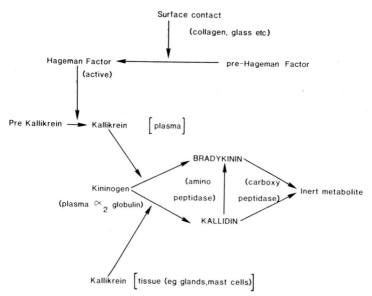

Fig. 17.4 The formation and degraclation of the plasma kinins

known as *prekallikrein* or *kallikreinogen*. Blood pre-kallikreins are converted to the active form by a variety of factors including exposure to foreign surfaces, blood dilution, blood coagulation (Hageman factor: see below) and plant and animal venoms. Kallikreins are also released from certain target cells, e.g. mast cells and leucocytes, during inflammation.

Bradykinin is the 'prototype' of the group: being a nine-amino acid polypeptide. Additional kinins include *kallidin* (or lysyl-bradykinin) which contains ten amino acids and *C-kinin*, a derivative of one of the early complement components (see below).

All kinins cause vasodilatation, increased venular permeability and oedema. They also evoke itch or pain by stimulating sensory nerves. Kinins act on most extravascular smooth muscle, generally causing contraction but occasionally causing relaxation. There is evidence that kinins are leucotactic, i.e. promote 'sticking' of leucocytes to endothelium and eventually their emigration. Kinins are believed to be among the more important general mediators of inflammation. They are rapidly broken down in tissue by kininases (carboxypeptidases) which split off the terminal amino acid from the molecule. It is now believed that bradykinin may act, in part, by activating prostaglandin pathways. This is a possible explanation for the fact that the non-steroidal anti-inflammatory drugs (e.g. salicylates), which inhibit prostaglandin synthesis, antagonise many of the effects of kinins.

Hageman factor (Factor XII) is a β-globulin of approximately 100,000 molecular weight. It is recognised as a blood clotting factor activated by contact with a variety of surfaces including collagen-containing basement membrane of injured vascular endothelium and antigen-antibody complexes. Activated Hageman factor can initiate four different systems relevant to inflammation: blood coagulation, plasminogen to plasmin conversion (fibrinolysis), complement-activation and kinin production. *Plasmin* (fibrinolysin), an enzyme of molecular weight 75,000, can cause the breakdown if fibrin 'clots' activate the first and third components of complement and lead to kinin formation.

Complement is a highly complex self-assembling series of enzymes which are involved in both immunological and non-immunological inflammation. The details of the system are well beyond the scope of this book. However, in essence the 'classical' sequences of biochemical events are as follows. In the presence of calcium the 3 subunits of the first component of complement, C1, are activated in sequence C1q, C1r, C1s, principally by immune complexes. The plasma substrates for activated C1 are C4 and C2 which, when activated (C42), in turn cleave C3 into two parts: C3a (a mast cell degranulator known as anaphylatoxin) and C3b which adheres to C42. This, in turn, splits C5 into C5a (another anaphylatoxin, like C3a) and C5b which adheres to C6 and C7. C5b67 can mediate cell lysis, particularly of erythrocytes. It is chemotactic for neutrophils. The final step in the sequence is the binding of C8 and C9. The ultimate complement complex, C56789, adheres strongly to cell membranes and may induce pore formation, osmotic fragility, cytolysis and cell destruction.

A non-immunological complement activating system, the so-called 'alternative pathway', exists. It may be activated by zymosan or by microbial polysaccharides. This pathway activates the terminal complement factors independent of early components C1, C4 and C2.

Eosinophil chemotactic factor (ECF) is composed of two tetrapeptides released in the preformed state from activated mast cells and basophils. This mediator is selectively chemotactic for eosinophils: cells which are believed to deactivate histamine, prostaglandins and leukotrienes.

Lysosomal enzymes from leucocytes and macrophages. A very large number of hydrolytic enzymes may be liberated from lysosomes following phagocytosis or cell death. Among these enzymes are phosphatases, saccharidases and phospholipases, kallikreins, collagenases, elastases, hyaluronidase and 'endogenous pyrogen'. Lysosomal enzymes directly damage tissue and lead to extensive inflammation.

Lymphokins (cytokines) are glycoproteins, derived from mononuclear cells, which participate in inflammation. Among the numerous factors are *macrophage migration inhibiting factor (MIF)* which immobilises macrophages and hence causes their accumulation at inflamed sites. *Cytotoxin*, a lymphocyte product, can destroy bystander cells. *Chemotactic factor(s)*, also derived from lymphocytes, may attract various classes of leucocytes to injured sites. *Interferon* is currently classified as a cytokine.

INFLAMMATORY MEDIATORS OF LIPID ORIGIN

Prostaglandins

In the 1930s there were several independent reports that seminal fluid possessed smooth muscle contracting and vasodepressor

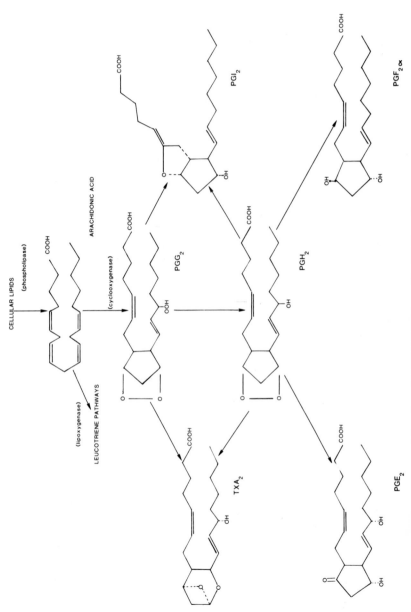

Fig. 17.5 Formation of prostaglandins and thromboxane A₂ by the cyclooxygenase pathway.

activity. Von Euler (1936) named the material *prostaglandin*, as it was thought to be derived from the prostage gland.

Many different prostaglandins have now been isolated as pure compounds. All are derived from 20 carbon fatty acids; the most important of which, in mammals, is *arachidonic acid*. This essential fatty acid is either found in the diet or may be liberated from cell membrane phospholipids by the enzyme *phospholipase A_2*. Arachidonic acid is converted by one of two oxygenating enzymes, *cyclooxygenase* and *lipoxygenase*, into biologically (pharmacologically) active compounds (see Fig. 17.5).

All the so-called 'primary' or 'classical' prostaglandins are products of *cyclooxygenase activity*. The first step is the creation of prostaglandins (PG) G and H, the cyclic endoperoxides, which are biologically active but chemically very unstable. PGG and PGH may subsequently be converted into PGD, E and F. *Classification of the prostaglandins is according to the letters of the alphabet and subscript numbers, depending on substitutions in the cyclopentane ring and the position of double bonds in the side chains.*

PGH_2 may also be converted by alternative pathways to *thromboxane A_2* (TXA_2) and *prostacyclin* (PGI_2). It appears that prostaglandins A, B and C, which are derived from PGEs, may be less important biologically than was originally believed.

Although small fractions of the prostaglandins may be excreted unchanged, the bulk is catabolized rapidly by oxidation at the 15 position by the universal enzyme: *15 hydroxy-prostaglandin dehydrogenase*. Further, several slower forms of degradation also occur.

Actions of prostaglandins

Prostaglandins have profound effects on most body organ-systems. The reader should refer to other chapters for further information. PGEs in the central nervous system cause pyrexia. This may explain the phenomenon of pyrogen-induced fever and the mode of action of anti-inflammatory drugs as antipyretics. PGEs and PGI sensitise peripheral sensory nerves which may contribute to pain production in inflammation.

In the cardiovascular system PGEs generally act as vasodilators. While their direct effect on vascular permeability is small they appear to potentiate other autacoids, e.g. histamine and bradykinin, and thus contribute to inflammatory exudation. Thromboxane A_2, released by platelets, causes the aggregation of platelets and platelet mediator release. Prostacyclin (PGI_2) produced by vascular endothelium in response to TXA_2, inhibits platelet aggregation. PGI_2, may be the natural physiological antagonist to the platelet.

Prostaglandins have powerful actions on smooth muscle. In the airways and gastro-intestinal tracts PGF's and TXA_2 generally cause contraction, whereas PGEs and PGI_2 produce relaxation. Their roles in inflammatory disease in these organs is not yet clear. PGE_1 and PGI_2 have been considered as potential therapeutic bronchodilators.

In addition, prostaglandins have important negative feed back, (i.e. counterinflammatory) effects. PGE's inhibit the release of chemical mediators from mast cells, of lysosomal enzymes from neutrophils and macrophages and of lymphokines from T-lymphocytes. PGE_1 suppresses humoral antibody synthesis.

Leukotrienes

A major alternative pathway of arachidonic acid metabolism is catalysed by *lipoxygenase*, an enzyme apparently confined in distribution to mast cells, macrophages, leucocytes and platelets. The primary step is the creation of hydroxy and hydroperoxytetraenoic acids (HETE and HPETE). These products are found in inflammatory exudates and, being strongly chemotactic for leucocytes, are presumed to participate in the cellular phases of inflammation (Fig. 17.6).

HETEs are subsequently converted into a series of non-cyclized, 20 carbon fatty acids called *leukotrienes* (LT) which, in the manner of the prostaglandins, have been classified alphabetically. LTA is an unstable intermediate. LTB_4 is one of the most potent leucotactic factors known and is presumed to have a key role in the cellular events of inflammation. LTC_4 and LTD_4 are now thought to represent slow-reacting substance of anaphylaxis (SRS-A). SRS-A was first reported in the 1930s as a powerful bronchoconstrictor released from lung along with histamine during anaphylaxis. LTC_4 and D_4 (SRS-A) also dilate and increase permeability of microvasculature. They are implicated in 'allergic' diseases such as atopic skin disease and obstructive pulmonary disease. Inhibitors of SRS-A are thus of considerable therapeutic potential. Paradoxically, inhibitors of prostaglandin synthesis, by blocking the cyclooxygenase pathway, divert arachidonic metabolism towards the lipoxygenase pathway and thus potentiate leukotriene production. The exact consequences of this phenomenon are not fully understood.

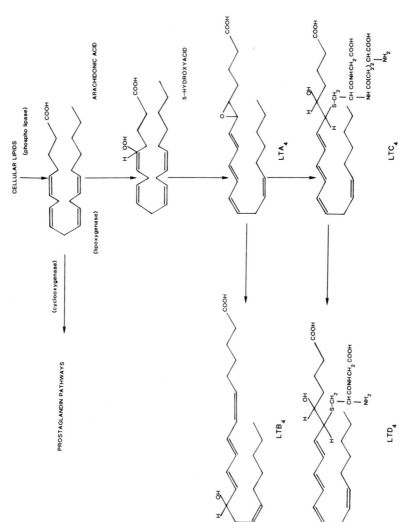

Fig. 17.6 Formation of leucotrienes by the lipoxygenase pathway.

Platelet-activating factor (*PAF*) is a lipid mediator of IgE-dependent reactions of mast cells and basophils. It is acetyl glyceryl ether phosphorylcholine. PAF causes a calcium-dependent aggregation of platelets and the secretion of 5-HT, histamine, thromboxanes and prostaglandins.

PAF is known to be involved in the pathogenesis of immune complex disease and in acute anaphylactic shock: contributing especially to both cardiovascular and pulmonary effects. These facts add yet another dimension to the participation of platelets in immunologically-mediated inflammation. So far there are no satisfactory means of antagonising PAF.

SUGGESTIONS FOR FURTHER READING

Blackwell G J, et al 1982 Glucocorticoid induced anti-inflammatory proteins. Br J Pharmac 76: 185–194
Douglas W W 1980 Autocoids. In: Gilman A G, Goodman L S, Gilman A The Pharmacological Basis of Therapeutics, 6th Ed. Macmillan Publishing Co, NY
Eyre P 1980 Pharmacological Aspects of Hypersensitivity in Domestic Animals. Vet Res Comm 4: 83–98; Elsevier Scientific Publ Co, Amsterdam

18

Antipyretics and anti-inflammatory agents

NON-STEROIDAL ANTI-INFLAMMATORY AGENTS

There is a considerable degree of arbitrariness in describing this group of pharmacological agents and an exact classification is essentially impossible. They are sometimes referred to as *non-steroidal anti-inflammatory agents* (NSAID), a term which will be used throughout this chapter. There are several general chemical classes within this group of drugs, all of which share, to varying degrees, antipyretic, analgesic and anti-inflammatory effects.

Unlike the narcotic analgesics, NSAIDs are relatively inactive when tested by a number of anti-nociceptive tests (described elsewhere in the text). Evidence suggests that NSAIDs act both centrally and peripherally. Their anti-inflammatory actions are essentially peripheral in origin; properties which are not shared by the narcotic analgesics. NSAIDs all share a common ability to block prostaglandin biosynthesis by inhibiting the essential enzyme cyclooxygenase, thus blocking the synthesis of intermediate endoperoxides and blunting the major inflammatory pathways which depend on prostaglandin activity. In addition, this class of drugs is also believed to inhibit kinin formation and to antagonise pharmacologically SRS-A on smooth muscle and vascular endothelium.

In veterinary medicine NSAIDs are used almost entirely for their anti-inflammatory properties and their principal utilisation occurs in the horse and dog.

Salicylates. *Salicylic acid* was first used in the form of bark from the Willow tree which contains a glycoside *salicin*. This glycoside yields salicylic acid on hydrolysis. It is now used in the form of white crystals of sodium salicylate which are very soluble in water.

Salicylates are quickly absorbed from the gut and excreted in all secretions. However, the greater portion is excreted in the urine partly unchanged, partly oxidised and partly combined with glucuronic acid. Since the cat lacks a glucuronide-forming enzyme, salicylates are potentially particularly dangerous in this species and toxic levels may be reached if large or continuous dosage is used. A single dose may take one to two days to be fully excreted.

There are marked differences in the manner in which various species metabolise salicylate and these are reflected to some extent by the varying times required for the concentration in plasma after an intravenous injection to fall to half its initial value. This figure is usually referred to as the plasma half life and for salicylates it is approximately one hour in horses, six hours in pigs, nine hours in dogs, and 36 hours in cats.

Salicylic acid is weakly bacteriostatic, and in concentrated solutions or ointments destroys the skin epithelium without pain. This kind of activity is called keratolytic.

The antipyretic action is seen only in animals with fever. It acts on the central nervous system, producing an increased heat loss by peripheral vasodilation. The analgesic effect is produced without the loss of other sensations. This action may be in part peripheral and arises from the anti-inflammatory action of salicylates, since they relieve the pain produced by the intra-arterial or intra-peritoneal injection of bradykinin. The anti-inflammatory properties of salicylates are possibly due, in part, to the drug inhibiting prostaglandin synthesis.

Salicylates are not devoid of toxic actions. Large doses may cause vomiting in the dog, dyspnoea and skin eruptions. The respiratory stimulation is due mainly to uncoupling oxidative phosphorylation leading to increased CO_2 production. Repeated large doses produce haemorrhages due to a fall in prothrombin. This can be remedied by giving vitamin K or an analogue.

Acetylsalicylic acid is a palatable substitute for salicylic acid, usually given in tablets because it is insoluble in water, unstable and incompatible with most drugs. Its use is confined to the dog and cat to produce analgesia. It is partly hydrolysed in the intestine, but some is absorbed unchanged. The actions of this drug differ from those of salicylic acid in several respects. Some individuals show an allergic response, and it causes hypoprothrombinaemia more easily than salicylic acid.

Methylsalicylate or 'oil of wintergreen' is a colourless liquid with a characteristic taste and smell. The main use of this oil is as a counter-irritant applied locally to the skin. However, it is readily absorbed from the skin and after absorption has an action like sodium salicylate.

Aniline and p. aminophenol have antipyretic activity but are too

Salicylates

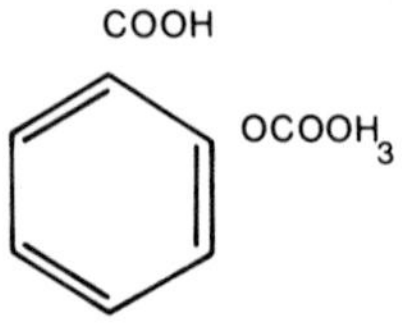

Acetyl salicylic acid

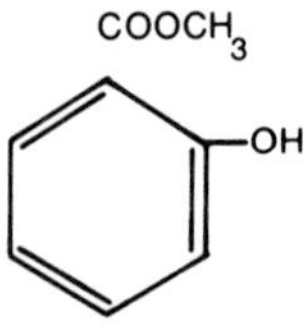

Methyl salicylate

Paraminophenols

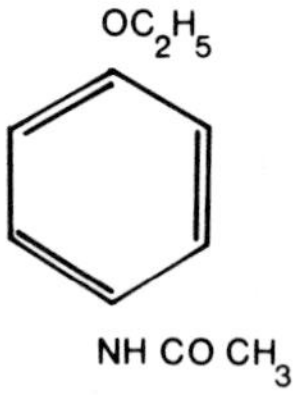

Phenacetin

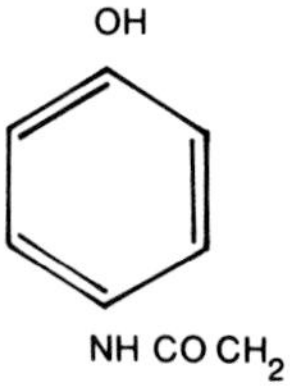

Paracetamol

Pyrazalon

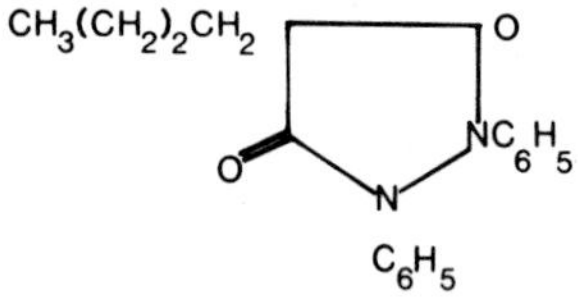

Phenylbutazone

Fig. 18.1 Formulae of some anti-pyretic analgesics

toxic for therapeutic use. However, both acetanilide and phenacetin have been used as anti-pyretics but are now replaced by paracetamol. When phenacetin is given to the dog it is deacetylated because the appropriate enzyme is present in the dog. This gives rise to the free amine. Since an acetylating enzyme is lacking in the dog, the free amine persists and this can give rise to toxic effects such as the formation of methaemoglobin. The replacement of phenacetin by paracetamol in man was due to the fact that the latter was the main active metabolite of phenacetin. The enzyme prostaglandin synthetase in the brain is especially susceptible to inhibition by paracetamol.

Phenylbutazone is a pyrazole derivative related to amidopyrine, used to relieve painful conditions affecting muscles and skeletal structures. It has also an antipyretic action. These, however, are not its sole properties as it influences the tissue reactions involved in inflammation and pain. The tubular re-absorption of sodium and chloride ions is increased by this drug, and may lead to oedema. Phenylbutazone should not be used where there is evidence of disease of the heart, liver or kidney. Horeover, it is advisable to reduce the salt intake of animals receiving phenylbutazone.

Phenylbutazone may be given by mouth; absorption from the gut being rapid. A peak concentration in plasma is reached in about two hours. Intramuscular injections give a peak plasma concentration in 6–10 hours because the drug is fixed to muscle protein and absorption delayed.

Phenylbutazone disappears from the body of the horse or dog within a few hours after absorption, but in man it is metabolised at the rate of about 10–15% per day, hence there is a much greater risk of chronic poisoning from this drug in man than in the horse or dog, and these are the species most likely to be given the drug in veterinary medicine.

The main toxic effects in the dog are nausea and oedema of the limbs, but in man there are many others, including skin sensitisation and damage to haemopoetic tissues.

Indomethacin is an agent with greater anti-inflammatory activity than hydrocortisone in equivalent doses. It is an indole compound

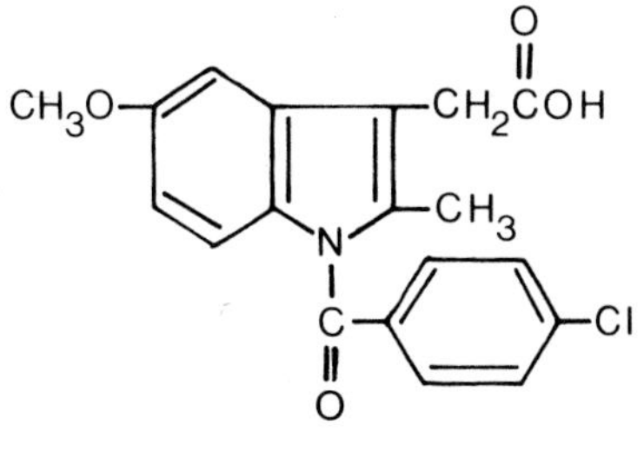

Fig. 18.2 Indomethacin.

which is well absorbed from the gut. The drug has not been widely accepted into veterinary medicine at the present time. This compound has been found particularly useful in osteoarthritis and ankylosing spondylitis. It is arguable that indomethacin is no more effective clinically than aspirin and certainly causes more toxic side effects. These include severe irritation of the digestive tract, depression and ataxia. Irritation of the stomach is extremely common and the drug must always be administered after food.

Meclofenamic Acid is yet another NSAID which, in some tests, has been reported to be up to 10 times as potent as phenylbutazone. As well as preventing prostaglandin release, meclofenamic acid inhibits the migration and phagocytic properties of mononuclear cells. Meclofenamic acid has been recommended as an oral treatment for chronic musculoskeletal inflammation, e.g. osteoarthritis, navicular disease, laminitis. The main toxic side-effect of this drug is gastrointestinal irritation, e.g. mild colic and diarrhoea. Meclofenamic acid is metabolised by the liver and is detectable in urine for 96 hours after cessation of treatment.

Flunixin meglumine is a recently-introduced NSAID which is significantly more potent than meperidine and pentazocine as an analgesic and four times more potent than phenylbutazone as an anti-inflammatory agent. In addition to its usefulness in alleviating musculoskeletal pain, flunixin in contrast to other NSAID, is efficient in controlling visceral pain, e.g. colic in the horse. As far as can be determined, acute and chronic toxicity phenomena are minimal unless the drug is inadvertently injected intra arterially when ataxia and inco-ordination will result. Flunixin is available in oral and injectable forms.

THE ADRENOCORTICAL STEROIDS

The body's responses to harmful stimuli depend on the integrity of the adenohypophseal–adrenocortical system. An interesting theory was put forward by Selye, in which he suggested that certain diseases of so-called 'adaptation' are the result of complex responses of susceptible tissues to the adrenocortical hormones. It is now well known that the corticosteroids alleviated the inflammatory changes in mesenchymal tissues.

Corticotrophin (ACTH)

The pharmacological effects of the corticosteroids may be produced by administering corticotrophin. This hormone of the anterior pituitary gland stimulates the adrenal cortex to release the cortico-steroids, mainly cortisone and cortisol. Corticotrophin is rapidly destroyed in the body and if it is used in treatment, it is necessary to give either frequent intramuscular injections or to use a long-acting preparation. Since the discovery of potent synthetic substitutes for the corticosteroids, there is less need to use corticotrophin, and it is now usual to use one of these potent synthetic analogues. More-over, by using corticotrophin it is impossible to separate the mineralocorticoid from the glucocorticoid effect.

Cortisone and cortisol

These hormones are synthesised from cholesterol by the adrenal cortex. The adrenocortical hormones used for their anti-inflam-matory properties are the glucocorticoids, so-called because they increase the deposition of glycogen in the liver. They are *gluconeo-genic* because they convert amino acids to glucose and decrease utilisation of glucose by the tissues. This may lead to hyperglycae-mia and even glycosurea. The conversion of amino acids to glucose by these compounds reduces the amount of amino acids which is available for conversion into protein. This leads to the defective repair of tissues and in young animals growth may be retarded by the prolonged treatment of an animal with glucocorticoids. The lack of amino acids may lead also to spontaneous fractures of bones be-cause the bones are weakened by this lack, which is often combined with an inhibition of osteoblast activity producing a condition called osteoporosis. Skeletal muscle may show a similar weakening. This condition is termed a 'myopathy'.

The classification of adrenocortical hormones into glucocorticoids and mineralocorticoids is not absolute and most of the hormones of the adrenal cortex have some of either activity; hence the glu-cocorticoids may cause sodium retention and loss of potassium in the urine. The glucocorticoids appear to be involved in the pro-motion of glomerular filtration and the maintenance of urine flow. It is, however, in alleviating inflammatory change that they find their main therapeutic employment.

The presence of glucocorticoids appears to increase the power of the body to withstand various stresses, such as those of trauma, infection and extremes of temperature. It is, however, important to realise that a situation which may be stressful to one species of animal is not necessarily stressful to another. The glucocorticoids suppress the inflammatory response and are used clinically for this effect. Although the exact mechanism whereby this response is produced is so far not fully understood, a number of actions are probably involved. The anti-inflammatory steroids cause the degradation of collagen by increasing the synthesis of certain proteases. They also stabilise cellular and lysosomal membranes which in turn inhibits the release of histamine and phospholipase A_2 and thus prevents the formation of prostaglandins in the area of the inflammation. The anti-inflammatory effect produced by cortisol is much greater than that of cortisone. This is because cortisone is active only after conversion in the liver to cortisol; hence cortisol is the more suitable preparation for local application to suppress the inflammatory response in tissues such as the conjunctiva. The anti-inflammatory effects appear to be due to a direct local action since certain glucocorticoids are effective when applied to skin or eye without there being any detectable systemic absorption. Several of the synthetic glucocorticoids are much more potent in their anti-inflammatory action than cortisol.

Since the glucocorticoids suppress the inflammatory response and fever, many of the objective clinical signs of infection may pass unnoticed and it is essential that a diagnosis should be reached before these drugs are adminstered. When the glucocorticoids are used therapeutically, especially in infective conditions, it is essential to give large doses of appropriate antibiotics simultaneously, both to control and prevent infection because the suppression of the inflammatory response greatly favours the spread of infection. The administration of these drugs may disturb the healing of surgical wounds and, although this could be a potential hazard, it has not so far proved an important contra-indication to the use of these drugs. It is important to realise that the continued administration of glucocorticoids suppresses the normal secretion of corticotrophin, and when the administration of the glucocorticoid stops, there may be signs of corticotrophin lack produced by this feedback mechanism. The signs of a too rapid withdrawal of glucocorticoid therapy are the same as those of acute adrenal insufficiency.

THE RELATION BETWEEN STRUCTURE AND ACTION OF THE CORTICOSTEROIDS

On studying the relationship between the activity of various corticosteroids and their chemical structure, it was found that certain features in the molecule were important in conferring anti-inflammatory activity. The conventional labelling and numbering of the steroid molecule is shown in Figure 18.3. The anti-inflammatory properties of cortisone appear to depend on the ketone group on carbon three; carbons four and five unsaturated; oxygen at carbon 11 and dihydroxyacetone chain at carbon 17. The introduction of a double bond between carbons six and seven pro-

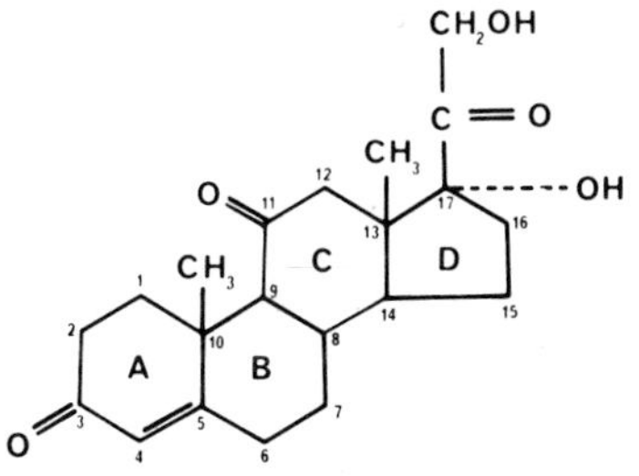

Cortisone

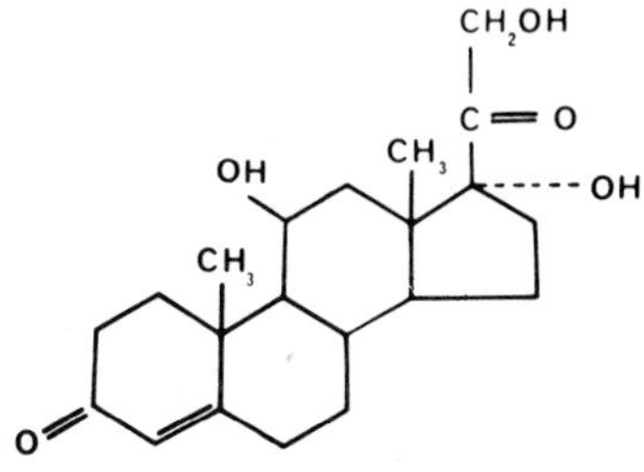

Cortisol

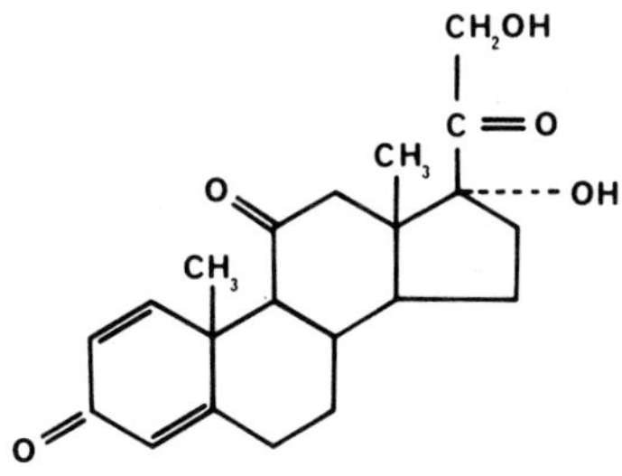

Prednisone

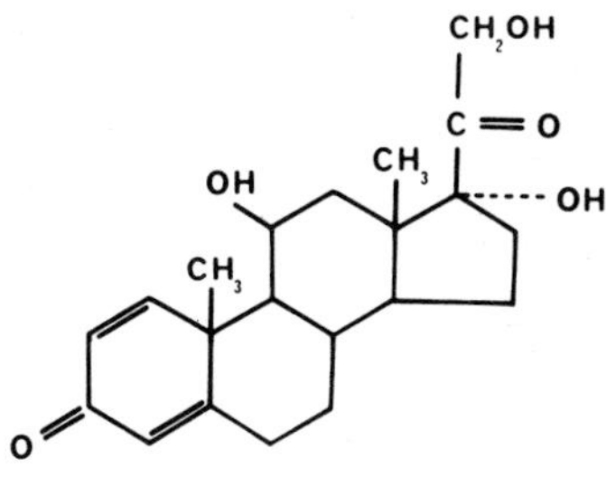

Prednisolone

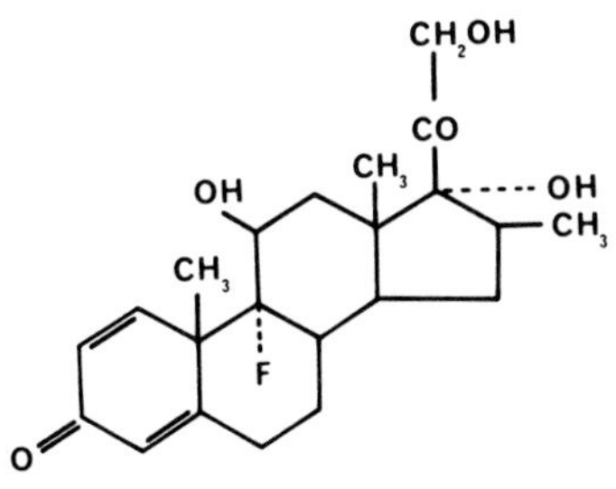

Betamethasone

Fig. 18.3 Adrenocorticosteroids

duced a loss in anti-inflammatory potency, whereas a double bond between carbons one and two increased anti-inflammatory activity without affecting mineralocorticoid activity.

Prednisone and prednisolone

These are synthetic analogues of cortisone and cortisol respectively. They have four to five times the anti-inflammatory activity of the naturally occurring glucocorticoids and have therefore the advantage of requiring a smaller dose to produce the same effect. This reduces the risk of salt and water retention. As with cortisone and cortisol, prednisolone is the main anti-inflammatory compound as prednisone is only active after conversion into prednisolone. These synthetic glucocorticoids are used as anti-inflammatory agents in the treatment of certain skin and orthopedic conditions. In the latter it is sometimes necessary to give them by intra-articular or peri-articular injection. Prednisone and prednisolone are powerful suppressors of the secretion of corticotrophin. Like cortisone and cortisol they are used for their gluconeogenic action in the treatment of ketosis in the dairy cows and as local applications in the treatment of inflammatory conditions of the skin of eye. Caution must be exercised in the application of glucocorticoids together with antibiotics to the eye in case the infection is not susceptible to the particular antibiotic. Moreover, there is evidence that glucocorticoids may induce increased intraocular pressure (glaucoma).

Betamethasone and dexamethasone

Glucocorticoid activity is greatly increased when a fluorine atom is introduced into the 9α position of the corticosteroids. Two such compounds are available for therapeutic use: they are the isomers betamethasone and dexamethasone. The anti-inflammatory activity of these substances is about 25 times as great as that of cortisol, and they are virtually devoid of mineralocorticoid activity. However, they may produce a negative calcium balance because they increase the loss of this element in the faeces. They are used for the same purposes as the other corticosteroids.

Triamcinolone and *Flumethasone* are also synthetic glucocorticoids containing fluorine. Their anti-inflammatory activity lies between that of cortisol and betamethasone. They are virtually devoid of mineral-corticoid activity.

Glucocorticoids have been administered for the induction of parturition in cows. This use arose from observations that not only were deficiencies in the foetal adrenal associated with abnormal or prolonged parturition but also that there was a rise in circulating corticosteroids shortly before parturition.

All corticosteroids can be administered orally, topically and parenterally. The latter includes intramuscular and intrasynovial injections. A single large dose is rarely harmful, and the administration over a few days in the absence of specific contraindications is unlikely to cause harm, but the abrupt termination of prolonged high dosage administration may cause adrenal insufficiency (Addison's syndrome).

When glucocorticoids are administered in large doses they are liable to suppress, but not prevent, skin test reactions. Their use may therefore, on occasion, confuse the results of allergy tests. Glucocorticoids suppress antibody production in some species such as the rabbit and rat but not in others, for example, man and guinea-pig. The situation in the domesticated animals is, as yet, unclear.

The adrenocorticosteroids are present in the plasma bound to the alpha globulin fraction. The half clearance time of cortisone from the body is approximately 30 minutes, whereas for prednisolone it is about 20 minutes. The corticosteroids are not stored in the tissues, but their metabolism may be delayed in liver disease, pregnancy and starvation.

DISODIUM CROMOGLYCATE

Disodium cromoglycate has been used in the management of bronchial asthma since the early 1960s. The drug acts by inhibiting the degranulation of mast cells and basophils which therefore prevents the release of a number of chemical mediators: principally histamine and leukotrienes. Disodium cromoglycate also inhibits cellular phosphodiesterase in a manner similar to the xanthines. In addition the drug protects against hypoxic bronchoconstriction and pulmonary oedema, and inhibits exercise-induced asthma. Clearly disodium cromoglycate has a complex mode of action. The drug is not a direct bronchodilator.

Disodium cromoglycate is used clinically as a prophylactic agent and is administered by inhalation of a powder or solution on a regular intermittent basis. The drug is not useful in controlling established acute asthma. Treatment with disodium cromoglycate is a promising method of controlling chronic obstructive pulmonary disease in horses.

SUGGESTIONS FOR FURTHER READING

Flower R G, Moncada S, Vane G R 1980 Drug Therapy of Inflammation. In: Gilman A G, Goodman L S, Gilman A The Pharmacological Basis of Therapeutics. 6th Ed., Macmillan Publ. Co. NY

Nickander R, McMahon F G, Ridolfo A S 1979 Non-steroidal anti-inflammatory agents. Ann. Rev. Pharmacology Toxicology, 19:469

19

Metals and metalloids of predominantly toxicological interest; chelation therapy

These are substances which do not occur in normal tissues, and have no role to play in normal living processes. At a time when a textbook of materia medica could state without further qualification that 'the bruised leaves (of rue) are put into horses' ears for the staggers', and that in the treatment of foot and mouth disease 'some cattle-masters give common salt in gruel with great success' (*The Druggist's General Receipt Book*, written by Henry Beasley and published by Churchill in 1861), the undeniable potency of the heavy metals must have been a welcome change and the incidence of deaths during therapy either a fair price to pay or, more likely, simply nothing out of the ordinary. Nowadays the maleficence of the heavy metals must be regarded as far outweighing their utility; they should be categorised, unequivocally in the great majority of cases, simply as poisons and their administration regarded as therapeutic atavism.

ARSENIC

Arsenic is the second commonest cause of poisoning in farm animals. The effects of the different arsenical compounds vary markedly, and the physical form may also be an important determinant of its toxicity.

Amongst the *trivalent* arsenical compounds **arsenic trioxide** (by convention As_2O_3, but actually As_4O_6) is probably the commonest in agricultural and domestic use; it has been used as a weedkiller and wood preservative. It was commonly used as an insecticidal preservative in taxidermy, and is still sometimes used as a sheep dip, especially in third world countries. It dissolves in water slowly and to a variable extent, depending on particle size; this greatly affects absorption from the gut. **Arsenites** can be formed by dissolving arsenic trioxide in strong alkalis; the sodium salt is the commonest, but the pigment usually known as **Paris green** is a complex copper aceto-arsenite and was widely used in victorian times in paints and wallpapers. Their pharmacological properties are similar to those of the trioxide, and their absorption is similarly variable, so that the toxicity to pigs of solid sodium arsenite in their feed is many times less than that of the same salt dissolved in their drinking water. Factors such as this may account for the myth of arsenic tolerance. Both trivalent and pentavalent inorganic arsenicals are also absorbed through skin and mucous membranes, especially if they are damaged or if the drug is in a lipid base. *Pentavalent* arsenic is much less toxic and its compounds show chemical resemblances to those of phosphorus (the next element in the periodic table). **Calcium** and **lead arsenates** have been used as insecticidal sprays on fruit trees.

Organic compounds of arsenic have been extensively investigated in an attempt to find chemotherapeutic agents which would moderate its intrinsic toxicity to the host, while still killing parasites (particularly spirochaetes and protozoa), by either concentrating or selectively releasing the inorganic ion in them. Success was never outstanding by modern standards, and with very few exceptions they are now obsolete; however some of them are still used as growth promoters in pigs, particularly phenylarsonic acids such as **arsanilic acid** and **3-nitro-4-hydroxy-phenylarsonic acid**, usually referred to (somewhat disingenuously) as '3-nitro'.

Arsenites bind strongly to proteins. Some 95% of absorbed arsenite attaches to globin molecules in red cells, and the rest to plasma proteins. During the subsequent 24 hours concentrations are particularly high in the liver and kidney, but arsenic is also present in lung, gut wall and spleen. Significant amounts are only found in skin, hair and bone after about 2 weeks. The arsenite ion is not filtered into urine to any great extent, and does not normally get into milk; it is mostly excreted slowly in bile. Because *arsenates* do not bind so avidly to tissues they do not accumulate, and are excreted much more rapidly, mostly in the urine.

Arsenites appear to owe their toxicity to their high affinity for thiol groups. They react particularly strongly with dithiols; their binding to lipoic acid, for example, blocks the oxidative decarboxylation of pyruvate and α-ketoglutarate, thus inhibiting cellular respiration (Fig. 19.1). Arsenates interfere with oxidative phosphorylation by substituting for phosphate to produce unstable high-energy arsenate analogues which then spontaneously break down. The tissue necrosis which follows inorganic arsenic ingestion usually results in acute gastroenteritis and dysentery which may be

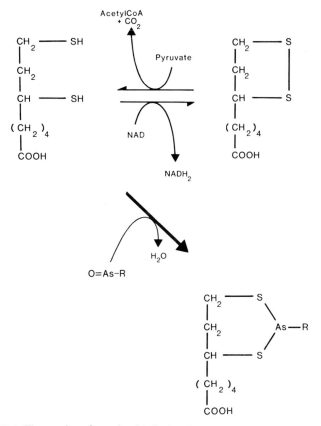

Fig. 19.1 The reaction of arsenic with lipoic acid.

so severe as to cause sudden death from circulatory collapse. More chronic poisoning is particularly manifested in capillary endothelial damage leading to engorgement of mucous membranes and oedema, especially in the splanchnic bed. Feed additive arsenicals are excreted fairly rapidly in the urine, and an adequate flow of urine is necessary for their safety; antidiuresis, whether due to diarrhoea or water deprivation, is often a major precipitating factor in their toxicity. The central nervous system is most obviously affected; incoordination (reversible) progresses to posterior paresis (the critical stage) and eventually quadriplegia (usually irreversible).

Treatment of arsenic poisoning

The existence of an arsenical military poison gas, Lewisite, led to

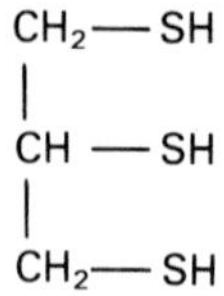

CH₂—SH
|
CH —SH
|
CH₂—SH

Dimercaptopropanol

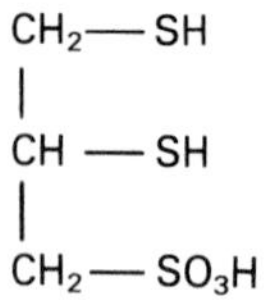

CH₂—SH
|
CH —SH
|
CH₂—SO₃H

Dimercaptopropanesulphonate

(DMPS)

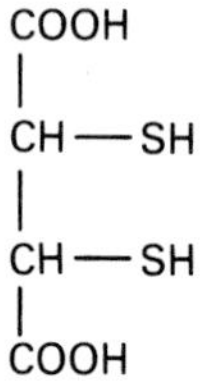

COOH
|
CH—SH
|
CH—SH
|
COOH

Dimercaptosuccinic acid

(DMSA)

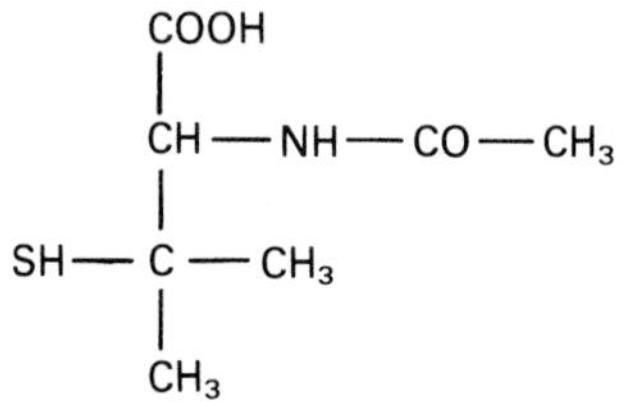

COOH
|
CH—NH—CO—CH₃
|
SH—C—CH₃
|
CH₃

N–acetyl–penicillamine

Fig. 19.2 Thiol-containing chelating compounds.

an energetic search for suitable antidotes during the years before the second world war. Of these the most promising was **2,3-dimercaptopropanol** (Fig. 19.2), also known as dimercaprol and BAL (British Anti-Lewisite). Because the thiol groups are on adjacent carbon atoms, arsenic binds so much more strongly to it than to lipoic acid that the activity of the latter is substantially restored. Agents such as dimercaptopropanol which form multiple bond complexes with heavy metals (or other reactive groups) are known as *chelators*, from the Greek word for a crab's claws.

Dimercaptopropanol is a viscous liquid with a vile smell of bad eggs. It is not well absorbed from the gut and is only slightly soluble, and rather unstable, in water. It is usually given as an intramuscular injection dissolved in peanut oil. It is rapidly excreted in the urine carrying with it its chelated load. As will be seen again with cadmium and mercury, dimercaptopropanol's binding of heavy metals is not always completely secure. This is usually a disadvantage, but **melarsoprol** (Fig. 19.3) is a combination of an organic arsenical with dimercaptopropanol which is valuable in the treatment of sleeping sickness for its outstanding ability to reach trypanocidal concentrations within the central nervous system

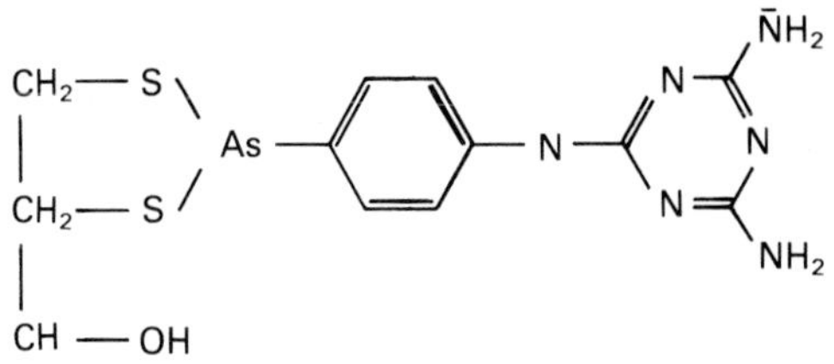

Fig. 19.3 Melarsoprol.

(CNS). On the other hand dimercaptopropanol's tendency to bind other metals, such as the iron and copper in cytochromes. makes it quite distinctly toxic in its own right. Signs of overdosage include vomiting, convulsions or coma, and capillary damage which may lead to cardiovascular collapse.

From the mid 1950s onwards chinese and russian work has demonstrated the clear superiority of **2,3-dimercapto-1-propanesulphonate** (DMPS) and **meso-dimercaptosuccinic acid** (DMSA) over dimercaptopropanol, but this has only gradually been appreciated outside the iron curtain. Their structures are shown in Figure 19.2; they are water soluble, and active following oral administration. Some 60% of an oral dose of DMPS is absorbed in dogs; it does not penetrate cells and is excreted unchanged in the urine over 24 hours. DMSA is less well absorbed and excreted; it appears to penetrate cells to some extent since a small proportion is metabolised. They are both only about a twentieth as toxic as dimercaptopropanol, but are more effective in mobilising arsenic from tissues and promoting its urinary excretion. Although DMSA is slightly less potent it is less toxic and can be given at a higher dose rate (approximately 100 mg/kg), which makes it clinically more effective.

As is often the case with chelating agents, the binding mechanism is less simple in practice than in theory, and molar binding ratios of DMPS to arsenic of approximately 3 : 2 have been reported. In addition, like most chelators, they bind several metals with varying avidities, and the *in vitro* stability constants rarely correlate with the clinical efficacies. When used as a prophylactic, DMSA was almost equally effective against poisoning with arsenic (As^{3+}), silver, mercury (Hg^{2+}) and lead, less so against copper and of only marginal value against cadmium. It was not significantly useful against poisoning with iron, selenium, barium, bismuth or thallium.

LEAD

Lead is still the commonest cause of poisoning in farm animals, and concern at contamination of the environment is, if anything, increasing as the less obvious effects of levels previously considered to be safe are demonstrated. Lead salts were once used as astringents and caustics; there are now no justifiable indications for lead compounds in veterinary therapy.

Lead used to be used extensively in building construction, as the elemental metal in water piping and roof flashings, and compounded in paints, linoleum and putty. Lead is less commonly employed for these purposes nowadays (although red lead paint is still sometimes used as a rust inhibitor), and poisoning by these materials is usually due to inadequate disposal of detritus resulting from building demolition or renovation. The major current sources of lead are mostly associated with the use of vehicles; old lead-acid accumulators, organic antiknock compounds of lead in petrol and discarded sump oil contaminated with lead from white-metal bearings account for the majority of agricultural poisonings. Less commonly spent ammunition (either ingested or accidentally administered parenterally), soft solder and contamination of pasture around mines and smelting works may cause trouble. Considerable interest is being taken in the possible toxic hazard to animals and humans near motorway junctions where the levels of lead (derived from burnt fuel) in grass and air may be twenty times normal; the evidence, although highly suggestive, is not yet clearcut.

The great majority of the sources of lead listed above contain inorganic plumbous (Pb^{2+}) compounds; the only significant exceptions are the petrol antiknock additives. These are covalent alkyl derivatives of plumbic hydride: **lead tetraethyl** and **lead tetramethyl**, which are volatile liquids insoluble in water. They break down to Pb^{2+} on combustion, but the metabolic and toxic properties of the undecomposed compounds are quite different from those of inorganic lead.

Over 70% of lead poisonings occur in cattle; the vast majority of them are in young calves, due to inappropriate transference of suckling reflexes but exaggerated by the unnatural conditions under which they are kept. Lead poisoning is fairly rare in pigs and cats, which are discriminating feeders, but is less so in horses, especially riding ponies confined on rubbish-strewn suburban pastures. The indiscriminate eating habits of most young puppies largely account for the frequency of lead poisoning in dogs (where it can be very difficult to distinguish from distemper). A surprisingly large proportion of water fowl suffer from chronic lead poisoning because they ingest shotgun pellets and fishing line sinkers in mistake for grit; the pellets are retained in the gizzard and slowly ground down.

Approximately 12% of an oral dose of an *inorganic* lead compound is absorbed, almost irrespective of its nature and formulation; the mechanism is unknown, although there appears to be some competition with calcium. Absorption of inhaled lead as a dust or vapour is much more efficient.

In the first instance virtually all the absorbed lead attaches to red blood cells, and there is rarely any in plasma. It subsequently redistributes to other tissues with little apparent preference, although the liver, bone marrow and kidney cortex are usually more heavily loaded than other tissues. This last tissue is probably the best to assay for lead content in a suspected case of recent poisoning. On any reasonable time scale the final resting place of lead is the bone marrow, where it may persist for years if the bone is not disturbed. However the therapeutic policy of encouraging this sequestration by feeding high calcium diets to poisoned animals is taking a risk which should at the least be a calculated one since subsequent bone resorption due to a fracture, calcium deficiency (for example in association with pregnancy or lactation), renal disease, or simply old age may release the lead and cause signs of toxicity.

The excretion of lead is partly urinary but, at least in the sheep, more is lost in the faeces. Excretion is so slow that exfoliation of skin and hair growth represent significant routes of loss. The maximum rate of loss is said to be 0.8 mg/day in sheep and 0.6 mg/day in man; if absorption exceeds this figure for the appropriate species accumulation and eventually toxicity will occur. As an example of this phenomenon a man who absorbed an estimated 2.5 mg/day from his diet took 4 years to develop clinical signs of lead intoxication.

Acute inorganic lead poisoning of cattle produces dysfunction of the gastro-intestinal tract (anorexia, salivation, pain or diarrhoea) in about 60% of cases, and of the nervous system in about 90%; in the latter group signs are highly variable, but blindness, muscle twitching, hyperexcitement or depression and convulsions are particularly common. Roughly a third of clinical cases show sudden death as the presenting sign. The effects of lead are similar in dogs, with a high proportion, especially of older animals, showing gastro-intestinal and nervous signs simultaneously. Horses often show signs of peripheral nerve involvement, including muscle weakness and recurrent laryngeal nerve paralysis. Sheep, as usual, show very few definite signs: anorexia and abortion, together with motor nerve disabilities in some of the surviving lambs may be suggestive.

Low levels of inorganic lead cause more subtle nervous damage in a number of species. There is strong evidence associating increased intake with low intelligence quotients in children, and lambs born of sheep given lead during the pregnancy are significantly slower at experimental learning tasks. In the developing rat very low doses of lead inhibit the proliferation of CNS capillaries, which may explain some of these effects.

Like arsenic, *inorganic* lead complexes thiol groups strongly, and the consequent enzyme inhibition is assumed to be an important factor in the mechanisms of its toxicity, although there is some evidence that it may also interfere with the movement of other metal ions, for example calcium entry at nerve terminals and iron transfer into mitochondria during haem synthesis. Lead inhibits at least two enzymes involved in haem synthesis; it is not therefore surprising that anaemia is an early and important sign of lead toxicity. There are also important diagnostic consequences: the inhibition of δ-aminolaevulinic acid dehydratase leads to increased levels of δ-*aminolaevulinic acid* (ALA) in plasma and urine, while at a later stage in the pathway the inability to form haem by incorporating Fe^{2+} into protoporphyrin IX leads to a build up of *coproporphyrin* in plasma, and also removes the normal feedback inhibition on ALA synthesis. The laboratory detection of these intermediates in urine or plasma is a useful aid to the diagnosis of lead poisoning. Blood samples for lead assay should not be taken through all-metal (soldered) needles, and EDTA should not be used as the anticoagulant.

Organic tetraalkyl lead compounds are rapidly absorbed from the gut and lungs and through intact skin. Organic lead is considerably more toxic than it is in inorganic compounds: the acute $LD_{50}s$ for the two forms in the rat being 10 and 70 mg of lead/kg respectively. Tetraalkyl lead is rapidly broken down to the corresponding trialkyl compound in the liver, and it is this which causes the damage (lead tetraethyl, for example, has almost no effect on isolated tissue respiration). Once dealkylated it causes severe central nervous stimulation, with results ranging from muscle tremors, hyperexcitement and hallucinations (at least in man) to convulsions and death. Blood cell abnormalities (such as stippled or nucleated erythrocytes) are much less common than in inorganic lead poisoning.

Treatment of lead poisoning

The classical treatment for *inorganic* lead poisoning is the chelating agent **ethylenediaminetetraacetate** (EDTA, Edetate, Versenate) which complexes a wide range of metal ions, forming bonds with the four carboxylic acid groups and the two nitrogen atoms (fig. 19.4). It strongly chelates zinc and cadmium (stability constant 10^{16}), copper and lead (10^{18}) and most strongly Fe^{3+} (10^{25}), although even this is inadequate to compete with binding by ferritin and transferrin. Amongst the physiologically important metals binding of sodium and potassium is virtually negligible, but it chelates calcium strongly enough (stability constant 10^{12}) to remove it from its physiological binding sites. For this reason it is usually administered as the disodium salt of its calcium complex (Fig. 19.4), by intravenous injection or infusion since its absorption from other parenteral sites is inadequate and from the gut almost non-existent.

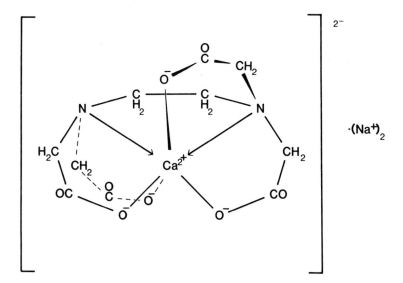

Fig. 19.4 Ethylenediaminetetraacetic acid and the calcium chelate of its sodium salt.

Its half-life in bovine plasma is approximately an hour, and it is rapidly excreted in the urine following glomerular filtration and extrusion into the lumen by the proximal tubular organic acid secretory mechanism. Its penetration of physiological barriers is not very good, and it is not metabolised to any appreciable extent. EDTA rapidly mobilises between a quarter and a third of soft tissue lead and promotes its urinary excretion. Unfortunately the binding of lead is only barely strong enough to compete with tissue ligands, and unless an excess of EDTA is maintained it may actually *increase* the effects of lead on the nervous system. The therapeutic desirability of continuous infusion over intermittent large injections is reinforced by the intrinsic toxicity of EDTA to kidney tubules (the acute LD_{50} is 440 mg/kg in cattle), which is probably due to binding of tissue metals such as zinc. EDTA can be incorporated in peritoneal dialysis solutions in the event of renal damage.

The clinical response to EDTA is considerably improved by concurrent injection of **dimercaptopropanol**, which removes more lead from erythrocytes and the CNS, but a number of the more recent dithiol chelators are more potent still. Amongst these **DMSA** is particularly effective; in a comparative study on mice at dose rates of 100 mg/kg it was found to remove between 70 and 300% more lead from most tissues, including bone and brain than did dimercapropropanol. **Diethylenetriaminepentaacetate** (DTPA) is closely related to EDTA; it has a higher affinity for heavy metals and has been more commonly used (with only limited success) in treating cases of contamination with radioactive heavy metals such as uranium and plutonium

Chelation therapy of *organic* lead poisoning is not usually a very rewarding exercise.

Other beneficial steps in the management of inorganic lead poisoned cases could rationally include the feeding of **magnesium sulphate** to precipitate any lead still in the gut and to speed its removal. **Thiamine** has been reported to reduce the lead content of soft tissues and to cause clinical improvement in poisoned domestic animals. Corticosteroids are specifically contra-indicated in animals receiving EDTA since they appear to increase the renal toxicity of lead-EDTA complexes. In view of the frequency of anaemia in lead poisoning it is perhaps worth noting that iron-containing tonics should not be combined with dimercaptopropanol therapy since the resulting iron complex is highly toxic, as well as being useless for chelating lead.

MERCURY

Mercury has been known since pre-Christian times, and its extraordinary physical properties, together with the undoubted power of its effects have ensured its widespread use in materia medica until only comparatively recently. The ancient Greeks used **mercuric sulphide** (cinnabar, HgS) as an eye ointment, and **mercurous chloride** (calomel, Hg_2Cl_2) must be one of the oldest purges. Whether Europe had the Arabs or Columbus to thank for the late 15th century epidemic spread of syphilis may never be decided, but the former were undoubtedly responsible for initiating four centuries of secondary mercury poisoning by ointments used to treat the cutaneous lesions, a practice only finally curtailed by the advent of penicillin. **Mercuric chloride** (corrosive sublimate, $HgCl_2$) and mercuric iodide have been used as counter-irritants and disinfectants, and organic mercurials such as **thiomersal** are still available for this latter purpose. Various organic mercury compounds have been used in the manufacture of mildew-proof paints and as 'slimicides' in paper manufacture. They are still widely used as antifungal seed-dressings; although alkoxyalkyl compounds such as **methoxyethylmercuric chloride** are being withdrawn under largely voluntary schemes and replaced by less acutely toxic compounds such as **phenylmercuric acetate**. Alkylmercurial compounds such as **methylmercuric chloride** were the original mercurial seed-dressing agents, but they were withdrawn after a series of disastrous poisonings. Their widespread occurrence in the environment is now due to metabolism of other mercury compounds particularly by microorganisms.

The absorption and distribution of mercury depends heavily on its chemical form. Clean liquid mercury metal is relatively safely ingested since little is absorbed from the gut. However it is dangerously volatile, and most of an inspired dose is retained; because of its high lipid solubility elemental mercury absorbed in this way is mostly taken up by the central nervous system and fixed there. Inorganic mercury compounds are approximately 7% absorbed from the gut; absorption of Hg^{2+} through skin may be only slightly less efficient. Elemental and monovalent mercury are rapidly oxidised in the blood to Hg^{2+}, which (by contrast with arsenic and lead) is about equally distributed between plasma and cellular protein binding sites. It subsequently accumulates to a considerable extent in the kidney cortex. Chronic administration of inorganic mercury leads to an increase in cellular content of *metallothionein*, especially in the kidney, which complexes Hg^{2+} and affords some protection.

Organic mercurial compounds have a high lipid solubility; they are well absorbed from the gut and through skin. Phenylmercuric compounds are fairly rapidly broken down to release Hg^{2+} and thus behave somewhat like inorganic mercury. Alkoxyalkylmercury is more slowly metabolised so that distribution into lipid-rich tissues such as the CNS is more likely. Alkylmercuric compounds are very stable and lipid soluble; although they, like Hg^{2+}, preferentially accumulate in the kidney, high levels are also reached in the CNS.

Inorganic mercury is very slowly excreted, mostly in the urine. Since virtually none is free in the plasma it is not filtered, and it is thought to accompany the breakdown products of the damaged tubules. Alkyl mercurials do not appear in the urine to any significant extent, and are mostly lost in the faeces through the exfoliation of gut mucosal cells. Their biological half lives are even longer than those of other mercury compounds. Both inorganic and organic mercurials appear in the bile in significant amounts, but are normally almost completely reabsorbed.

The toxic effects of mercury are believed to be due to its great affinity for thiol groups (their alternative name 'mercapto-' celebrates this property), but so many enzymes and other proteins are thereby inhibited and denatured by it that the precise mechanisms of its clinical effects remain obscure. Organic mercurial compounds are also highly potent mutagens, damaging chromosomes in somatic and germ cells, and causing foetal abnormalities and death. Acute poisoning with ingested soluble *inorganic* mercury compounds can produce death from circulatory collapse with no impending clinical signs at all, but severe abdominal pain and bloody diarrhoea are more commonly seen first. The kidney is the main target organ after absorption, and the immediate effect is anuria which gives way, if the animal survives, to a prolonged diuresis. Signs of muscle weakness, emaciation, skin and mucosal degeneration (including pruritus, loss of teeth and chronic diarrhoea) and excessive salivation ('mercury ptyalism') may also be seen in chronic cases. Inhalation of mercury metal vapour can lead to massive dissolution of lung tissue and death from pneumothorax and haemorrhage; in less severe cases it is notable in man for its neuropsychiatric effects, which include the well-defined mood and personality changes known as 'erethism'.

Poisoning with *organic* mercurials also produces predominantly neural toxic signs, but these are usually sensori-motor; paraesthesia is the most sensitive response, but tremor is usually present at higher doses. These signs progress to blindness, coma and death, they often continue to intensify for some time after removal of the source of mercury, and are frequently irreversible. Chapter 14 in Oehme (1978) gives futher details of the horrifying incidents which finally forced the abandonment of alkylmercury seed-dressings, but other mercury compounds are still in use. These are, of course, still highly toxic if seed treated thus is ingested; in addition their bio-conversion to alkylmercurials has been clearly demonstrated, not only in free-living microorganisms (especially in low pH environments such as acid rain polluted waters), but also in domestic food-producing animals.

Treatment of mercury poisoning

Chelating agents such as EDTA are of very little use, probably because Hg^{2+} has a bond angle of 180°, and hence does not readily form ring structures. However a number of compounds containing thiol groups have been shown to form complexes with mercury sufficiently strongly to influence its distribution. Of these **dimercaptopropanol** is only slightly useful in clinical cases of inorganic mercury poisoning, and ineffective in removing organic mercury from the CNS; indeed it may even transport mercury *into* it.

D-penicillamine has been largely superceded by its derivative **N-acetyl-DL-penicillamine** (Fig. 19.2), which is less toxic and more slowly metabolised. It has been suggested that these compounds are effective in removing even alkylmercury compounds from tissues because they help to disrupt the carbon-mercury bond as well as complexing the resulting Hg^{2+}. Both **DMSA** and **DMPS** have been found to be more effective than N-acetyl penicillamine (at equimolar dose rates) in removing both alkyl and inorganic mercury from tissues in experimental animals; DMPS was up to four times as good, although the lower toxicity of DMSA gave it a slight advantage when used at maximum tolerated dose rates. Very recently dithiol compounds have. been developed which are excreted in the bile, and which thus greatly increase faecal loss of mercury.

CADMIUM

Cadmium is a metal closely related to zinc. It has achieved its greatest notoriety as an environmental pollutant around zinc mining and processing works, most notably in Japan where contaminated water was used for irrigating staple food crops; cadmium also occurs at high concentrations in association with old lead mining works. It has been used as a cheap rust-inhibiting plating on steel articles, when it imparts a distinctive blue tint; its presence on food containers and implements has caused poisoning. It is one of the reactants in some types of alkaline voltaic cell, and cadmium salts have been used as pigments and as anthelmintics.

Cadmium only exhibits one valency state in its compounds (Cd^{2+}) and it does not form covalent organic compounds. Its strong acid salts are water soluble, but its oxide, hydroxide and carbonate are not. Up to 10% of an ingested dose is absorbed, apparently in part attached to calcium binding protein; so that calcium deficiency increases cadmium absorption. Like copper, zinc and mercury it induces metallothionein synthesis in almost all cells. In the gut the cadmium–thionein complex is re-excreted; in other cells it accumulates, sometimes taking many years to reach toxic levels. Particularly high levels are found in liver and kidney, although whether this is due to their metallothionein content is not known. Excretion is extremely slow, and appears to be mainly *via* the urine in man and faeces in experimental animals.

In high doses cadmium seems to interfere with zinc metabolism and causes direct tissue irritation: vomiting and diarrhoea follow oral administration, with subsequent kidney failure. Inhalation of dust causes acute and severe pulmonary oedema. Chronic poisoning with low doses causes deminerallisation of bone, leading in man to excruciating bone and joint pain and multiple spontaneous fractures.

Treatment of cadmium poisoning is difficult. Both dimercaptopropanol and EDTA mobilise cadmium from tissues and promote renal excretion, but their ability to protect the kidney from cadmium's toxicity is entirely inadequate; the procedure merely accelerates the onset of renal failure and in fact increases the final mortality rate. Even the newer dithiols DMSA and DMPS have only a slight effect on cadmium toxicity. Dietary supplementation with **selenium** has been claimed to reduce the severity of clinical signs, and large doses of **vitamin D** have been found helpful in reversing the skeletal lesions during the recovery phase in chronic cases.

GOLD

In view of its value it is perhaps not surprising that accidental poisoning or environmental pollution with gold is rare, and the only real danger from it is iatrogenic. Gold salts, particularly **sodium aurothiomaleate**, are sometimes used in human practice as a palliative treatment for chronic arthritis, and unfortunately hope and alchemy occasionally triumph over experience in veterinary practice as well. It rapidly enters the circulation after intramuscular injection, and becomes extensively bound to plasma proteins, with a plasma half-life of several weeks. It slowly redistributes into arthritic tissues, liver, kidney and spleen, where high levels persist for up to a year. Excretion seems to be mostly urinary.

Side-effects are very common and appear to be related to therapeutic efficacy, so that clinical improvement can be regarded as the first sign of impending toxicity, soon to be followed by pruritus and albuminuria; at this point therapy should be stopped completely. Further poisoning leads to dermatitis, mucosal inflammation and blood dyscrasias. Death usually results from thrombocytopenia.

Dimercaptopropanol hastens gold excretion, but only at near-toxic dose rates; the penicillamines are ineffective. **DMPS** has been reported as an effective means of mobilising gold from tissues in experimental rats.

ANTIMONY

Antimony is very similar in most respects to arsenic. In bygone centuries lumps of antimony metal were used as recyclable purging pills; more recently ionic compounds such as **antimony potassium tartrate** (tartar emetic) and covalent ones such as **stibophen** were used to treat schistosomiasis, leishmaniasis and other (mainly tropical) parasitic diseases. The metal is still used alloyed with lead in type metal (which expands slightly on cooling) and in bearing surfaces.

Compared with arsenic it is more slowly absorbed and excreted, and causes more local irritation. Dithiol compounds such as **dimercaptopropanol** are more effective against trivalent antimony compounds than against pentavalent ones.

BARIUM

Barium is in the same group of the periodic table as calcium, and most of its effects can be ascribed to its blockage of calcium fluxes and channels and its inhibition of calcium-dependent cellular processes. Some studies have suggested that it may also be an essential trace element. **Barium sulphate** is used as a digestive tract X-ray contrast medium, and is non-toxic because of its almost complete insolubility. **Barium carbonate** is sufficiently soluble to cause toxicity, and is sometimes used as a rodenticide, even although it is more toxic to humans than to rats.

Barium causes gastroenteritis, paralysis of skeletal muscle and bradycardia leading to ventricular fibrillation and cardiac arrest. A high extracellular K^+ concentration antagonises the cardiac effects (as it does those of hypercalcaemia); hence intravenous **potassium chloride** is said to be beneficial, although risky since it also stops the heart in overdosage. Purgation with **magnesium sulphate** reduces the absorption and hastens the elimination of any barium left in the gut.

THALLIUM

Thallium salts have been used as depilatories and, more commonly, as rodenticides. Large doses cause severe gastroenteritis followed, if the animal survives long enough, by signs of cardio-vascular and CNS involvement due to interference with potassium metabolism. More chronic poisoning causes hair-loss, paralysis due to central nervous necroses and damage to liver and kidney.

Although these signs are thought to be due to the combination of thallium with mitochondrial enzyme thiol groups, dithiol chelators, including dimercaptopropanol and DMSA, are ineffective in alleviating them.

SUGGESTIONS FOR FURTHER READING

Aposhian H V 1983 DMSA and DMPS — water soluble antidotes for heavy
    metal poisoning. Annual Review of Pharmacology and Toxicology 23: 193–215
Hammond P B, Beliles R P 1980 Metals. In Doull J, Klaassen C D, Amdur M O
    (eds) Cassarett and Doull's Toxicology, 2nd Edn. MacMillan, New York,
    ch 17, p 409–467
Jones M M, Basinger M A, Weaver A D, Davis C M. Vaughn W K 1980
    Comparison of standard chelating agents for acute mercuric chloride poisoning
    in mice. Research Communications in Chemical Pathology and Pharmacology
    27: 363–372
Oehme F W (ed) 1978 Toxicity of heavy metals in the environment, part 1.
    Dekker, New York.
WHO 1976 Environmental health criteria. 1. Mercury. World Health
    Organisation, Geneva
WHO 1977 Environmental health criteria. 3. Lead. World Health Organisation,
    Geneva

20

Chemotherapy drug resistance

This term could include the whole of pharmacology but is usually restricted to mean the destruction of obnoxious parasites within the animal body. The most famous name associated with this branch of science is that of Ehrlich, who in fact invented the term 'chemotherapy'. His idea was to discover a substance which would combine with the tissues of the parasites and kill them but would not affect the host's tissues. He termed substances which combined with the parasite's tissues 'parasitotrophic' and those combining with the host's tissues 'organotrophic'. This concept has been modified to a large extent, because it is realised now that the tissues of the host are essential to combat diseases caused by pathogenic organisms.

Ehrlich's histological experiments on the vital staining of tissues led him to study the staining of bacteria. He developed a method of staining the tubercle bacillus with an acid-fast stain which forms the basis of the Ziehl-Neilson stain. Ehrlich also introduced a method of staining bacteria which involved the use of an aniline dye, usually methyl violet. This technique was further developed by Christian Gram and is known as Gram's stain. Whether or not a bacterium is stained by Gram's method indicates to some extent the organism's susceptibility to drugs. The differences between the responses of Gram-positive and Gram-negative organisms to drugs are usually correlated with the presence or absence of lipid in cell wall which is said to impair penetration of the organism by the drug. The Gram-staining properties of some bacteria of veterinary importance are shown in Table 20.1.

Because a drug in low concentration will kill parasites in test tubes it does not follow that it will be effective in curing animals suffering from disease caused by the same parasites. There are several reasons for this anomaly. For example, some drugs act slowly on the parasite whereas the life of the parasite in the test tube may be too short for the drug to exert its effect. This difficulty may be

Table 20.1 Bacterial Genera

Gram-positive	Gram-negative
Staphylococcus	Pseudomonas
Streptococcus	Vibrio
Micrococcus	Spirillum
Sarcina	Escherichia (Bacterium)
Corynebacteria	Aerobacter
Listeria	Proteus
Erysipelothrix	Haemophilis
Bacillus	Actinobacillus
Clostridium	Neisseria
Mycobacterium	Spirochaetes (where stainable)
Actinomyces	All generic names ending in ella
Nocardia	e.g. Salmonella
Streptomyces.	Shigella
	Klebsiella
	Brucella
	Pasteurella
	Moraxella
	Veillonella
	Campylobacter
	Legionella

overcome by improving culture methods and prolonging the in vitro life of the parasite.

Another reason for discrepancy between in vivo and in vitro tests may be due to the conversion of the drug into a therapeutically active substance by the tissues, or, conversely, the body may inactivate a drug shown to have activity in vitro.

Whilst test tube tests are valuable in searching for new chemotherapeutic agents, it is not always easy to interpret the results of such tests. They are complicated by the fact that the host's tissues do not behave as a passive vehicle for the parasites but act on them by phagocytosis and by forming antibodies. However, such tests can give fundamental information about the action of some chemotherapeutic agents, especially when the reason for their failure is studied. For example, sulphanilamide stops the growth of streptococci in test tubes but does not kill them, whereas streptococcal infections in animals are cured by this drug. The reason for this difference is that sulphanilamide stops the growth of streptococci in the body and this allows the phagocytes time to remove them.

Chemotherapeutic agents are used in veterinary medicine to treat diseases caused by worms, insects, bacteria and fungi.

DRUG RESISTANCE

Following the introduction by Ehrlich of effective drugs for the treatment of trypanosomiasis, it was noticed that after a period of use these drugs ceased to cure certain cases of trypanosomiasis. Furthermore, arsenical compounds which had been used as dips in the control of certain ectoparasites were found also to have ceased to be effective against some strains of ticks which were formerly susceptible. These are examples of drug resistance. This phenomenon has been observed with many protozoa, bacteria, fungi, viruses and insect parasites. Certain strains of the worm *Haemonchus contortus* are resistant to phenothiazine and others require greatly increased doses of thiabendazole. Similarly some strains of *Fasciola hepatica* require greatly increased doses of hexachlorophene for their elimination. Resistance is largely specific; for example, trypanosomes resistant to suramin are not resistant to organic arsenicals and vice versa. However, strains of trypanosome resistant to Homidium are, unfortunately, also resistant to Quinapyramine despite these drugs being chemically quite dissimilar. This latter phenomenon is termed cross-resistance. Drug resistance may be described as the temporary or permanent capacity of an organism to remain viable or multiply in the presence of concentrations of a drug which would destroy or inhibit other similar organisms. Drug resistance may be either natural or acquired. Natural organism resistance is intrinsic in the particular species or strain of organism regardless of whether the organism has been exposed to the drug or not. Although the occurrence of drug resistant strains of pathogenic micro-organisms is of undoubted clinical importance the incidence is by no means uniform. Resistant strains of *Pasteurella, Erysipelothrix rhusiopathiae, Corynebacterium pyogenes* and most *Streptococci* have not emerged to any significant extent, despite the widespread use of drugs in the treatment of diseases of animals caused by these organisms. Despite being used for more than 30 years penicillin is still effective against infections caused by *Streptococcus pyogenes*. Similarly, *Streptococcus agalactiae* has remained susceptible to penicillins and this has resulted in a marked decline in the importance of this organism as a causal agent of bovine mastitis. Unfortunately, *Staphylococcus aureus* has largely replaced the streptococcus as the most important causal organism of bovine mastitis and important penicillin-resistant strains of *S. aureus* from cases of bovine mastitis have shown a steady increase in frequency of occurrence from around 40% in the mid 1950s to over 70% by the 1960s. Drug resistance also presents a problem in animal diseases caused by *Mycoplasma gallisepticum* and certain strains of *Clostridium welchii*. Drug resistance is a common phenomenon in members of the *Enterobacteriaceae*, such as *E. coli* and *Salmonellae* where it shows important characteristic properties, in particular, transmisability.

Transferable resistance

This phenomenon was first noticed in Japan. Most of the information about transferable resistance has been obtained by work on the **enterobacteriaceae** (*Salmonella, Escherichia, Shigella*).

It has been shown that resistance to antibiotics can be transferred from one organism to another by so-called resistance factors or R factors. The R factor consists of R-determinants which are genetic

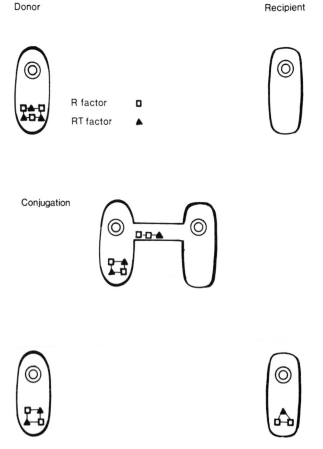

Fig. 20.1 A schematic representation of transferable resistance.

features and RT (resistance transfer) factors which are present in the bacterial cytoplasm. The RT factor is involved in the transference of resistance from one organism to another.

There appear to be at least three ways in which genes can be transferred between bacterial cells all involving the passage of DNA. The three processes are termed conjugation, transduction and transformation. In **conjugation** the DNA passes from the donor to the recipient cell through a bridge formed during the actual contact between bacteria. For this type of transfer to occur the donor bacterium requires the necessary surface structure to form the bridge, this protuberance is sometimes called a pilus. The transference of R factors by conjugation occurs mainly amongst Gram-negative organisms and can take place not only between different strains of the same organism but even between different *genera*. The genetic material transferred consists of plasmid DNA which confers on the recipient organism resistance which is usually multiple, often to six or more drugs. The recipient organism can then act itself as a donor spreading resistance to pathogenic and non-pathogenic organisms so that bacteria never exposed to any drug can acquire multiple resistance. It was to avoid this hazard that the decision was made to restrict the antibiotics which may be added to the food of pigs and poultry to a very limited number which are not required for use in therapy.

Experimental work has shown that the R factor consists of a portion conferring the metabolic ability to inactivate the drug, namely, the R determinant, and a portion responsible for the conjugation process, the RT (resistant transfer) factor. Incubating a strain of *E. coli* which had a non-transferable R determinant for resistance to ampicillin with an ampicillin/sensitive strain of phage type 29S *typhimurium* which had an RT factor, lead to the acquisition of the RT factor by the *E. coli* which then could transfer its R factor back to the S. *typhimurium* or to any other suitable recipient organism the result being that both species of bacteria possessed transferable resistance to ampicillin.

Some resistant strains of bacteria carry genes for resistance on the chromosome. However, most high-level resistant types of organism are associated with resistant plasmids. Some of these resistance plasmids whilst not self transferable can be mobilised by other plasmids. Sometimes the resistance genes may be located on discreet movable DNA elements called transposons. These transposons possess the ability to move from plasmid to plasmid or plasmid to chromosome. Bacteriophages may also be involved in the spread of transposons. The transposon can remain stable in different species even if its vector is lost since the resistance transposon can be incorporated into a stable resident plasmid or chromosome of the new host. The discovery of transposable resistance has helped in understanding the rapid spread of resistance throughout the bacterial kingdom.

Mechanisms of bacterial resistance

Chromosomal resistance other than from transposon insertions is usually due to a simple low level, non-enzymatic mechanism. In many instances this involves a decreased permeability of the cell membrane. Plasmid or transposon-mediated resistances are of a higher level and involve more active processes. Many of these types of resistance involve the extracellular inactivation or degradation of the drug by various enzymes. Examples of these are the β-lactamases which destroy the β-lactam ring of the penicillins and cephalosporins and those which inactivate chloramphenicol in many cases the cell itself remains susceptible to the drug. Various enzymes inactivate the aminoglycosides (aminocyclitols) by acetylation, nucleotidation or phosphorylation. They do not act on the drug outside the cell. A small amount of inactivated drug fails to inhibit protein synthesis and stops ribosomal binding and the cellular uptake of the unchanged drug.

Tetracycline resistance is associated with a decreased accumulation of the drug mediated by an energy dependent efflux of the drug specified by the resistance determinant. The drug is not degraded. The anti-folates such as the sulphonamides and trimethoprim, show resistance due to an enzyme which substitutes in the folic acid synthesis pathway and is unaffected by the drug. There have been marked increases in the incidence of resistance genes in reservoirs of non-pathogenic bacteria and of the emergence of resistance amongst previously susceptible pathogens.

Transduction is the term applied to the transfer of resistance by a bacterial virus, bacteriophage, through the phage's apparatus for the insertion of DNA into recipient bacteria. Usually phage DNA is transferred in this manner but sometimes DNA from the bacterial cell on which the virus was grown takes the place of the phage DNA. This type of transfer occurs mainly in staphylococci but may occur between both Gram-positive and Gram-negative organisms. Phage transmitted resistance usually is confined to only one or two drugs. In **transformation**, DNA seems to pass from donor to recipient through the growth medium and may be a process confined solely to the laboratory.

SUGGESTIONS FOR FURTHER READING

Anderson E S 1968 The ecology of transferable drug resistance in entero-bacteria. Annual Review of Microbiology 22:131

Levy S B 1982 Microbial resistance to antibiotics. Lancet ii:83

Linton A H 1982 Problems of antibiotic resistance in animals and their public health significance. Vet. Ann. 22:45

Oppenoorth F J 1965 Biochemical genetics of insecticide resistance. Annual Review of Entymology 10:185

Whitehead J E M 1973 Bacterial resistance. Changing patterns of some common pathogens. British Medical Journal 31:224

Williams Smith H 1971 The effects of the use of antibacterial drugs on the emergence of drug-resistant bacteria in animals. Advances in Veterinary Science 15:67

21

Chemotherapy of bacterial infections

SULPHONAMIDES

Despite the introduction, in the early years of this century, of drugs effective against pathogenic protozoa and spirochætes, the treatment of acute bacterial infections was symptomatic until the mid 1930s. In fact many authorities felt that only in sera and vaccines lay any hope of combating such diseases, and the announcement by Domagk in 1935 that mice, treated with an azo dyestuff 'Prontosil', survived many times the lethal dose hæmolytic streptococci, was received with some scepticism. In the same year Trefouel, Trefouel, Nitti and Bovet showed that para-amino benzene sulphonamide had the same effect and concluded that prontosil was broken down to this simpler compound in the body. However, it was the publication of the results of an extensive clinical trial one year later which established the drug. Puerperal septicæmia in women is caused by hæmolytic streptococci. Colebrook and Kenny treated alternate cases of this disease with para-amino benzene sulphonamide, the remaining cases receiving the same care but not the drug. The death rate in the cases receiving the sulphonamide was 3% and in the others 20%. These facts placed the value of the drug in this and similar infections beyond question.

Thousands of compounds modelled on sulphanilamide have been made and some are of greater value. Drugs in which the amino group is substituted are broken down in the body to a form with a free amino group and sulphur linked directly to the benzene ring because this is essential for anti-bacterial activity. Prontosil is an example of this type of compound as are *succinylsulphathiazole* and *phthalylsulphathiazole*. The last two compounds are very poorly absorbed from the gut, but the succinyl and phthalyl groups are split off in the intestine liberating sulphathiazole to exert its antibacterial activity. Sulphanilamide will be considered in detail to provide a basis for discussing the other more therapeutically important sulphonamides.

Sulphanilamide is completely absorbed from the small intestine and distributed throughout the whole of the body water. It is acetylated in part mainly in the liver. The acetylated compound has no bacteriostatic powers. The degree of acetylation varies between species, the domestic animals can be arranged in descending order of acetylation thus: cow, rabbit, sheep, horse, cat. The dog does not acetylate sulphonamides. Both free and acetylated sulphonamides are excreted in the urine, and about one-third of the dose is metabolised in the body.

Binding with the plasma proteins takes place to a varying extent with all the sulphonamides. The binding is not firm and the bound sulphonamide is released continually. It is usually considered that only the unbound fraction is available for urinary excretion and antibacterial action. Sulphonamides enter the pleural, peritoneal, synovial, ocular and similar fluids.

Sulphanilamide may be used locally as it dissolves slowly in serum and so maintains a steady concentration. The other sulphonamides are too insoluble except as the sodium salts which are strongly alkaline. The alkalinity of the soluble sodium salts of sulphonamides may cause considerable tissue damage and pain if they are injected subcutaneously. The intravenous route is safest for parenteral administration but care must be taken not to allow the solution to leak around the vein. *Sulphacetamide* is an exception in forming a sodium salt which is nearly neutral and is suitable to use as an antiseptic in the eye.

Sulphanilamide prevents the growth of certain bacteria and so allows the phagocytes of the body to destroy them. This bacteriostatic effect is antagonised by para-amino benzoic acid or material containing it, such as pus, necrotic tissue, extracts of microorganisms and yeast. Para-amino benzoic acid will antagonise 1600 times its weight of sulphanilamide. Substances such as methionine have a similar but weaker effect. Certain drugs such as procaine which have a free amino group attached to a benzene ring will also produce antagonism. It is probable that sulphanilamide acts by competing for the same enzyme receptors on the bacteria as para-amino benzoic acid. When the chemical structure of folic acid was established it was realised that it contained a *para-aminobenzoyl* group derived from para-amino benzoic acid which supported the hypothesis that sulphonamides inhibited the biosynthesis of folic acid.

Sulphonamides act in part by being used within the bacterium as substrates instead of the normal substrate paraaminobenzoic acid

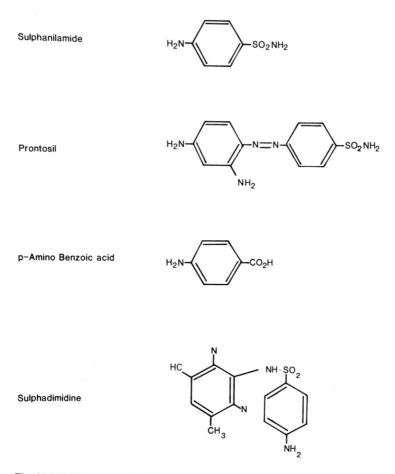

Fig. 21.1(a) The structural relationship between some sulphonamides of veterinary importance and para-amino benzoic acid.

resulting in the formation of false folic acids. Animal cells are un-affected by sulphonamides because these cells receive folic acid already formed and do not have to manufacture their own. Both the sulphonamides and para-aminobenzoic acid can enter the bacterial cell freely whereas most biosynthetic intermediates formed on the way to the production of folic acid carry phosphoric acid groups which inhibit their movement from the medium into the bacterium and hence cannot take the place of the need for the bacterial cell forming its own folic acid.

Sulphanilamide inhibits the enzyme carbonic anhydrase which, amongst other important actions, appears to be involved in the for-

Sulphacetamide

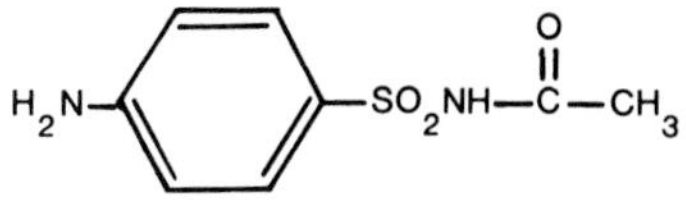

Sulphadiazine

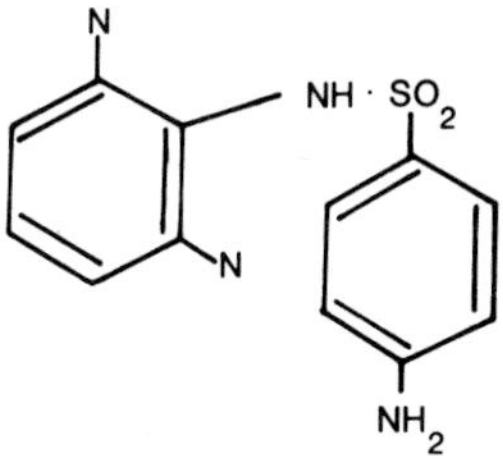

Phthalylsulphathiazole

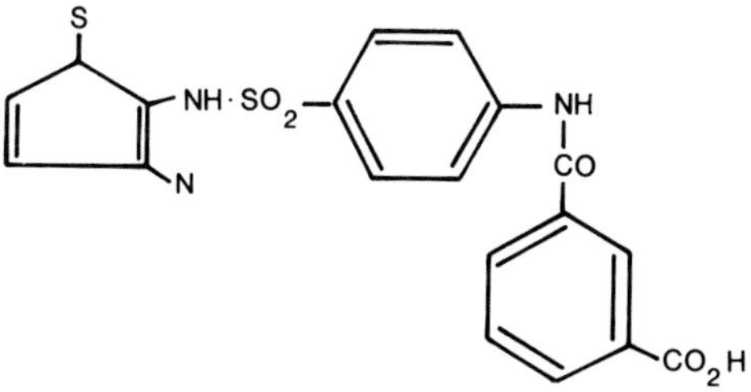

Succinylsulphathiazole

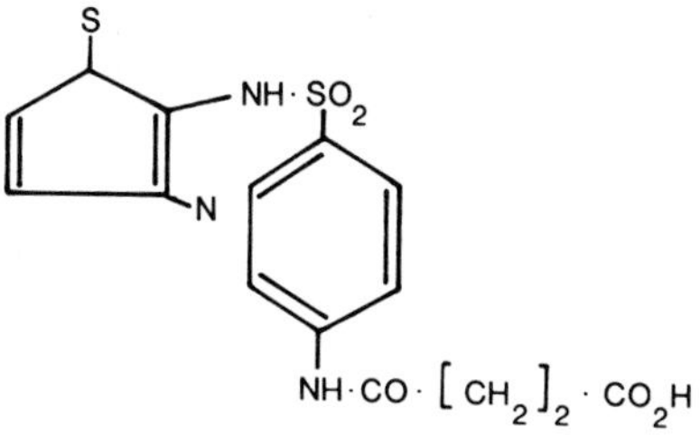

Fig. 21.1(b)

mation of egg shells, hence hens on sulphanilamide lay soft-shelled eggs. The other sulphonamides do not have this action.

The differences between the various sulphonamides are quantitative rather than qualitative. They are very active against *hæmolytic streptococci*, less so against *pneumococci* and even less against *staphylococci*. The *anthrax bacillus, Brucella abortus* and *Streptococcus fæcalis*, are unaffected by sulphonamides.

Organisms exposed to sulphonamides but not killed by them may become resistant to these drugs. Fortunately, such organisms remain sensitive to other substances, such as penicillin and acriflavine. These resistant organisms often make more para-amino benzoic acid than non-resistant organisms.

Sulphadimidine is quickly absorbed and relatively slowly excreted. This is because about 80% of the drug filtered through the glomerulus is reabsorbed by the tubules. It is acetylated to a less extent than sulphanilamide. The acetyl derivative is more water soluble. It is a useful sulphonamide in veterinary practice, both in treating infections caused by susceptible organisms and in cæcal coccidiosis in chickens. This latter disease is treated by giving sodium sulphadimidine in the drinking water. This effect is antagonised by para-amino benzoic acid.

Sulphadiazine is probably the most active sulphonamide. It is well absorbed from the gut, a varying proportion is acetylated depending on species and it is readily excreted by the kidney. The high concentration produced in the urine is useful in the treatment of urinary tract infections. A substantial proportion is reabsorbed by the renal tubules. **Sulphamerazine** is often combined with other sulphonamides. It is well absorbed from the gut but is excreted more slowly than sulphadiazine hence can be given in smaller doses at longer intervals. A greater proportion is acetylated and reabsorbed from the renal tubules as compared with sulphadiazine.

Sulphafurazole has properties similar to the other sulphonamides but has the advantage of acting against certain Gramnegative bacteria. This compound is particularly effective against infections with *E. coli. Proteus vulgaris* and *Pseudomonas aeruginosa*, coccal and mixed infections are less susceptible. It is excreted rapidly, but the excretion products are more soluble in urine than those of the other sulphonamides. This makes it very useful in treating urinary infections.

Succinylsulphathiazole and **Phthalylsulphathiazole** are poorly absorbed from the gut. This is probably because these compounds are almost completely ionized in the gut. With succinyl sulphathiazole 0.1% is un-ionised at pH 7, whereas nearly all the sulphanilamide is un-ionized at pH 7, hence it is sulphanilamide which is almost completely absorbed. Succinyl and phthalylsulphathiazole are slowly hydrolysed in the intestine to liberate sulphathiazole and are useful in treating intestinal infections.

A development of recent years has been the introduction of sulphonamides which are well absorbed from the gut and slowly excreted. These compounds give a concentration of sulphonamide in the plasma which will persist at a reasonably high level for one or more days, hence they have potential advantages in veterinary therapeutics. However, generally speaking, they should not take the place of the quickly absorbed and quickly excreted sulphonamides in the treatment of acute infections as their persistence in the body is a disadvantage if there are any toxic effects. Moreover, towards the end of their time in the body, the concentration may fall below a bacteriostatic level and yet be sufficient to allow resistant strains of organisms to develop.

Sulphamethoxypyridazine is a member of this group. It may be given by all routes but the same objections to parenteral administration exist as with the other sulphonamides. The explanation of the persistence in the body of this compound is partly because of the proportion which is bound to plasma proteins, and partly due to the very effective tubular reabsorption of the free drug. Of the animals so far studied, protein binding is highest in the cow. The bound drug is inactive.

Sulphamethylphenazol is a sulphonamide which persists in the body substantially longer than does sulphamethoxypyridazine. Resistance to the sulphonamides may be due to an alteration in the enzyme using para-amino benzoic acid, an increased ability to destroy the drug, the development of an alternative metabolic pathway or an increase in the production of re-essential metabolites.

TOXIC EFFECTS

The low solubility of the acetyl derivatives in acid or neutral fluids such as dog or cat urine may cause the deposition of crystals of these compounds in the renal tubules. This may produce renal irritation leading to hæmaturia and even anuria. A plentiful supply of liquids together with sodium citrate or bicarbonate to make the urine alkaline will reduce this risk. The urine of herbivores is usually alkaline. In an attempt to reduce the likelihood of a crystalurea, mixtures of sulphonamides have been used. The basis of the employment of such mixtures depends on the fact that substances can exist in solution without interfering with each others solubilities, hence it is possible by using a mixture of sulphonamides to obtain a higher concentration of total sulphonamide without reaching a level at which any individual sulphonamide would crystallize out. Such mixtures commonly contain three sulphonamides usually including sulphacetamide and sulphadimadine.

Cyanosis may occur during sulphonamide therapy due to the formation of sulphaemoglobin or methæmoglobin; this is rarely serious. The most serious complication is the production of an agranulocytosis due to bone marrow damage, and characterised by the disappearance of polymorphonuclear leucocytes from the blood. This is a rare complication, especially when the treatment lasts less than ten days as is usual in veterinary practice.

SULPHONAMIDE SYNERGISTS

When the relationship between the sulphonamide's para-aminobenzoic acid and folic acid was established a search was made for compounds which would interfere with bacterial metabolism. Some of these were structural analogues of folic acid, most were highly toxic because folic acid is important in the metabolism of animal cells being necessary for the synthesis of nucleic acids.

An essential difference between animal cells and bacterial cells lies in the former obtaining their folic acid from external sources, whereas the bacterial cell manufactures its own from para-aminobenzoic acid. An important step in this reaction involves the reduction of dihydrofolate to tetrahydrofolate. This is accomplished through the medium of an enzyme dihydrofolate reductase. Fortunately this enzyme in different organisms differs in structure hence, specific antagonists can be made for the various enzymes.

Trimethoprim antagonises dihydrofolate reductase, the bacterial enzyme being inhibited by concentrations tens of thousands of times less than are required to antagonise the enzyme in mammalian tissues. It can be administered to all the domesticated species by mouth or by injection. Sometimes local reactions take place at the site of injection and depression has been noticed in dogs and cats.

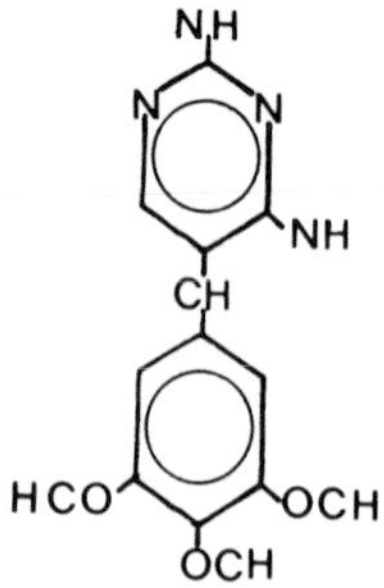

Fig. 21.2 Trimethoprim

So far, haematological changes such as have been recorded in man have not been noted in domesticated animals.

There is a marked difference in the rate at which trimethoprim is removed from the body of different species, and in every case it is much faster than with man. The time for half-clearance is less than four hours in the case of the horse and dog, less than two hours for chickens, cattle, and pigs, and less than one hour for sheep and goats. Most of the drug is metabolised and in the horse about 10% appears in the urine unchanged. Trimethoprim is unevenly distributed in the tissues, the highest concentration occurring in the kidney and liver. It is recommended that milk from cattle treated with this drug should not be used for human consumption for at least 72 hours after the last oral administration, and 7 days after the last injection. Animals for slaughter after administration of trimethoprim should be allowed 28 days after the last injection or 5 days after the last oral administration.

Although trimethoprim has an anti-bacterial activity in its own right it is used in conjunction with a sulphonamide usually sulphadiazine, the action of which is greatly potentiated when the two drugs are given together. This mixture is effective against a wide range of organisms including both Gram-positive, and Gram-negative bacteria. Strains of organisms resistant to sulphonamides are frequently susceptible to the addition of trimethoprim. Sensitivity tests of this drug can be carried out in vitro using a similar technique to that employed for the demonstration of antibiotic sensitivity. Organisms resistant to trimethoprim have been identified and transferrable resistance to this drug has also been found.

SUGGESTIONS FOR FURTHER READING

Finland M, Cass E H 1973 Trimethoprim-sulfamethoxazole. Journal of Infectious Diseases 128:S433
Hawking F, Lawrence J S 1950 The sulphonamides. Lewis, London
Neipp, L 1964 Anti-bacterial chemotherapy with sulphonamides. In: Schnitzer R J, Hawking F (eds) Experimental chemotherapy, Vol 2. Academic Press, New York

22

Chemotherapy of bacterial infections

ANTIBIOTICS

This term is used to describe substances produced by micro-organisms which inhibit bacteria. The first useful antibiotic was penicillin, and the astonishing success of this substance stimulated an intensive search for other antibiotics; only a few of those discovered have proved clinically useful.

Functional classification

It is possible to classify antibacterial agents into three groups on the basis of their activities. Group one includes drugs active mainly against Gram-positive organisms. These have a narrow range of activity and include such drugs as benzylpenicillin, the semi-synthetic penicillinase resistant penicillins and the macrolides.

The second group includes drugs active against aerobic Gram-negative organisms, the amino glycosides, and the polymixins.

The third group includes a wide range of drugs active against both Gram-positive and Gram-negative bacteria such as the broad spectrum penicillins, ampicillin, cephalosporins, the tetracyclines, chloramphenicol and the mixture of sulphonamide with trimethoprim.

The main modes of action

1. The drugs act by interfering with enzymes involved in cell wall formation. Examples of this are the penicillins and cephalosporins.
2. Drugs which affect the permeability of the cell membrane causing leakage of the contents. This group includes detergents, polymixins and nystatin.
3. Drugs which inhibit protein synthesis by acting on the bacterial ribosomes. Examples of such are chloramphenicol, the macrolides.

4. This group includes agents which bind with three OS ribosomal units causing protein synthetic initiation complexes and misreading of the mRNA code and the production of abnormal polypeptides. This group includes the amino-glycosides.
5. Drugs which inhibit DNA-dependent RNA polymerase. An example is rifampin.
6. Certain antimetabolites which block specific essential metabolic steps. These include the sulphonamides and trimethoprim.

Penicillin

In 1877 Pasteur and Joubert discovered the fact that certain common air bacteria stopped the growth in culture of the anthrax bacillus. The most important of these air bacteria was (*B. pyocyaneus*) *Pseudomonas aeruginosa* from which in later years the enzyme pyocyanase was extracted. However, this growth inhibiting property was of no clinical value because the substance responsible was too toxic to use on animals.

In 1928 Fleming found that the growth of staphylococci was inhibited when the cultures in which they were growing became contaminated with the mould *Penicillium notatum*. A substance inhibiting their growth passed into the medium; Fleming called this substance penicillin and showed that it was non-toxic and could be used successfully as an antiseptic. Unfortunately, early attempts to purify this substance failed, and it was not until 1940 that Florey, Chain and their colleagues succeeded in isolating a concentrated preparation of penicillin which was stable when dried. They were able to extract penicillin because when it is acid it passes into an organic solvent from which it can be recovered by shaking with water and alkali.

Several strains of *P. notatum* and various culture media have been used to produce Penicillin, and it was soon realised that a number of penicillins were produced. They differ in their activity on microorganisms and in the rate of absorption and excretion.

Penicillin chrysogenum is used now rather than *P. notatum* because it gives a better yield. In the presence of phenylacetic acid *P. chrysogenum* produces benzylpenicillin and in the presence of phenoxyacetic acid, phenoxymethyl penicillin. A great advance resulted from the discovery that a strain of *P. chrysogenum* produced 6-amino-penicillanic acid, the nucleus of penicillin, which permitted the synthesis of a large number of new penicillins. some of these compounds have great therapeutic value. These manufactured peni-cillins are usually called semi-synthetic.

Benzylpenicillin is widely used in veterinary therapeutics. It forms calcium and sodium salts which are very soluble in water and a procaine salt which is relatively insoluble. The potency of peni-cillin can be expressed either in terms of the weight of the pure substance or with reference to a standard preparation. The standard consists of pure sodium benzyl-penicillin and contains 1670 units per mg.

The sodium and calcium salts of penicillin are stable when dry but aqueous solutions lose their strength. Penicillin is destroyed by acids, alkalies and heat. The optimum pH is 6.5, but solutions at this pH are stable for only about one week even when kept at 4 °C. Oily solutions are quite stable. Some organisms which are often present in non-sterile distilled water secrete an enzyme penicillinase which quickly inactivates penicillin. It is important that solutions of penicillin should be sterile. Since penicillin is destroyed by acids it cannot be given orally.

Aqueous solutions of penicillin are quickly absorbed after sub-cutaneous or intramuscular injection and quickly removed from the body, about 60% of a single dose being excreted in the urine, most of this taking place in the first hour. This rapid urinary excretion shows that the renal tubules excrete a considerable proportion; glomerular filtration as the sole mechanism would be slower. After absorption, penicillin can be detected in bile and saliva. It enters the foetus across the placenta but only a little passes into serous sacs. Penicillin does not enter the cerebro-spinal fluid, and when given parenterally only small amounts are secreted in milk. At-tempts to prolong the effect of a single dose have been directed at either delaying absorption or blocking tubular excretion.

Absorption is prolonged after a suspension of the insoluble pro-caine penicillin in oil or water has been injected intramuscularly or subcutaneously. A further delay in absorption can be produced by adding a water repellant such as aluminium stearate. Preparations such as these only provide a low blood level of the drug and are useless when high concentrations are required.

The excretion of penicillin can be delayed by giving at the same time substances such as diodone and para-amino-hippuric acid which are excreted by the tubules. *Probenecid* is the most effective drug of this kind and acts by blocking the mechanism which con-trols the tubular excretion of penicillin and reabsorption of uric acid but does not affect other renal functions.

Penicillin is most effective against Gram-positive bacteria such as *Staphylococci, Streptococci, Leptospira, Anthrax, Actinomyces, Clostridium tetani* and *Cl. welchi*. It is ineffective against Gram-negative bacteria, *E. coli, Brucella abortus, viruses, protozoa* and *moulds*. Penicillin is a bactericidal antibiotic. The primary mechanism of its action is due to interference with the formation of the bacterial cell wall which it does by inhibiting the synthesis of a mucopolypeptide. It has no effect on formed cell walls, hence it is only active against actively growing bacteria.

Early studies showed that giant forms of bacteria were produced when organisms grew in concentrations of penicillin too weak to kill them. When *Staphylococcus aureus* grew in the presence of penicillin, uridine diphosphate derivatives of muramic acid and muramic acid peptides accumulated. It was then observed that the cell walls of Gram-positive bacteria contained a muramic acid derivative and certain amino acids in the same proportions as they occurred in the aforementioned peptides. This led to the idea that these peptides were the precursors of the cell wall. Penicillin was found to inhibit the incorporation of four cell wall amino acids into the cell wall fraction of *S. aureus* but not into cytoplasmic proteins. Lastly, a good correlation was found between the growth inhibiting concentrations of various penicillins and the inhibition of mucopeptide synthesis in *S. aureus* and *Escherichia coli*.

The intracellular osmotic pressure in bacteria is high because the organism can assimilate and concentrate many soluble substances obtained from the medium in which it is growing. Protection from this high osmotic pressure is provided by a strong cell wall due to the presence of a tough outer coat. The division of organisms into those which stain by Grams' method and those which do not has a greater significance than mere staining. Gram-positive organisms have exacting nutritional requirements with less developed synthesizing abilities, they require amino acids, vitamins and growth factors. Gram-negative organisms on the other hand are highly adaptable organisms with strong synthetic powers. The strength in the wall is provided by a substance murein which is a tough fibrous mucopeptide or glycopeptide. In Gram-negative organisms the murein layer is much thinner and hence the wall is weaker.

Evidence for the action of antibiotics being on murein biosynthesis lies along the following lines: (1) bacteria allowed to grow in a medium of high osmotic pressure are protected from concentrations of antibiotic which would cause lysis and death if they were growing in a normal medium. Bacteria in these conditions lose the stiffening of murein in their walls and become spherical, the cytoplasmic membrane being undamaged but the wall deficient. (2) L-forms of bacteria are deficient in murein and are not susceptible to antibiotics which interfere with murein synthesis. (3) This group of antibiotics act only on growing cells. (4) Bacterial growth in the presence of sub-lethal concentrations of these antiobiotics causes the accumulation of uridine nucleotides of N acetylmuriamic acid with attached amino acid residues. These compounds represent intermediates in early murein synthesis.

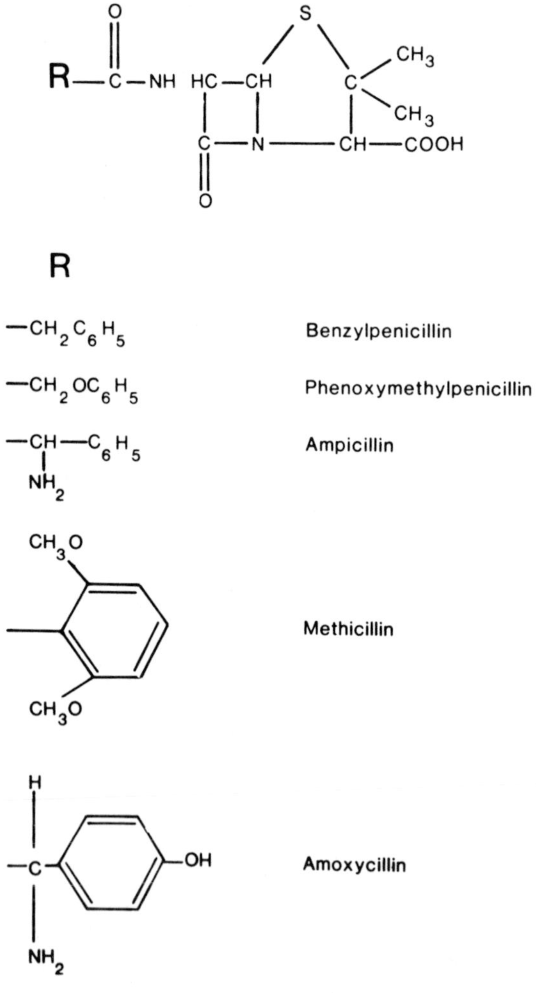

Fig. 22.1 The chemical formulae of some penicillins.

Penicillin, cephalosporin and bacitracin are antibiotics which affect the synthesis of the bacterial cell wall. Penicillin acts at the stage of transpeptidation bringing about the cross-linking of two linear peptido-polysaccharide chains. Penicillinase (β lactamase) converts penicillin to the inactive penicillinoic acid.

Acquired resistance may be induced in some bacteria as a result of exposure to penicillin stimulating the production of penicillinase. Unlike the sulphonamides the action of penicillin is not impaired by blood, pus, tissue autolysates or large numbers of bacteria.

Penicillin is notable for its lack of toxic effects although crude preparations may contain impurities. An untoward effect may arise in veterinary practice due to the widespread use of penicillin as an intramammary injection. Milk containing penicillin is unsuitable for cheese making as the bacteria responsible are often sensitive to penicillin, and milk after intramammary injections may contain enough to prevent the cheese bacteria acting. Very large doses given parenterally may produce the same effect by some of the penicillin being excreted in milk. Intramammary injections of antibiotics to cows may cause illness in babies whose diet consists largely of milk. Milk should not be fed to babies for at least 48 hours after the last intramammary injection. A small proportion of the human population shows a sensitivity reaction to penicillin, and this can be caused by ingesting food stuffs containing even small amounts of this antibiotic. The presence of penicillin in milk is detected by means of a dye test. The dye used is triphenyl-tetrazolium chloride (TTC). This dye changes from colourless to red in the presence of a growing organism (*Str. thermophilus*). This organism fails to grow in the presence of antibiotic and hence the dye fails to change in colour. This test will detect 0.03 μg/ml. of penicillin.

Bacillus subtilis has also been used as a test organism for the detection of antibacterial residues in milk, however, *Bacillus megaterium* is claimed to be better requiring only an incubation of 4–5 hours and being sensitive to a number of different antibiotics and other antibacterials.

SEMI-SYNTHETIC PENICILLINS

Benzylpenicillin has the following shortcomings: (1) it is unstable in acids and, therefore, cannot be given orally. This is, however, of little importance in veterinary medicine. (2) Penicillinase-producing organisms are resistant and such organisms are not uncommon. (3) It is active against only a narrow range of organisms.

Since the introduction of penicillin into medicine, a search has been made for derivatives which overcame these various drawbacks. The first disadvantage was overcome fairly quickly by a relatively simple modification of the benzylpenicillin molecule and phenoxymethyl-penicillin was introduced. This derivative has a sole virtue of being stable in acid medium and hence is suitable for oral administration to dogs and cats. **Phenethicillin potassium** was developed as an improvement on phenoxymethylpenicillin. This derivative is also acid stable and gives almost twice the concentration in blood after oral administration. It is slightly resistant to penicillinase and is given by intramammary injection in the treatment of bovine mastitis when the disease is due to strains of streptococci and staphylococci which are susceptible to this antibiotic.

The search for new penicillins was greatly facilitated when the penicillin nucleus, 6-amino-penicillanic acid, was isolated. This compound greatly increased the number of side chains which were available for substitution and hence the number of possible derivatives. Some of these derivatives have proved of great therapeutic value.

Methicillin

This important derivative of 6-amino-penicillanic acid is resistant to penicillinase. However, it can only be given by injection. Methicillin should never be used in the treatment of infections caused by organisms susceptible to benzyl-penicillin because Methicillin is much less potent and may give rise to strains of organisms which show penicillin resistance not due to the production of penicillinase. Moreover, Methicillin stimulates the production of penicillinase and may increase the number of resistant strains of organism which are resistant by producing this enzyme.

Cloxacillin is resistant to penicillinase and is stable in acid medium. It is a potent drug for inducing the production of penicillinase by organisms which already produce a little of this enzyme.

Ampicillin is an important member of the new penicillins because it is active against both Gram-positive and Gram-negative organisms. This compound is especially useful against coliform organisms which have become resistant to tetracyclines, and strains of *Proteus*, *Pseudomonas*, *Salmonella*, *Shigella* and *Pasteurella* which are not readily treated by other antibiotics. Ampicillin is less potent than benzyl-penicillin against bacteria susceptible to the latter drug. Ampicillin is not resistant to penicillinase and is, therefore, not active against organisms which owe their penicillin resistance to the production of this enzyme. It is acid stable.

Amoxycillin is a semi-synthetic penicillin with similar properties to ampicillin, but is more rapidly and completely absorbed from the gut. It has the same half life as ampicillin but about 60% is excreted in the urine as compared with about 35% of ampicillin. Hetacillin has properties similar to those of ampicillin.

Naphcillin is a semi-synthetic penicillin resistant to penicillinase and inactivated by gastric juice. It must therefore be given parenterally. It produces a lower concentration in the blood than an equivalent dose of cloxacillin because part of the dose is sequested in the liver and a large part excreted in bile.

Flucloxacillin has actions and uses similar to those of cloxacillin. When given by mouth it produces higher concentrations in the blood than an equivalent dose of cloxacillin. It is sometimes used for intra-articular injections.

Oxacillin, dicloxacillin and floxacillin have similar properties to cloxacillin.

Carbenicillin is a semi-synthetic penicillin with similar antibacterial properties to ampicillin but is especially active against *Pseudomonas* and *Proteus*. It must be given by injection as it is unstable in an acid medium. Nearly the whole of a single dose can be recovered from the urine, and it has a plasma half life slightly longer than either penicillin or ampicillin.

Benethamine penicillin is a long-acting preparation which, given by intramuscular injection as an insoluble suspension, slowly releases benzylpenicillin.

Benzathine penicillin has similar properties. However, benzathine penicillin is acid stable and can be given to dogs and cats by mouth.

β-Lactamase inhibitors

Drugs which inhibit a number of β-lactamases have been introduced. These are given in combination with a β-lactamase susceptible penicillin, thus preventing its destruction by the enzyme and permitting the pencillin to produce its usual anti-bacterial action. Clavulanic acid which itself is a β-lactam inhibits a number of β-lactamases in classes II, III, IV, and V. The inhibition produced is irreversible. The Olivanic acids are a group of chemicals which also inhibit a number of β-lactamases. The inhibition is irreversible.

THE CEPHALOSPORINS

This group of antibiotics was derived originally from a strain of *Cephalosporium acremonium* but now an increasing number of semi-synthetic Cephalosporins have been produced. Chemically they are closely related to the penicillins having a nucleus of 7-amino-cephalosporanic acid.

Cephaloridine is one of the principle semi-synthetic cephalosporins which can be used clinically as an alternative to ampicillin because it is bacteriocidal to both Gram-positive and Gram-negative organisms. It is inactive against *Pseudomonas* and fungi. This drug is given by intramuscular injection because it is not absorbed from the gut. It is excreted by the kidney mainly by glomerular filtration. Renal damage has been produced in animals. As with the penicillins these compounds act by interfering with bacterial wall synthesis. They are also similar in producing hypersensitivity reactions.

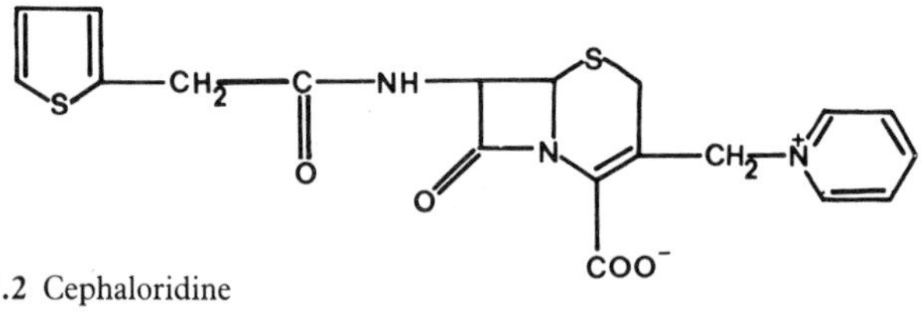

Fig. 22.2 Cephaloridine

THE AMINOGLYCOSIDES

Although chemically it would be more correct to call the antibiotics in this group the aminocyclitols, the older name is more widely used. The antibiotics in this group include *streptomycin, neomycin, dihydrostreptomycin, gentamycin, kanamycin, paromomycin, framycetin, tobramycin* and *amikacin*. Although spectinomycin does not contain an aminoglycoside group it is very similar to the other antibiotics in this category.

Streptomycin

Streptomycin was discovered in a search for antibiotics active against Gram-negative bacteria. Hydrogenation produced dihydrostreptomycin which has similar properties but is more toxic to the cochlea nerve and should not be used systemically.

Streptomycin acts on the bacterial ribosome inhibiting protein synthesis and the fidelity of translation of the genetic code. To reach

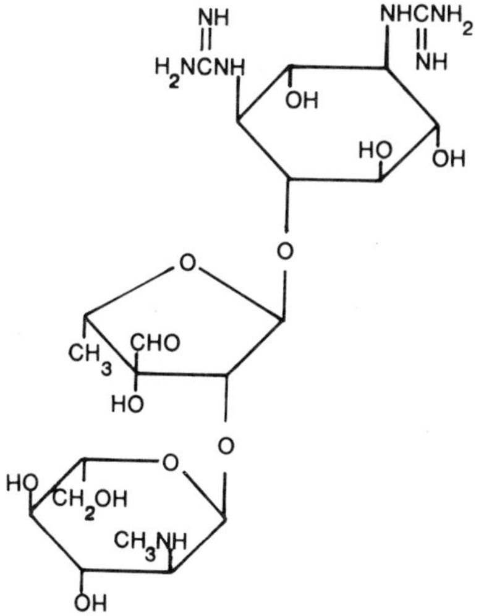

Fig. 22.3 Streptomycin

the ribosome streptomycin must cross the cell membrane and because it is a highly polar compound this requires an active process involving electron transport, oxidative phosphorylation and the respiratory quinones in the cell membrane.

Streptomycin is poorly absorbed from the intestine and is not inactivated in the gut. It has been used to modify the gastrointestinal flora of poultry, pigs and ruminants.

Administration may be also by intramuscular injection or local application. Between 50 and 60% of the absorbed drug is excreted by glomerular filtration through the kidneys. About a third of the drug is bound to protein and hence cannot pass through the glomerulus and between 2 and 5% is excreted in the bile.

Streptomycin is active against most penicillin-sensitive organisms, and some Gram-negative bacteria including *Brucella abortus,*. *E. coli, Proteus sp.* and *Pseudomonas aeruginasa.* It acts also against *Mycobacterium tuberculosis*, but this is only of importance in human medicine as veterinary policy is directed to the eradication of this disease.

The great disadvantage of this antibiotic is the ease with which resistant strains are produced. Resistance to this antibiotic may be due to its failure to permeate the bacteria or to inactivation by microbial enzymes.

The newer amino glycides are much less bound to protein than streptomycin of the order of 10% rather than 30%. The volume of distribution of the aminoglycosides approximates to that of the extra-cellular fluid because their highly polar nature excludes them from most cells. Prolonged treatment with streptomycin may cause renal and hepatic damage and, in dogs and cats, cerebellar and labyrinth disturbances.

Neomycin

Neomycin is obtained from *Streptomyces fradiae* and is a water-soluble basic compound. This antibiotic is similar to streptomycin chemically, pharmacologically and in antibacterial activity. It is active against *Streptococci, Staphylococci, Anthrax, E.coli* and *Proteus* and this activity is unaffected by pus. Neomycin is poorly absorbed from the gut. In some severe infections by bacteria resistant to other antibiotics it may be given by intramuscular injection, intramammary injection or applied locally. It has proved useful in enteritis in foals and calves and in some cases of bovine mastitis.

Spectinomycin acts mainly against Gram-negative organisms and mycoplasma. It inhibits the biosynthesis of protein but is bacteriostatic rather than bacteriocidal in action.

Framycetin has very similar properties to the other aminoglycosides such as neomycin. Its main use is in the treatment of intestinal infections of pigs, calves, and poultry. It has been used against coccidiosis in poultry. This drug is too toxic to administer parenterally, and when organisms show resistance to Framycetin they usually show cross-resistance to the other aminoglycosides.

Gentamycin is an important antibiotic used against Gram-negative organisms. **Tobramycin** given in combination with Penicillin is active against *Pseudamonas*. **Amikacin** is similar to the other amino glycosides pharmacologically but has the widest range of antibacterial activity. Moreover, it resists destruction by the aminoglycosides inactivating enzymes.

The amino glycosides produce a neuromuscular block. Neomycin has the greatest neuromuscular blocking activity followed in descending order of activity by kanamycin, amikacin, gentomycin and tobramycin. They appear to inhibit the pre-junctional release of acetylcholine. This effect is overcome by calcium ions and intravenous calcium is the best treatment if neuromuscular block occurs from the therapeutic use of the amino glycosides.

Novobiocin

This antibiotic which is related chemically to dicoumarol resembles benzylpenicillin in its antimicrobial activity. There is some evidence that novobiocin acts by interfering with bacterial cell membrane synthesis but this is by no means established. It can be used in the treatment of systemic infections and locally. In veterinary therapeutics its main use is in the form of an intramammary injection along with other antibiotics for the treatment of mastitis. It is used in this way to treat staphylococcal infections which are resistant to other antibiotics. In the treatment of infections with *P. vulgaris*, particularly those involving the urinary tract it is to be preferred to neomycin because it is safer. This antibiotic is also active against Gram-negative cocci but it induces resistance in micro-organisms very readily.

TETRACYCLINES

The *tetracylines* were discovered as a result of a search for antibiotics active against a wider range of bacteria than penicillin. **Chlortetracycline** was obtained from *Streptomyces aureofaciens*, **oxytetracycline** from *Streptomyces rimosus* and **tetracycline** is semi-synthetic. More recent introductions have been demethyl-chlortetracycline, methacycline, doxycycline and minocycline.

The tetracyclines form odourless, yellow bases, insoluble in water but soluble as the hydrochloride. Solutions lose their activity in a few days.

These drugs inhibit a wider range of Gram-positive and Gram-negative organisms than penicillin or streptomycin, and have the additional property of acting against certain protozoa such as the *Anaplasma* and *Theileria*, as well as *Rickettsia* and some *Mycoplasma*.

The tetracyclines only inhibit rapidly growing organisms and can give rise to resistant strains, but less readily than streptomycin and erythromycin. Unfortunately, when resistance to one tetracycline develops, the organism is usually resistant to all the tetracyclines; this is called cross-resistance. *Proteus* and *Pseudomonas* organisms are unaffected by the tetracylines.

The tetracyclines may be given by mouth except to ruminants. In carnivores a peak concentration in the blood occurs in two to four hours after oral administration and lasts about six hours. They are widely distributed, entering the CSF and crossing the placenta. Excretion is partly in the urine and bile and part is destroyed in the body. An oral dose takes 3–4 days for its excretion. Because the absorption of tetracyclines from the gut is incomplete and some

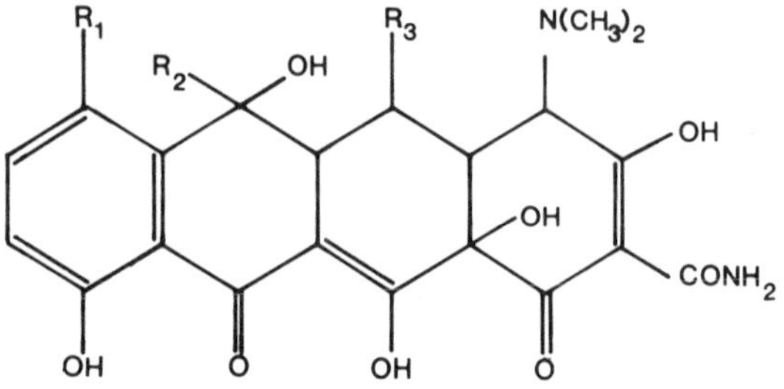

Fig. 22.4 The chemical formulae of some tetracyclines.

	R_1	R_2	R_3
Tetracycline	H	CH_3	H
Chlortetracycline	Cl	CH_3	H
Oxytetracycline	H	CH_3	OH
Demethylchlortetracycline	Cl	H	H
Methacycline	H	CH_2	H
Doxycycline	H	CH_3	OH
Minocycline	$N(CH_3)_2$	H	H

may also be excreted into the intestine, these drugs are usually present in the faeces of animals receiving tetracycline therapy. The daily dose should be divided and given 6-hourly.

The tetracyclines are bacteriostatic excepting in concentrations higher than are produced in the tissues by the usual therapeutic doses. They act on the bacterial ribosome. This involves two processes, firstly passage of the drug through hyrophilic pores and secondly, an energy dependent pump. They inhibit protein synthesis by the micro-organisms, bind to 30S ribosomes preventing access of tRNA to its site on the mRNA ribosome. This prevents the addition of amino acids to the growing peptide chain.

They have also a chelating action in binding the metallic ions, calcium, magnesium and manganese, and so inhibit a number of essential enzyme systems. Moreover, because of this chelating property the tetracyclines are deposited in bones and teeth as a bright yellow fluorescent calcium complex. There is some evidence that in young animals this deposition of the tetracyclines may affect the growth of teeth and bones.

Minocycline is metabolised to a greater extent than the other tetracyclines and persists in fatty tissues.

Doxycycline is not excreted in the urine to the same extent as the other tetracyclines but is excreted mainly in the faeces as an inactive conjugate. It is therefore the safest tetracycline to use for the treatment of extra-renal infections in cases of renal failure. It has the least effect of any of the tetracyclines on the gut flora.

The oral administration of these drugs even in dogs and cats may suppress the normal flora of the digestive tract and allow resistant bacteria, moulds, and fungi to grow, causing several gastro-intestinal disturbances. Chlortetracycline was used as a food supplement. It may now be used only for therapeutic purposes. It improves the growth rate in pigs, chickens and rats, but causes deaths when fed to guinea-pigs over a period of weeks. This shows the dependence of a herbivore on the bacteria of the digestive tract.

The tetracyclines are irritant, and if it is necessary to inject them subcutaneously the injection should incorporate procaine hydrochloride. Apart from these risks the tetracyclines have a low toxicity.

Demethylchlortetracycline is a member of the group of demethyltetracyclines which have been introduced into therapeutics. It is well absorbed from the gut and persists in the body for nearly twice as long as the other tetracylines. This persistence is not due to protein binding because the proportion of demethylchlortetracycline which is protein bound is not substantially different from other tetracyclines. It is equally active to the other tetracyclines but may have some action on *Ps. aeruginosa* and *P. vulgaris*. In man photosensitisation has been reported as occuring after the administration of this tetracycline.

Methacycline is a synthetic derivative of oxytetracycline. It gives a higher concentration of antibiotic in the blood than demethylchlortetracycline and is more slowly excreted in the urine. The persistence in the body may be due to the fact that a greater proportion of methacycline is bound to plasma protein. This compound has a similar range of antibacterial activity to demethylchlortetracycline. However, the most important use of methacycline in veterinary medicine is probably in the treatment and prevention of chronic respiratory disease (CRD) in poultry, as it appears to be particularly effective against the mycoplasma.

Chloramphenicol

Chloramphenicol was first isolated from *Streptomyces venezuelae* as a crystalline compound, which proved to have a simpler structure (Fig. 22.5) than most antibiotics and was soon synthesised. It is poorly soluble in water but dissolves in several organic solvents.

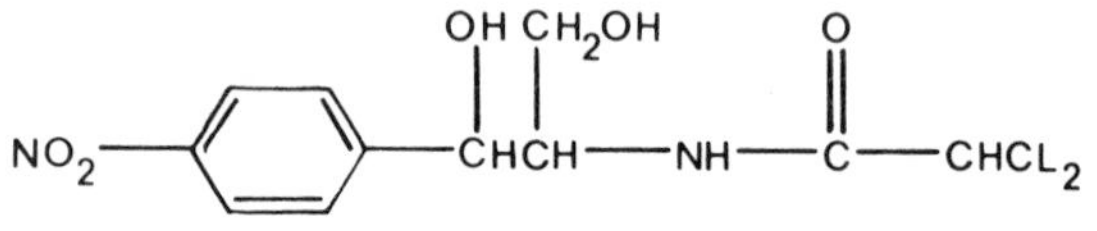

$$NO_2 \text{—} \bigcirc \text{—} \underset{\underset{\text{CHCH}}{|}}{\overset{\overset{\text{OH CH}_2\text{OH}}{|\ \ \ |}}{}} \text{—NH—} \overset{\overset{O}{\|}}{C} \text{—CHCL}_2$$

Fig. 22.5 Chloramphenicol.

When given by mouth, chloramphenicol is well absorbed in dogs and horses but not in cattle or goats. In these latter species it is probably destroyed by rumen bacteria. In the body it is inactivated by conjugation with glucuronic acid. Since cats are deficient in glucuronyl transferase chloramphenicol presents additional hazards in this species. The rate of removal of chloramphenicol varies between the species. The plasma half clearance time ranges from less than an hour in ponies to more than five hours in cats. Dogs have a plasma half clearance time of over four hours. In goats, cats and dogs, the volume of distribution is much greater than one, indicating tissue fixation. About one-third of the drug is bound to plasma protein, the percentage varying between species. The concentration of chloramphenicol in milk resembles that in plasma, and there is some evidence of the excretion of chloramphenicol into the gut through the bile. This is of more than theoretical importance because not only are there glucuronidases which can free the conjugated drug after excretion into the bowel, but the presence in the bowel increases the chance of resistant organisms arising, and also of transferable resistance taking place. The commonest cause of chloramphenicol resistance is from the organism acquiring the resistance factor from other bacteria by conjugation.

Chloramphenicol is active against many Gram-positive and Gramnegative organisms, *Rickettsia*, *Chlamydia* and *Mycoplasma*. The organism involved in swine erysipelas, *Erysipelothrix rhusiopathiae*, is unaffected. Chloramphenicol has been used to combat salmonellosis and CRD infections in poultry. For these purposes it is given in the drinking water. Although it was not detectable in muscle and liver 48 hours after administration ceased, detectable levels were present in the kidney 72 hours after administration and since this organ is usually left in the carcass there is a possible hazard. Moreover, when this drug was given to laying hens the yolks of eggs produced by these birds contained the drug for more than four days after treatment ceased.

Chloramphenicol inhibits the microsomal drug metabolising enzymes and thus prolongs the effects of drugs normally removed from the body by oxidation. The effect of barbiturates on dogs undergoing treatment with chloramphenicol is prolonged.

It is bacteriostatic acting by interference with protein synthesis. This drug blocks the transfer of amino acids from tRNA to the polypeptide chain on the ribosome and interferes with mRNA. Mammalian cells are much less affected than bacterial cells because of their much slower turnover of mRNA.

In man chloramphenicol is an important specific treatment for typhoid and the increase in chloramphenicol resistant strains of the organism causing this disease has given rise to concern. Because of this and the risk of bone marrow damage producing an aplastic anaemia the use of this drug in man is restricted to conditions for which no other microbial agent is available.

Since transmissible resistance is the main type of chloramphenicol resistance, to safeguard the use of this drug for conditions for which no other is suitable, and in particular the treatment of human typhoid, it should be used in veterinary practice with great discretion. However, the use of chloramphenicol in veterinary practice could probably be justified for the treatment of systemic salmonellosis in cattle, respiratory infections in calves and feline panleucopenia. It is probably also the drug of choice for infections of the eye caused by *Moraxella spp.* in cattle and sheep.

Chloramphenicol has caused bone marrow damage in the cat similar to that recorded in man and this may be associated with the inability of the cat to conjugate drugs with glucuronic acid. This drug has also caused death in newborn calves due to kidney damage which may be due to failure of conjugation or inadequate renal excretion of the unconjugated drug.

Lincomycin is an antibiotic with a narrow range of activity exerted mainly against Gram-positive organisms and *Bacteroides*. It is bacteriostatic and acts by interfering with DNA synthesis. It is well absorbed from the gut and has a half clearance time from the plasma of several hours. It is only weakly bound to plasma proteins and enters all tissues including the milk and bile, but excepting the brain and CSF. It also crosses the placenta. This drug has the un-usual property of penetrating bone and is used in the treatment of osteomyelitis. Resistance to this organism is easily induced but cross-resistance only occurs with erythromycin. It is sometimes used as an adjunct to other drugs in the treatment of mycoplasma infections in poultry. It should not be given to laying hens, the treatment should be discontinued at least 48 hours before slaughter.

Clindamycin resembles lincomycin and acts mainly against Gram-positive cocci. It is well absorbed from the gut and may also be given by injection. It is widely distributed entering bone but not cerebrospinal fluid. Most of the absorbed drug is inactivated and little is excreted in the urine. In man it may give rise to disorders of the gastro-intestinal tract.

THE MACROLIDE ANTIBIOTICS

This large group of antimicrobial agents are called Macrolides be-cause one of their chemical characteristics is the possession of a large lactone ring. They are active against most Gram-positive or-ganisms and, in addition, the *Mycoplasma* (PPLO; pleuropneu-monia-like organisms), Rickettsia and certain large viruses. The macrolides are mainly bacteriostatic but, depending on the number of microorganisms and concentrations of antibiotic, they may be bactericidal. These antibiotics inhibit protein synthesis by binding to the ribosomal sub-unit and interfering with the transfer of amino acids from tRNA. There is some degree of cross-resistance between the various members of this group. The macrolides of veterinary importance include **Erythromycin, spiramycin, oleandomycin** and **tylosin**.

Erythromycin

Erythromycin is an antibiotic obtained from *Streptomyces erythreus*. It is selective in action. The susceptible organisms of veterinary im-portance include *Streptococci, Staphylococci, Corynebacteria, Erysi-pelothrix, Clostridia, B. anthracis,* and *Brucella abortus suis*. The *Salmonella, Escherichia, Proteus* and *Br. abortus* are not susceptible. This antibiotic is used only when penicillin-susceptible strains have developed resistance to penicillin. Resistance to erythromycin de-velops quickly. It is relatively non-toxic. Erythromycin probably acts by interfering with the movement of tRNA.

Erythromycin when given by mouth to dogs and cats is rapidly absorbed, giving effective blood levels for six hours. It is widely distributed and excreted in the urine and bile. It also enters the prostatic fluid. Since erythromycin is destroyed by acid gastric juice it is given as enteric coated pills or a suspension of an insoluble preparation. It is too irritant for parenteral administration, although it is sometimes stated that it can be given to all species by intramuscular injection and to poultry subcutaneously.

Oleandomycin is used mainly for the treatment of infections due to staphylococci and streptococci which are resistant to penicillin. It is relatively non-toxic and when given by mouth to rabbits produces a peak concentration in the serum after one hour but the level falls to a low concentration in five hours.

Spiramycin has a range of antibacterial activity similar to that of the other macrolides but has greater in vivo activity. This is probably because spiramycin persists longer in the tissues and at higher concentration than the other macrolides. Spiramycin is probably concentrated and excreted in the bile, hence the faeces have antibiotic activity. The main use in veterinary medicine of this drug is in the prevention and treatment of mycoplasmosis (*M. gallisepticum*) in turkeys. It is also used in the treatment of mastitis due to penicillin-resistant staphylacocci.

Tylosin is a macrolide antibiotic which is absorbed from the gut and excreted in the urine and in bile. It is not very toxic and is active against a large number of Gram-positive organisms, a few Gram-negative organisms and the mycoplasma (PPLO). The main use of this drug in veterinary medicine is in the prevention and treatment of chronic respiratory disease (CRD) caused by mycoplasma in poultry. Tylosin is given for this purpose in the water or poultry feed. It is useful also in the treatment of vibrionic dysentery in pigs. Sometimes pigs react to treatment with tylosin. Oedema of the rectal mucosa and anal protrusion are features of this reaction, the animals also show erythema and pruritus.

POLYPEPTIDE ANTIBIOTICS

Polymyxins

Polymyxins are polypeptide antibiotics like neomycin and bacitracin and are obtained from *Bacillus polymyxa*. There are several polymyxins. They are basic polypeptides which give salts with mineral acids which are water-soluble and stable.

Polymyxin B is the least toxic and only member of the group

suitable for clinical use. It is water-soluble, stable in acids and destroyed by alkalies. It has a selective action on a narrow range of Gram-negative bacteria especially *E. coli, Haemophilus, Salmonellae, Pasteurellae, Brucellae, Shigellae,* and *Vibrio.* It is also active against many strains of *Pseudomonas aeuginosa* but its activity against *Brucella* is limited. The *Staphylococci, Streptococci, Corynebacteria, Proteus, Clostridia* and *Anthrax* are unaffected by this antibiotic. In general polymyxin is regarded as too toxic to administer parenterally and it is used mainly as a local application. It is not absorbed from the gut and is used very occasionally in the treatment of certain intestinal infections. In rare cases of infections of the urinary tract, where the organism is not sensitive to any other antibiotic, it is justifiable to give polymyxin by intramuscular injection. It is excreted in the urine.

Polymyxin is strongly bacteridical, acting on growing and non-growing cells, and its effectiveness depends on the number of organisms present. Polymyxin is a surface-active agent and substances which are antagonistic to the cationic detergents also inhibit polymyxin. This activity does not completely explain the antibacterial action of polymyxin which is restricted to Gram-negative organisms whereas the cationic detergents are effective against both Gram-positive and Gram-negative organisms. This drug is strongly bound to bacteria and causes the release of cytoplasmic solutes by increasing the permeability of the cell membrane. It also has an inhibitory action on oxidative metabolism. The surface activity shown by polymyxin on bacterial cells can also affect the cells of the host, and polymyxin is known to cause the release of histamine from cells containing this active substance. Resistance to polymyxin is infrequent, hence this drug is often combined with other antibiotics. Polymyxin is used in veterinary therapy in local applications to the skin, mucous membranes, the external ear and intramammary injections.

Bacitracin

Bacitracin is an antibiotic obtained from a strain of *B. subtilis.* This bacterium was found on the infected wounds of a patient, Miss Tracy, after whom the antibiotic was named. It is active against Gram-positive organisms including some *Clostridia* and *Actinomyces bovis.* It is poorly absorbed from the gut and in fact is destroyed in the alimentary tract. This antibiotic blocks the incorporation of nucleotides into the cell wall.

Since bacitracin is one of the few antibiotics which is permitted in the United Kingdom to be used as a food additive for growth promoting purposes without the need of a prescription it would be wise to restrict its use to this purpose.

Nystatin and Griseofulvin are antibiotics active against yeasts and fungi and are considered later (p. 404).

Sodium fusidate is a bacteriostatic agent active against both Gram-positive and Gram-negative cocci. It is useful against penicillin resistant staphylococci and as an ointment in skin infections. It is well absorbed from the gut and may be administered topically when it penetrates the skin especially when given dissolved in dimethyl sulphoxide. It is widely distributed but does not enter the CSF or cross serous membranes. However, it crosses the placenta and is excreted in milk. Large amounts are protein-bound but small amounts are excreted unchanged in the urine and bile.

CHOICE OF ANTIBIOTICS

The *selection* of antibacterial agent depends on the infecting organism and its sensitivity to the various drugs. However, it is often essential to begin the treatment without this knowledge, and it is necessary to act on the assumption that the organism will be sensitive to a particular antibacterial drug. Should there be no response to treatment within two days, or laboratory tests show the organism more sensitive to another drug, the treatment can be changed accordingly.

The most commonly used test for determining the sensitivity of a pathogenic organism to antibiotic is to spread the infective material on suitable plate of agar culture medium and to place on the surface discs of filter paper which have been soaked in the various antibiotics under test. When an organism is sensitive to an antibiotic, tested in this way, there is a clear zone around the filter paper indicating the absence of bacterial growth. The size of the clear zone does not necessarily indicate relative potency of the antibiotic as the clearing can be influenced by factors such as the size of the inoculum and the rate at which the antibiotic diffuses through the agar. However, it serves as a crude test of sensitivity and the results of such tests should be treated in this light. It is sometimes possible by the use of tests of this kind to determine in a matter of a few hours whether or not a particular organism is antibiotic sensitive and, using such relatively rapid tests, to initiate

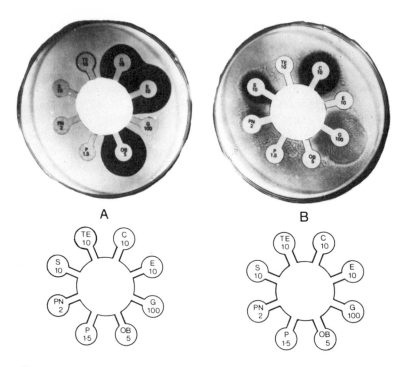

Fig. 22.6 An antibiotic sensitivity test. Dish A: *Staph. pyogenes aureus*. Dish B: *Proteus mirabilis*. The clear zone around the disc indicates antibiotic sensitivity. This strain of staph pyogenes is resistant to benzylpenicillin.

C = chloramphenicol 10 μg;   OB = cloxacillin 5 μg;
E = erythromycin 10 μg;   PN = ampicillin 2 μg;
G = sulphafurazole 100 μg;   S = streptomycin 10 μg;
P = penicillin G 1.5 μg;   TE = tetracycline 10 μg.

treatment, in cases such as bovine mastitis, sufficiently quickly to prevent the loss of a quarter of the udder.

Occasionally in vitro tests do not correlate with in vivo sensitivity.

Antibacterial drugs fall into two categories when classified according to their mode of action, that is they can be considered as either bacteriostatic or as bactericidal agents. In general, it is better to use a bactericidal rather than a bacteriostatic antibiotic. However, even when using such a compound complete bactericidal action may be cancelled by the presence, of organisms which are sometimes called 'persisters'. These organisms represent a small proportion of dormant bacteria which, although potentially sensitive to the drug, survive the effect of the bactericidal drug and may give rise to a subsequent infection. Such organisms are common in old bacterial populations, inside cells and in pus. The common bactericidal antibiotics are penicillins, streptomycin and polymyxin. The sulphonamides, tetracyclines, chloramphenicol, erythromycin and novobiocin are bacteriostatic agents. In severe infections it is better if possible to use a bactericidal rather than a bacteriostatic antibacterial agent as it is possible that the hosts immunosuppressive mechanism may be impaired and the bacteriostatic drugs depend greatly for their action on the hosts defence mechanism.

The importance of the phenomenon of antibiotic resistance has already been discussed. There are, however, two further categories of resistance worth mention, the phenomenon of so-called 'multiple resistance' and that of 'one step' resistance. It has been shown in the laboratory by repeated exposure of organisms to drugs that the induction of resistance to penicillin is a slow or step-wise process, whereas the repeated exposure of organisms to an antibiotic, such as streptomycin, results in a very rapid increase of resistance; this is sometimes called multiple resistance. The drugs against which multiple resistance is most likely to occur are streptomycin, erythromycin, and novobiocin. It is considered usually a sound general principle that the drugs which show multiple resistance should be used in conjunction with at least one other drug which is effective against the particular organism to be treated. This procedure is adopted because it is hoped that the second drug of the combination will affect not only all the organisms sensitive to the first drug, but will include a small proportion of the mutants which are naturally resistant to the first drug.

The site of the infection together with the fate of the drug in the body and the possibility of producing undesirable side effects have also to be considered in selecting the drug. Sometimes antibiotics may act synergistically; those acting as bactericides, such as penicillin, bacitracin and neomycin, may potentiate each other, but when combined with the tetracyclines and chloramphenicol which are bacteriostatic may produce antagonism. This can be appreciated when one considers that a bactericidal drug, such as penicillin, which exerts its effect on actively growing organisms cannot do so if the growth of the organism is suppressed by a bacteriostatic agent. The difficulty of measuring the effectiveness of antibiotic combinations clinically, coupled with the risk of producing drug-resistant strains, make it advisable to begin treatment with one antibiotic and to change only when laboratory tests or lack of clinical response show it to be unsuitable.

Synergism between antimicrobial drugs is uncommon. The combination of sulphonamide and trimethoprim, and possibly the combination of penicillin with streptomycin are examples. However, antimicrobial combinations are sometimes used with the intention of delaying the development of drug resistance; to broaden the range of antibacterial activity; or to reduce the incidence of adverse reactions. It is difficult to find evidence to justify combinations which achieve these ends. Moreover, when antimicrobial agents are given in combination then the dose of one determines the amount of the combined drugs, whereas by administering each drug separately greater latitude in dosage is allowed.

The misuse of antibiotics

In order to limit the rate of increase of antibiotic resistant strains of bacteria every effort should be made to limit the use of these drugs, and in particular to avoid their misuse. Among the common misuses are procedures such as using them to treat untreatable infections such as viruses or using them indiscriminately to treat fevers of unknown origin. The administration of improper doses may also lead to trouble. If too much is given toxic effects may be produced. Conversely, too little for too short a time may be ineffective and also help in the production of resistant strains. Chemotherapy without appropriate surgery is also inadvisable. For example, in the treatment of abscesses. The lack of adequate bacteriological information may also lead to the misuse of antibiotics.

EFFECTS OF ANTIBIOTICS ON GROWTH RATE

Very small amounts of antibiotics when fed to chickens produce an increase in growth. Food conversion is increased and a reduction in mortality in growing chickens is also produced. It is now common practice to add an antibiotic to poultry foods. Similar but more variable results have been obtained with fattening pigs. In ruminants antibiotics in food may be used up to the onset of rumination to produce a similar effect.

There have been a number of theories which attempt to explain the growth-promoting action of antibiotics but the evidence, so far, is inconclusive. It has been suggested that the growth-promoting antibiotics affect the intestinal flora in such a way as to increase the synthesis of certain growth factors essential to the host. Another suggestion has been that these antibiotics, by inhibiting certain organisms which compete for growth factors produced in the gut allow these growth factors to become available to the host. A third theory proposes that the antibiotics act by inhibiting organisms which produce toxic substances deleterious to the host.

A further theory which is supported by some experimental evidence implicates pathological changes in the intestinal epithelium. In this theory it is suggested that, in the absence of antibiotics, organisms in the gut cause damage to the epithelium which impairs absorption. The antibiotics by inhibiting these organisms prevent the damage and thus facilitate the absorption of nutrients. In support of this theory, it has been shown that the intestinal epithelium of antibiotic-fed animals is thinner than in untreated animals. There is also evidence that some antibacterial agents depress the body metabolism and thus allow more of the absorbed nutrients to be used for building tissues.

However, probably the most widely accepted explanation of the growth-promoting activity of antibiotics is that these drugs produce this effect by curing sub-clinical infections. These infections are not such as to produce obvious clinical signs of disease but are, nonetheless, present, hence are termed sub-clinical. The best evidence for this type of drug-promoting action has been obtained from experiments with chickens. It has been shown that the droppings of untreated fowls apparently contain growth-suppressing agents which are not present when antibiotics are added to the diet. Moreover, the better the general management and hygiene of the animals the less effect antibiotics have on food conversion and mortality.

The increasing incidence of resistance to antimicrobial agents has been the cause of some concern. This concern was increased as the potentialities of transferable resistance became widely appreciated. In the United Kingdom a Government Committee was set up to study the hazards which might arise from using antibacterial agents to promote growth in food producing animals. This Committee recommended, and their recommendations were later implemented in law, that antimicrobial agents should be separated into two classes so that those of major therapeutic importance would not be used for growth promoting purpose. As a consequence a limited number of antimicrobial agents are available as food additives without prescription for the purpose of promoting growth. At present these comprise Flavomycin for calves and pigs and non-laying poultry; Virginiamycin for pigs and non-laying poultry; and Bacitracin for pigs and non-laying poultry. In addition to these antibiotics two nitrofurans with antimicrobial activity namely: Nifursol and Nitrovin are available without prescription for the same purpose. Carbadox is a quinoline antibacterial agent used as a growth promoter. Zeranol given as an implant has both anabolic and eostrogenic actions which promote carcase growth.

SUGGESTIONS FOR FURTHER READING

Edwards S J 1964–1965 Antibiotics as supplements in the food of calves. Vet. A. 6:22

English P B 1965 Antibiotics in veterinary practice. Australian Veterinary Journal 41:80

Franklin T J, Snow J A 1971 Biochemistry of microbial action. Chapman & Hall, London

Gale E F 1963 Mechanism of antibiotic action. Pharmacological Reviews 15:481

Pratt 1977 Chemotherapy of infection. Oxford University Press, New York
  Schnitzer R J, Hawking F 1964 Experimental Chemotherapy, Vols. 2 & 3.
Academic Press, New York

Stratton J 1964–1965 Sulphonamides, antibiotics. Vet. A. 6:268

Wallace H D 1970 Biological responses to antibacterial feed additives in diets of meat producing animals. Journal of Animal Science 31:1118

23

Chemotherapy of protozoal infections

PROTOZOA are the causal agents of many diseases of domestic animals, and drugs are available for both the prevention and treatment of several of these diseases. Probably the commonest protozoal diseases in the United Kingdom are caused by coccidia, and although most species of domestic animal are affected it is a particularly serious problem in poultry.

ANTI-COCCIDIAL DRUGS

There are many species of coccidia of which those of importance in veterinary medicine infest the epithelium of the gut, biliary tract or the urinary system, causing damage to capilliary vessels and a consequent loss of blood. The organism is transmitted from animal to animal by faecal contamination and thus attention to hygiene is important in the control of this disease.

Although the second generation schizont is the most pathogenic stage of this disease it is also the phase most susceptible to the actions of drugs for example, the sulphonamides. Probably only six species of cocoidia are of economic importance namely; *Eimeria acervulina*, *E. brunetti*, *E. maxima*, *E. mivati*, *E. necatrix*, and *E. tenella*. *E. necatrix* and *E. tenella* can cause death, the other species impair the maximum growth rate of the bird. Drugs which act against coccidia are frequently called coccidiostats, it is probably preferable to use the term anticoccidial which does not distinguish between coccidiostatic and coccidiocidal activity. The ideal anticoccidial agent should show a high level of activity against most species of coccidia, it should leave no residue of either the parent drug or metabolite in the carcase and should be cheap. The available drugs suppress coccidial development and the first generation schizont stage, and this also suppresses the development by the bird of resistance to coccidial infection.

The sulphonamides were the first effective drugs used in the

329

treatment of coccidiosis in chickens (*Eimeria tenella*) and are still valuable for this purpose. Probably the most widely used is sulphaquinoxaline. Sulphadimidine is also employed. These drugs are usually given as their sodium salt in the drinking water.

Sulphadimethoxine and sulphachlorpyridazine appear to be more effective against coccidia than sulphaquinoxaline. The therapeutic effect depends upon the maintenance of an effective concentration of sulphonamide in the blood which is similar to that required in bacterial infections, 5–10 mg/100 ml blood. Para-amino benzoic acid antagonises this effect of the sulphonamides.

The nitrofurans

One of the earliest coccidiostatic agents introduced into veterinary medicine was a member of the group of mononitro compounds, the **nitrofurans**. The nitrofurans also show marked antibacterial activity against a wide range of organisms.

Nitrofurazone is a nitrofuran used to prevent and treat caecal coccidiosis in chickens. It is less effective in duodenal coccidiosis or in coccidiosis in turkeys. This drug is effective also in infections due to Gram-positive and Gram-negative organisms and is used externally to treat such infections. When used to prevent caecal coccidiosis it is given in the dry mash because it is insoluble in water. Five parts nitrofurazone per 1000 parts feed do not interfere with

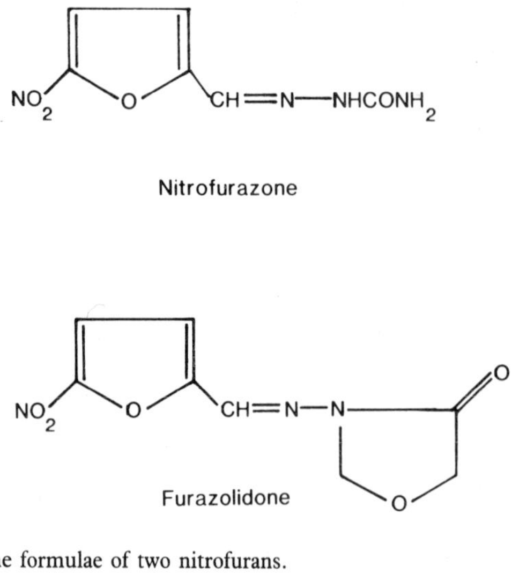

Nitrofurazone

Furazolidone

Fig. 23.1 The formulae of two nitrofurans.

growth. However, toxic effects may arise due to errors in mixing or feeding or to individual birds being especially susceptible. Birds so affected lose their appetite and appear bedraggled and motionless, small numbers show excitement. On post-mortem a patchy enteritis and cardiac degeneration are found. Toxic signs and pathological changes are occasionally produced by feeding at the rate of one part per thousand. A particularly important toxic effect is the reversible arrest of spermatogenesis which is associated with testicular changes and occurs after the prolonged prophylactic use of nitrofurazone. Ducklings appear to be particularly susceptible to its toxicity. Resistant strains of coccidia have appeared after the prophylactic use of nitrofurazone. These nitrofurazone-resistant strains of coccidia do not show cross-resistance and are usually susceptible to treatment with a sulphonamide.

Furazolidone is a nitrofuran which is active against a number of pathogenic protozoa, in particular, *coccidia, hexamita, histomonas* and *trichomonas*. It is effective also against many Gram-positive and Gram-negative organisms and, in particular, it is used to control the mortality in fowl typhoid (*Salmonella gallinarum*) and pullorum disease (*S. pullorum*). It has an inhibitory action on the protozoa causing blackhead in turkeys (histomoniasis), and is used also for the treatment of infectious sinusitis in turkeys. A preparation is available which can be injected into the sinuses. This drug should not be fed to breeding stock because changes in the testicular tissue may be produced, although egg production and the fertility of eggs are unaffected. Calves are particularly susceptible to nitrofuran poisoning. Although furazolidone is effective in producing a clinical cure of certain *Salmonella* infections of large animals, a bacteriological cure does not always occur and organisms may persist especially in the gall bladder. Moreover, certain *Salmonella* of the large animals present a potential hazard to humans and it is doubtful whether the treatment of animals used for food is justified.

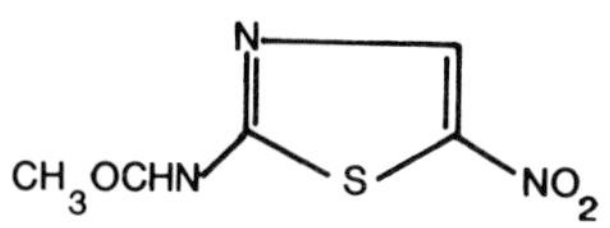

Fig. 23.2 Acinitrazole.

A related compound METRONIDAZOLE is used in infections with trichomonas and studies of the mode of action of this compound have shown that it inhibits the synthesis of DNA. It is rapidly metabolised by trichomonads probably to form a reactive derivative which is preferentially absorbed through the cell membrane and binds to DNA, thus inhibiting a synthesis of further DNA. Metronidazole is also useful in the treatment and prevention of infections involving anaerobic bacteria.

Dimetridazole is used to prevent and treat infections with *Histomonas meleagridis* infections in turkeys. It is also used to treat dysentry in pigs caused by spirochetes, vibrios, bacteroides and some protozoa. Pigs excrete 80% of a single dose within 2 days and turkeys 90% in 3 days. It is of low toxicity.

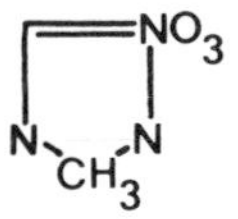

Fig. 23.3 Dimetridazole.

Acinitrazole has replace aminonitrothiazole for the treatment and prevention of blackhead (histomoniasis) in turkeys. This is because acinitrazole is almost free from toxic effects even when fed to breeding birds over long periods. For the prevention of histomoniasis, acinitrazole is given continuously in the feed. When thus fed for very long periods it may cause a loss in weight. Testicular atrophy has also been reported.

Dinitro compounds

Nicarbazin is a complex of two chemical compounds used in the prevention of coccidiosis in poultry. The morbidity and mortality from *Eimeria acervulinum*, *E. necatrix* and *E. tenella* and from mixed infections are prevented. Moreover, strains of coccidia resistant to other coccidiostatic drugs may be susceptible to nicarbazin. The drug is fed continuously as 0.0125% of the ration. It is usually diluted with an inert vehicle before mixing with the food. The administration of nicarbazin may reduce egg production and the hatchability of fertile eggs. It may increase the incidence of eggs with mottled yolks but it does not appear to affect the quality of the semen. De-pigmentation of the shell has been recorded, and when given in excessive doses a reduction in food consumption and growth occurs. This drug has now been superseded by other anticoccidial agents.

Vitamin Antagonists

Amprolium hydrochloride is a coccidiostatic agent whose action depends on the fact that it is antagonistic to thiamin, hence. high concentrations of aneurin prevent amprolium exerting its anticoccidial activity. It is considered that amprolium, by antagonising thiamin, denies thiamin to the coccidia and since the requirements of the coccidia for thiamin are greater than those of the host, the coccidia suffer more from this deprivation.

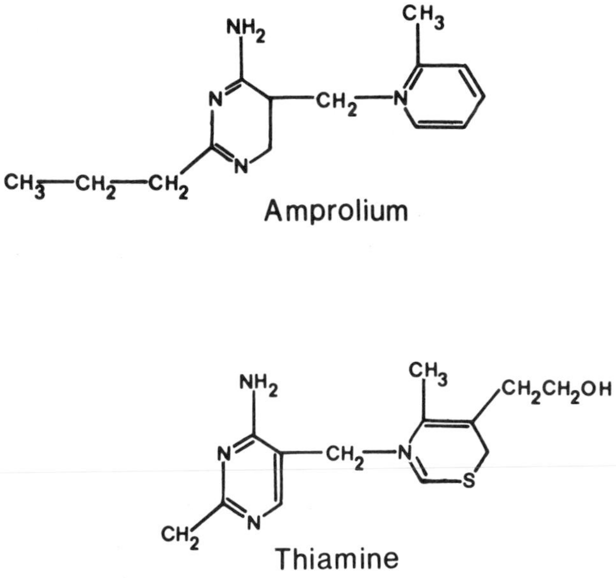

Amprolium

Thiamine

Fig. 23.4 The vitamin thiamine and its anti-coccidial antagonist.

Amprolium is used prophylactically to prevent coccidiosis in chickens and turkeys and for this purpose it is given mixed in the feed as a continuous medication. Amprolium is often combined with other coccidiocidal and coccidiostatic agents such as sulphaquinoxaline and sulphadimidine. It is regarded as having a satisfactory degree of activity against *E. tenella* and *E. acervulina* but not against *E. necatrix*, *E. brunetti*, *E. maxima* and *E. mivati*.

The toxicity of amprolium is due to the antagonism of thiamin and the signs of amprolium poisoning are those of thiamin deficiency. Although in the concentrations usually fed, amprolium has no effect on the fertility of poultry, a proportion of the chickens hatched from eggs produced by hens treated with this drug may be found dead within the shell.

Diaveridine is an analogue of the antimalarial pyrimethamine and like this compound is a folic-folinic acid antagonist. Although diaveridine possesses bacteriostatic properties, it is primarily a coccidiostatic agent used to prevent coccidiosis in poultry. It is given together with sulphaquinoxaline because there is a degree of synergism in the coccidostatic action of these two drugs. This synergism results from each of the two drugs influencing a different phase of the folic acid metabolism of the coccidia. The sulphonamide interferes with the p-aminobenzoic acid metabolism which is concerned in the production of folic acid whereas diaveridine interferes with the actual folic acid metabolism. The life cycle of the parasite is not completely interrupted by diaveridine and sufficient coccidial development takes place to produce a high degree of immunity in birds exposed to infection whilst these drugs are being given. Diaveridine itself has a very low toxicity. This toxicity is increased by the addition of the sulphonamide but not until four times the recommended prophylactic dose is given. Egg production, fertility and hatchability appear to be unimpaired by diaveridine.

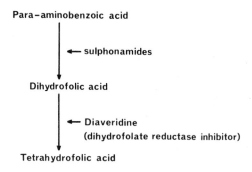

Fig. 23.5 A diagram to illustrate the points at which sulphonamides and dihydrofolate reductase inhibitors such as diaveridine interfere with the formation and metabolism of folic acid by micro-organisms.

Ethopabate is a para-aminobenzoic acid antagonist which is coccidiostatic against most coccidia with the important exception of *Eimeria tenella*. It is active against strains of *E. brunetti* which are very resistant to sulphonamides. Ethopabate potentiates pyrimethamine, a folic-folinic acid antagonist and may be combined with it or with its analogue diaveridine in a coccidiostatic mixture.

The quinolates

Methyl benzoquate is a comparatively new coccidiocidal agent which appears to act when the sporozoites penetrate the epithelial cell. It is active against all the common species of coccidia which infest poultry and no ill effects have appeared after the continuous feeding of this drug. It is claimed that **Methyl benzoquate** is more active than many other anticoccidial agents on a weight basis. Less than 0.3% of an oral dose is absorbed hence residues are very low, a little being detected in the liver. Chemically methyl benzoquate is a quinolate. Two other quinolates are *decoquinate* and *clopidol*. These quinolates resemble methyl benzoquate in coccidiocidal activity. They are insoluble in water and their activity is influenced by particle size the smaller particle showing greater activity.

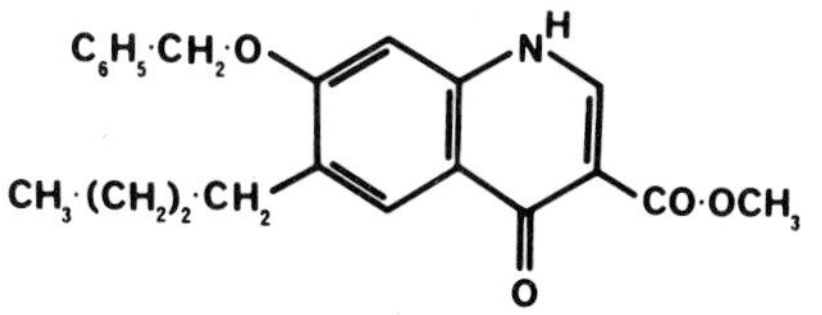

METHYL BENZOQUATE

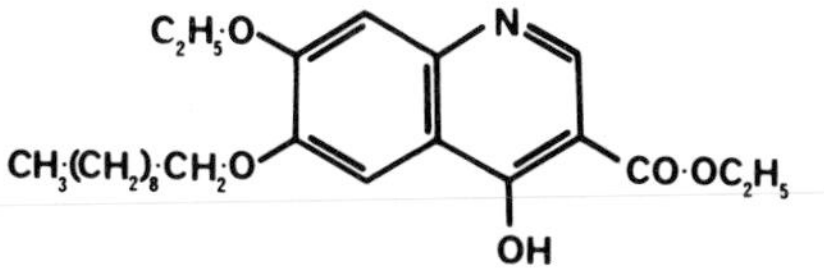

DECOQUINATE

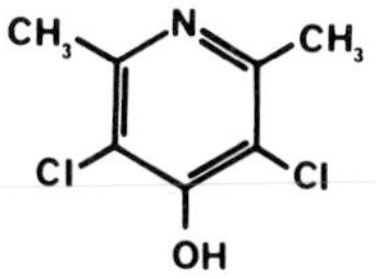

CLOPIDOL

Fig. 23.6 Three quinolate coccidiocidal drugs.

The quinolates permit some occyst production and seem to have a greater tendency than many other anti-coccidial drugs in allowing the development of drug resistant strains.

Methyl benzoquate inhibits but does not kill coccidia and only inhibits parasites in epithelial cells being unable to reach organisms in the deeper tissues.

Decoquinate is known to be the most active quinolate and to have the largest margin of safety.

Robenidine is an anti-coccidial which has proved effective against a number of strains of coccidia resistant to one or more of the older drugs. It has been claimed to give complete suppression of oocyst production but has the disadvantage of tainting the flesh in at least a proportion of birds and, if fed to laying birds tainting the eggs. It has so far proved impossible to separate the anticoccidial activity in closely related compounds from the taint producing property and the only way whereby this drug can be used is to withdraw medicated feed at least seven days before slaughter.

Aprinocid. This anti-coccidial appears to act by inhibiting nucleic acid formation. It is rapidly metabolised in the chick and at the recommended doses does not appear to produce adverse effects.

Halofuginone. Weight for weight this is one of the most active anti-coccidial agents known, but the separation of activity from toxicity is minimal. However, it is chemically different from the other anticoccidial agents and may provide a basis for the synthesis of new and better agents.

A recently introduced anti-coccidial is a premix containing salinomycin-sodium. It is used in the prevention of coccidiosis in chickens caused by *Eimeria acervulina, E. brunetti, E. maxima, E. mivita, E. necatrix* and *E. tenella*. This preparation is only suitable for use in broilers. Care should be taken to prevent horses gaining access to feed containing this drug as it has caused fatalities. Operators handling the product should wear suitable protective clothing and wash thoroughly after handling the substance. Birds fed this drug should not be slaughtered for human consumption until at least 5 days have elapsed since the last treatment. It should not be used in conjunction with any other anti-coccidial nor in breeding birds.

THE IONOPHOR ANTICOCCIDIALS

Monensin is a member of this group of agents which is probably the most widely used anticoccidial for prophylaxis in the USA. As a therapeutic agent it compares unfavourably to most of the other established anti-coccidials. Part of its action in promoting weight gain especially in ruminants may be due to its ionophor action on the rumen fermentation in facilitating the production and movement of proprionate through the cell wall of the ruminal and intestinal epithelium. It is a specific ionophor for Na ions.

Lasalocid is an ionophor with some relationship to monensin. It appears to have a greater separation of activity and toxicity than does monensin and although it has proved superior to monensin in laboratory studies there is insufficient evidence as yet from the field to see whether it may replace monensin. However, monensin is a most economical prophylactic anticoccidial and the price of any replacement would be an important factor.

BABESIOCIDAL DRUGS

The babesia or piroplasmata are protozoal parasites which multiply in the red blood cells of various mammals or birds and are transmitted by ticks. They cause disease in the domesticated animals as, for example, in British redwater (*Babesia divergens*). A useful drug in the treatment of this disease is **quinuronium sulphate**, a compound of quinoline and urea (Fig. 23.7). It is effective against all babesia but does not completely eradicate all the parasites, and animals which clinically appear to have recovered may still harbour parasites. This drug must be given by subcutaneous injection as it is dangerous to inject it intramuscularly or intravenously. Shortly

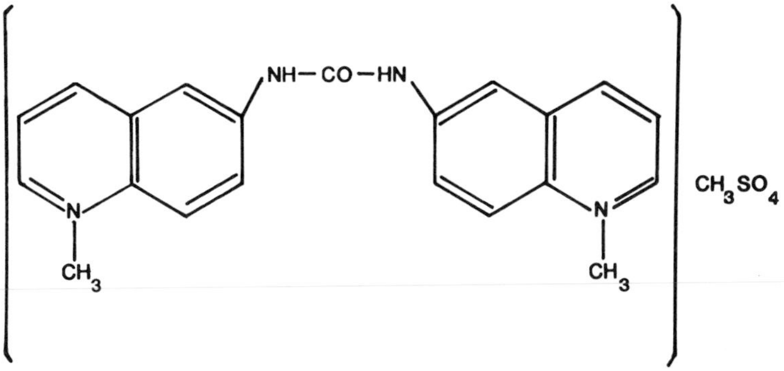

Fig. 23.7 Quinuronium sulphate.

after the injection the animal salivates, defaecates and may stagger and fall. The drug causes a fall in blood pressure, increases testinal contractions and salivation. Species differ in their susceptibility to these side effects and, arranged in decreasing order of susceptibility, they are dog, horse, cattle, sheep and pig. These effects are due mainly to the potent anticholinesterase activity of quinuronium and they can be alleviated but not completely prevented by giving a large dose of Atropine before the administration of quinuronium (Fig. 23.8). Quinuronium also releases histamine and depresses cellular oxidation but these various actions probably do not account for all the pharmacodynamic effects of this drug.

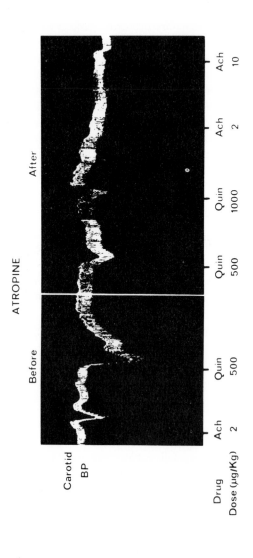

Fig. 23.8 The antagonism by atropine on the fall in blood pressure produced by Quinuronium. The effect on the blood pressure of a sheep of the administration of acetylcholine and quinuronium is shown before and after atropine. (Courtesy of P. Eyre.)

Amicarbalide (3 : 3-diamidinocarbanilide) has replaced quinuronium to a large extent for the treatment of babesiasis. However, it is less effective against other species. Amicarbalide is much less toxic; for example the L.D.50 of amicarbalide in mice is 15 times that of quinuronium. Moreover, the only untoward effect reported as occurring in animals treated with amicarbalide has been a mild ataxia. Amicarbalide given by intramuscular injection caused only a transitory swelling, but a severe local reaction followed the subcutaneous injection of this drug. Some of this reaction may be due to the histamine releasing action of amicarbalide. In horses there is evidence that this drug can damage the liver as a rise in serum glutamic oxalacetic transaminase, sorbitol dehydrogenase and serum urea nitrogen followed its administration. This has been supported by histopathological studies. There is also evidence of necrosis of the muscle around the site of injection. It has been suggested however, that certain strains of *Babesia* are resistant to amicarbalide and this may reduce the usefulness of the drug.

Imidocarb is chemically related to amicarbalide also being a carbanilide. It was selected from a series of these compounds because it had a good therapeutic index. It is effective in cattle against *Babesia bigemina* having both curative and prophylactic properties and consistent with the latter, residues persist in the liver and kidneys. It is recommended that animals should not be slaughtered within three months of treatment. It is also effective in *B. divergens*. In dogs (*B. canis*) and the babesia of the horse respond to imidocarb.

This drug may give rise to a local reaction at the site of subcutaneous or intramuscular injection. The higher doses of this drug produce untoward effects in all species reminiscent of an anticholinesterase action. In the dog the cardiovascular and neuromuscular effects predominate, whereas in the horse, a species in which marked reactions have been observed, these take the form of salivation, colic, diarrhoea, and loss of weight.

Phenamidine has been used occasionally to treat babesiasis in horses and dogs.

Diminazene is an active babesiacidal agent and is of value in the treatment of clinical babesiasis in cattle, sheep, horses, and dogs. It is mainly used for its trypanocidal actions and is considered later (p. 345).

ANAPLASMOSIS

The tetracyclines are well established in the treatment of clinical cases and the eradication of the carrier state of this condition. However. the expense prevents their use on a large scale. Moreover intramuscular or intravenous injections with these compounds are time consuming and add to the expense. Although it is possible to administer tetracyclines orally to infected carrier cattle, this does not greatly reduce the cost. Some dithiosemicarbazones have shown activity against *Anaplasma marginalae* they have to be given by intravenous injection and only after daily administration for 10 days was it possible to eliminate the parasite completely. Moreover degeneration of the vagus nerve and the development of tympanities have been recorded. There appears to be a degree of synergism between the dithiosemicarbazones and oxytetracycline, this would allow the employment of small amounts of the first drug and presumably the reduction of the toxic effects. The babesicide imidocarb has proved effective against *Anaplasma marginalae*. However, it requires at least three injections at intervals of 24 hours to eliminate the carrier state.

TRYPANOCIDAL DRUGS

The trypanosomes are flagellates which live in the blood and tissues of vertebrates and are particularly important because they cause disease in livestock. They are transmitted by tsetse flies (*Glossina*). Since the recognition of these protozoa as pathogenic organisms, attempts have been made to devise drugs to kill them.

The discovery by Ehrlich that certain dyestuffs, first used as stains, had a specific affinity for these parasites led eventually to the discovery of the trypanocidal action of the organic arsenicals. In recent years many hundreds of compounds have been tested for trypanocidal actions and substances which are more effective and less toxic than the organic arsenicals are now available.

Quinapyramine

It has been shown that quinapyramine has moderate trypanocidal activity in vitro in addition to its in vivo action against these parasites, but the most significant property of this drug lies in its power to destroy the infectivity of trypanosomes. This is shown by its action in mice infected with trypanosomes. The trypanosomes in the mice continue to multiply for one to two days after treatment with quinapyramine. However, during this period these trypanosomes are no longer infective and after this initial multiplication the trypanosomes in the blood diminish and ultimately disappear. Quinapyramine has a curative action against infections of *T. congolense* and *T. vivax* in cattle. This drug will cure *T. evansi* in horses and is the only effective drug against *T. simiae* in pigs.

Quinapyramine is available as the chloride and as the methyl sulphate (Fig. 23.9). The chloride is only 0.12% soluble in water whereas the methyl sulphate is 33% soluble. The difference in solubility is reflected in the rates of absorption, the methyl sulphate being quickly and the chloride slowly absorbed from sites of subcutaneous or intramuscular injection. The slightly soluble chloride forms a depot in the tissues from which absorption proceeds over several weeks. Quinapyramine chloride is unsuitable as a general prophylactic in cattle and it is better to use the so-called 'pro-salt'. This 'pro-salt' is a mixture of two parts quinapyramine chloride and three parts quinapyramine methylsulphate and is used because the initial sterilising action of the methylsulphate on the trypanosomes is required.

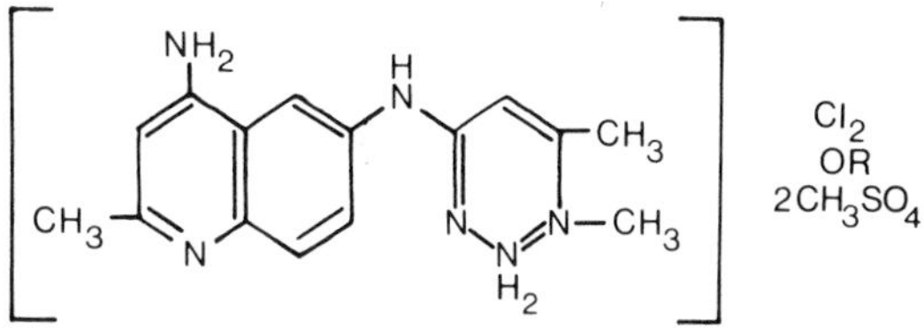

Fig. 23.9 Quinapyramine chloride or methylsulphate.

It has been found that the trypanosomes appearing towards the end of a period of prophylactic treatment are resistant to the drug. Therefore, unless the challenge to the prophylaxis is very light the period between prophylactic doses should not be more than 2–3 months. Trypanosomes which have become resistant to quinapyramine are usually resistant also to homidium and prothridium but not to diminazene or to suramin. There is evidence that the more trypanosomes there are present the more drug will be required.

Toxic effects are not uncommon after the administration of quinapyramine. The maximum dose of the methylsulphate is 5 mg/kg and this produces increased salivation, sweating, tremors. even loss of consciousness and sometimes death two to six hours after the injection. These untoward effects may be due in part to released histamine since quinapyramine is a drug with this property; there may be also an anticholinesterase action. Some animals develop a gastro-enteritis forty-eight hours after the injection and may die six to twelve days later. The local reaction produced by the injection is rarely serious, excepting in the horse. In this species the local reaction, which may be severe. can be reduced by dividing the dose and injecting in two or three different sites. The quinapyramine chloride in the 'pro-salt' causes a hard swelling at the site of injection which may persist for months or even years.

Phenanthridinium compounds

In 1938 trypanocidal activity was discovered in a series of phenanthridinium compounds (Fig. 23.10), and in 1944 one of these, *Dimidium bromide*, was shown in field tests to be effective against *T. congolense*. However, animals treated with this drug showed delayed toxic effects which presented a serious disadvantage. The methyl group of Dimidium was replaced by an ethyl group giving a less toxic trypanocide which is called *homidium*.

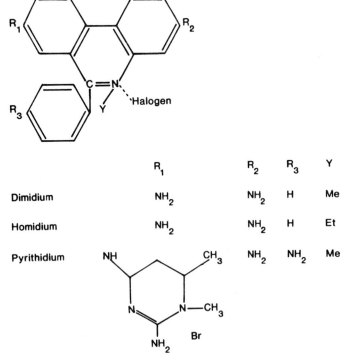

	R_1	R_2	R_3	Y
Dimidium	NH_2	NH_2	H	Me
Homidium	NH_2	NH_2	H	Et
Pyrithidium		NH_2	NH_2	Me

Fig. 23.10 Some phenanthridinium trypanocidal compounds.

In recent years two other trypanocidal properties, *pyrithidium* which has a pyrimidine moiety as in quinapyramine and metamidium which has a pyrimidine moiety as in quinapyramine and metamidium which has a substituent which corresponds to the meta version of diminazene. This development whereby portions of known trypanocides are combined has been termed 'hybrid synthesis'. Although these compounds have some virtues as trypanocides, cross resistance frequently arises between drugs structurally related and this is an obvious danger of such hybrid synthesis.

Homidium is eliminated fairly rapidly from the body but Pyrithidium and Metamidium persist and are of value in prophylaxis. The phenanthridinium compounds are active mainly against *T. congolense* and *T. vivax* but are not equal and even different strains of *T. congolense* vary in their response to these trypanocidal compounds.

The mode of action of the phenanthridiniums is not understood but an interesting hypothesis has been put forward. It has been suggested that the phenanthridinium compounds are fixed by the trypanosomes in very small amounts and this small amount of drug inhibits the factor required for division of the trypanosomal cytoplasm. When the store of this factor has been exhausted, the trypanosomes cease to multiply and disappear. This factor may be a substance required for the synthesis of DNA as it is known that homidium inhibits the synthesis of DNA in a flagellate *Strigomonas oncopelti* and moreover, the antibacterial activity of this phenanthridinium compound is antagonised by DNA.

Homidium bromide was introduced in 1952 to replace dimidium bromide. Homidium causes only transient liver damage but there is an appreciable local reaction at the site of either intramuscular or subcutaneous injection. It is ten times as active as dimidium against *T. congolense* infections in mice. In the field homidium is active against *T. congolense* and *T. vivax*, less so against *T. brucei* and inactive against *T. evansi*. Homidium is rapid in action and acts prophylactically for about a month. Less local reaction is produced by intramuscular than subcutaneous injection. It is dangerous to give intravenously.

Pyrithidium bromide (Prothidium) is chemically like quinapyramine but has a phenanthridinium instead of a quinoline nucleus. This compound was introduced as a prophylactic drug, a single dose given subcutaneously or intramuscularly. it is claimed, gives protection to cattle exposed to a moderate infection for six to eight months. However, resistance to pyrithidium appears to occur fairly readily. This prophylactic action in cattle probably depends on the persistence of the deposit of the drug at the site of subcutaneous injection and this may last for several weeks. About half the pyrithidium present in the blood is bound to plasma protein which explains in part the persistence in the body of this compound. After absorption the highest concentration of the drug is found in the liver and a substantial proportion is excreted in the bile. Occasionally cases of delayed poisoning have been reported after the administration of pyrithidium. *Metamidium* is a phenanthridinium compound introduced for its prophylactic properties. It owes its prophylactic activity to being deposited at the site of subcutaneous or intramuscular injection from which there is a slow absorption.

The diamidines

Trypanosomes require a great deal of glucose for their activities and their multiplication in vivo is decreased by the administration of insulin. A guanidine which lowers the blood sugar called '*Synthalin*' was tested and found to be trypanocidal in vivo. However, this drug was an equally effective trypanocide in vitro thus demolishing the hypothesis of trypanocidal activity being related to hypoglycaemia.

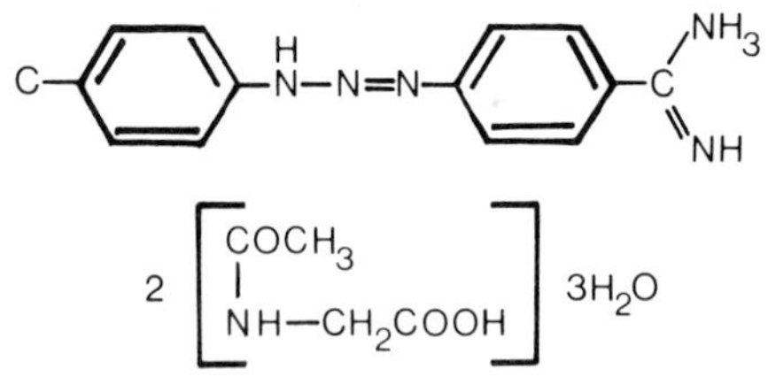

Fig. 23.11 Dimanazene aceturate.

This discovery led to the study of a series of related diamidine compounds such as propamidine, pentamidine, phenamidine and diminazene. Metamidium, which has been discussed with the phenanthridium trypanocides has the meta version of diminazene as a substituent of the phenanthridinium nucleus.

The diamidines are not well absorbed from the gut. After intraperitoneal or intravenous injection the concentration in the blood falls rapidly. Propamidine and pentamidine are retained in the body for a relatively long period probably due to their fixation in the liver.

Diminazene is an active trypanocide, babesiocide and bactericide which appears to act directly on the parasites. This drug kills a number of different bacteria but is particularly active against *Brucella* and *streptococci*. In trypanosomiasis a single dose of diminazene usually gives a clinical cure within 24 hours and recovery is followed by a degree of premunity. It is given by subcutaneous or intramuscular injection and produces a local reaction at the injection site. In cattle most of a single dose of diminazene is metabolised or excreted in the urine within 24 hours. Experimentally. subeffective doses of this drug fail to produce resistance in *T. congolense*; hence, diminazene differs from other diamidines in this respect. The rapid clearance of diminazene from the body probably accounts for the relative freedom from producing resistant strains although the plasma of cattle given diminazene intramuscularly showed anti-trypanosomal activity three weeks after the dose was given. Recently, however, reports have been made of the existence of certain strains of trypanosomes which are resistant to this drug. It is interesting to note that, despite the similarities in chemical structure between diminazene, homidium and metamidium, trypanosomes resistant to the last two compounds remained susceptible to diminazene. Diminazene resistance against T. congolense has been produced in mice. The sensitivity to diminazene of these trypanosomes returned in six months and no cross-resistance to other anti-trypanosomal agents was shown.

The toxic effects attributed to diminazene involve the central nervous system and are manifest as ataxia and convulsions. This drug, however, appears to be both ineffective and toxic when used in camels infected with *T. evansi*. Reports of chronic toxicity have not appeared which is unremarkable in view of the rapid clearance of this drug. It has been used successfully in the field against *T. congolense* and *T. vivax* infections.

A nitrovinylfuran derivative has been found to have trypanocidal activity in mice infected with *T. rhodesiense* when given by mouth. A single intramuscular injection of this compound had prophylactic properties. It appears to inhibit various nucleic acid and carbohydrate metabolic pathways.

Prophylactic complexes

Suramin is one of the older trypanocides which is still used against *T. evansi* infections in camels. It is effective also against *T. brucei*, *T. equinum* and *T. equiperdum* but not against *T. congolense*, *T. vivax* or *T. simiae*. This substance is given by intravenous injection, because it is too irritant for intramuscular or subcutaneous injection. Suramin is exceptional amongst the trypanocides in being an acidic substance, hence it combines firmly with the plasma proteins and persists for many weeks in the body. Since quinapyramine, the phenanthridiniums and diminazene are basic substances the acidic suramin will combine with them to form an insoluble complex. These complexes, when injected, form depots from which absorption proceeds very slowly. They are of particular value in prophylaxis. An important disadvantage possessed by these suramin complexes is the intense local irritation they produce which may be sufficiently severe to cause sloughing and loss of the deposit. There is, of course, no longer any prophylaxis if the deposit has been lost. The complex which appears to cause the least irritation is that between pyrithidium and suramin. Protection of seven months' duration has been obtained using a suramin–homidium complex. Suramin may cause degenerative changes of the liver, kidneys and, especially in horses, the adrenals.

Suramin, whilst effective in killing trypanosomes, does not show this effect until after a latent period of 7 trypanosome divisions. It appears to act by disrupting and eventually preventing cell division. The phenanthridinium compounds and quinapyramine also have this type of action. Homidium and suramin inhibit the enzymes concerned with RNA and DNA metabolism. Suramin is an effective compound for killing the adult worms of *Onchocerca* and *Litomosoides* but its lethal action is not shown until after five weeks of treatment.

SUGGESTIONS FOR FURTHER READING

Baines E J, McFadzean J A 1981 The action of metronidazole on anaerobic bacilli and similar organisms. Advances in Pharmacology and Chemotherapy 18:224
Fitzgerald P R 1980 The economic impact of coccidiosis in domestic animals. Advances in Veterinary Science 24:121
Hawking F 1978 Suramin: with special reference to onchocerciasis. Advances tn Pharmacology and Chemotherapy 15:289
Newton B A 1974 The chemotherapy of trypanosomiasis and Leishmaniasis. Ciba Foundation Symposium 20:285
Ryley J F 1980 Drug resistance in coccidia. Advances in Veterinary Science 24:99
Ryley J F 1980 Screening for the evaluation of anticoccidial activity. Advances in Pharmacology and Chemotherapy 17:1
Ryley J F, Betts M J 1973 Chemotherapy of chicken coccidiosis. Advances in Pharmcology and Chemotherapy 11:221
Schnitzer R S, Hawking F 1962 Experimental chemotherapy, Vol 1. Academic Press, New York

24

Chemotherapy of helminth infections

ANTHELMINTICS

The drugs in this group kill or remove parasitic worms from the animal. As no single drug has so far been discovered which is effective against all species of worm it is convenient from the therapeutic point of view to consider worms as falling into three groups: cestodes, nematodes and trematodes. The first and second group are the tapeworms and roundworms which live mainly in the alimentary canal. The third group represents the flukes which live mainly in the biliary tract. Some nematodes live in the lungs and in other tissues and certain flukes inhabit the rumen and kidney.

One of the first attempts to study the actions of anthelmintics was made by von Schroeder in 1884. He investigated the effect of various drugs on ascarids in vitro. More recent elaborations involving hanging segments of worm in a constant temperature bath in physiological saline and recording the movements of the worm have been developed. It has been found that certain anthelmintics inhibit the movement of these segments but that others are without effect. This kind of experiment is of little value in discovering whether a new chemical will be a good anthelmintic but may be useful in studying how various known anthelmintics work.

Female worms in the gut, lungs or bile ducts lay eggs which are passed out into the faeces. This fact has been made use of in testing anthelmintics since worms which are killed can no longer lay eggs. However, some drugs merely inhibit egg-laying, hence the results of such tests of anthelmintic activity can be misleading. The best evidence of anthelmintic activity is supplied by using the 'critical test' devised by a United States veterinarian called Hall, in 1918. In this test, which was intended for assessing the activity of anthelmintics against gastro-intestinal worms, each animal infested with the worm or worms under study is given the drug; after dosing, the faeces are collected and the worms in the faeces counted and identified. The host animal is then killed and the gut examined. The worms remaining in the host are counted and identified. Adding together the worms of each species in the faeces to those remaining in the gut gives the number of worms in the host at the time of treatment. The worms in the faeces together with dead worms in the host expressed as a percentage of the initial infestation shows the efficiency of the particular anthelmintic for the worm infestation studied. The efficiency of an anthelmintic should be in the region of 90%. A deficiency of this test is that it fails to take account of worms killed in the first part of the gut being digested and therefore not appearing in the faeces. With suitable modification this test can be applied to the study of drugs acting on liver flukes and lung worms.

The critical test used directly on parasitised animals of the species in which the anthelmintics are ultimately intended to be used is expensive and time consuming. It is not well adapted to the development of new anthelmintics. To overcome this difficulty laboratory rodents infected with their specific helminths have been used. Such animals are sometimes called the 'primary screen'. These screening tests are based on the belief that the parasites which are systematically related have similar chemotherapeutic responses. Unfortunately, this belief is not wholly true but is, nonetheless, a useful working premise. It has been shown, for example, that the nematode of mice, *Nippostrongylus muris*, the trichostrongyles of sheep and cattle and hookworms of the dog all respond to bephenium compounds, hence mice infected with *N. muris* provided a suitable primary screen for anthelmintics against certain worms infesting ruminants and dogs. Unfortunately, a similar relationship does not apply to phenothiazine or certain organophosphorus compounds.

Dichlorophen is active against a tapeworm of mice, *Hymenolepis nana*, and the larger tapeworms of domesticated animals hence, this mouse parasite can be used for screening taenicides. However, hexachlorophene is active against the chicken tapeworm *Raeillietina cesticillus* and not against *H. nana*. It is advisable, therefore, where possible, to test drugs which have been developed for their anthelmintic activity against a diversity of parasitic helminths in the primary screen. However, a secondary screen, whereby the drug is tested against the parasite in the normal host, is necessary before proceeding to clinical trials.

Assays of anthelmintic activity which depend on counting worm eggs in faeces have only a limited place as such; results can be very misleading. Certain anthelmintics are particularly active in depressing the egg-laying of the worm without killing the worm, hence the administration of such a compound could cause a complete absence of worm eggs from the faeces for several days, only for them to return once the worm has been removed from the effect of the drug. Such tests have a place when advancing from anthelmintic tests on parasites of rodents to those on the more definitive species, especially when the larger farm animals are concerned and the consequent expenses. Clearly, unless a compound does not cause a dramatic fall in the faecal egg count when tested on species on which it is intended to be used and against the worms for which the anthelmintic is required the compound is of no value.

In a clinical trial the parasitised animals are divided by a process of randomisation into two groups, one receiving the drug and the other group is left untreated. After a suitable interval, all the animals in both groups are killed and the number of worms remaining in each animal counted, the various species present being enumerated separately. It is thus possible to determine the proportion of each species of worm removed by the drug under test. However, before the drug can be marketed it is necessary to carry out toxicity tests and any drug to have prospects of wide use as an anthelmintic must be shown to have very limited toxic effects. It is now advisable to obtain information about the possibility of residues of anthelmintics remaining in the tissues of the host, since many of the species in which the anthelmintics are used are animals whose carcase and organs are likely to be used for human consumption.

The legislation of many countries now necessitates comprehensive studies on the toxic effects and metabolism of drugs particularly those used in the food producing animals. The possibility of harmful residues of either the drug itself or a metabolite have to be eliminated in so far as possible. All new anthelmintics are subject to such studies. However, comparatively few studies are made into the mode of action of anthelmintic drugs. Such studies as have been made seem to indicate that the chemotherapeutic effects of the anthelmintics are due either to the interference with the muscular activity of the worm or with the energy supplying mechanisms.

Resistance to anthelmintics is now recognised in an increasing number of nematode species in domestic livestock and is a major concern. Resistance to all known benzimidazole anthelmintics for *Haemonchus contortus* and *Trichostrongylus colubriformis* now indicates a limit to their potential usefulness. There is even laboratory evidence of co-resistance to thiabendazole, levamisole, and morantel.

It may emerge as a field problem in the near future. It will therefore be important to pay more attention to the possibility of the development of resistance to anthelmintics.

DRUGS ACTING ON TAPEWORMS

Arecoline hydrobromide

This drug has been given by mouth and has been shown by critical tests of dosing infected dogs to be a most effective anthelmintic. This drug stimulates the secretion of glands and plain muscle innervated by the parasympathomimetics. The anthelmintic effects are probably due to a combination of increased intestinal secretions and movements together with some action on the worm. This latter action is shown by the fact that arecoline given by mouth is between 75 and 80% effective, given by subcutaneous injection only 0.1% of the worms are expelled. Arecoline has a depressant effect on the segments of tapeworms suspended in an isolated organ-bath. It is used only in dogs and it is usually given after withholding food overnight. Vomiting after dosing only reduces the efficiency of the drug if it takes place within the first few minutes after administration. This drug is an effective anthelmintic only when it produces purgation. Unfortunately purgation may sometimes be severe and this constitutes a marked disadvantage to the use of the drug. It is a most effective drug against *Echinococcus granulosus*, a tapeworm of dogs with public health importance because man can provide an intermediate host and suffer serious consequences.

Preparations are available in which the acetarsol, a pentavalent organic arsenical, has been added to the arecoline. There is no evidence that such preparations are more effective than arecoline. They are more expensive. Arecoline should never be administered to cats as in this species the gastro-intestinal stimulation is particularly severe and may cause death.

Dichlorophen

This is used to treat dogs and cats affected with tapeworm. This drug is also fungicidal and bacteriostatic. The tapeworm becomes detached from the intestinal wall within 30–40 minutes after dosing, it then disintegrates in the gut, hence treated animals do not pass segments of worm in the faeces. The main advantage in the use of dichlorophen is that it is unnecessary to withhold food before administering the drug. Dichlorophen does not cause the very severe purgation which may be produced by arecoline. Unfortunately, dichlorophen is relatively ineffective against *E. granulosus* and *Dipylidium caninum*. It has, moreover, disadvantages; vomiting, colic and occasionally diarrhoea may be produced. Furthermore, the dose is very bulky and this presents difficulties in administration. The drug is alleged to be more effective in cats than dogs; it is no doubt preferable in cats. The fringed tapeworm of sheep is not affected by dichlorophen.

Bunamidine hydrochloride

In critical tests bunamidine has been shown to be effective in the treatment of infestations of *T. pisiformis*, *D. caninum* and *E. granulosus* in the dog and *H. taeniaeformis* in the cat. This drug is also effective against *Moniezia* species in lambs and *Raillietina* species in chickens. Egg production was unaffected and there was no untoward effects in the birds.

Bunamidine is about 90% effective against *E. granulosus* in dogs and may be slightly better than arecoline. However, arecoline hydrobromide is of diagnostic value for *E. granulosus* infections when administered to groups of dogs.

Bunamidine is given in cachets or tablets and it seems important that when the tablets are given, the formulation should be such as to allow rapid disintegration; otherwise the effectivity of the drug is decreased. When bunamidine is given as a drench, inflammation of the buccal mucous membrane is caused. The toxic effects so far described include vomiting and diarrhoea in certain dogs. In addition, deaths have been reported which may be due to ventricular fibrillation since bunamidine sensitises the heart to catecholamines.

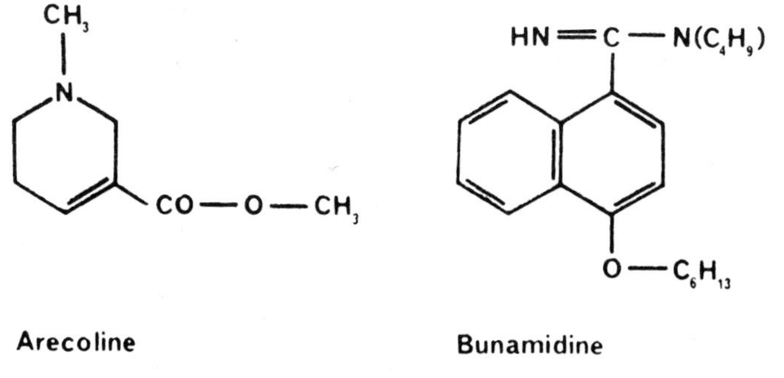

Arecoline   **Bunamidine**

Fig. 24.1 The structural formulae of two anti-tapeworm drugs.

The hydroxynapthoate is less likely to cause diarrhoea than the hydrochloride.

Niclosamide

This drug was introduced for the treatment of *T. pisiformis* in dogs and *T. taeniaeformis* in cats. It is also effective against D. caninum in the dog. Infestations with *E. granulosus* in the dog should be treated with four times the recommended dose. Niclosamide is also effective in sheep infected with *Moniezia* species and in birds infected with *Raillietina* species. Niclosamide is apparently safe to treat young and pregnant animals. However, it should not be used in cases of intestinal atony or acute diarhoea.

Nitroscanate

Nitroscanate is a broad spectrum anthelmintic for use in dogs. It is effective against both nematodes and cestodes including *Toxicara canis*, *Toxascaris leonina* and *D. caninum* but at recommended doses it gives limited control of *E. granulosus*. For best effects nitroscanate should be given with a small quantity of food on an empty stomach and food should then be withheld for a further 8 hours. Because nitroscanate may be irritant it is given as film coated tablets which should not be divided. Side-effects include vomiting after administration.

Praziquantel

Praziquantel has been shown to be effective against both immature and mature forms of adult tapeworms in dog and cats. It is effective against *E. granulosus*, *D. caninum*, and *Taenia* species. It may be given either in tablet form or by intramuscular or subcutaneous injection. Praziquantel is rapidly absorbed and metabolised by the liver. It is excreted rapidly and entirely as metabolites in the urine and bile. Praziquantel is known to impair the normal tegument function of the tapeworm making it permeable to excessive glucose loss and more easily attacked by proteolytic enzymes. As a result of this whole tapeworms including the scolex are very rarely passed in the faeces following administration of the drug. Praziquantel may be given by either subcutaneous or intramuscular injection. Intramuscular injection is preferred when ever *E. granulosus* infestations are suspected.

Few toxic effects of praziquantel are recorded. It can be administered to pregnant females and is safe to the pregnant female herself as well as to the unborn foetus and newborn young. It is well tolerated by both dog and cats so that withholding of food is not necessary.

Resorantel

This compound is effective against *Moniezia* species in both cattle and sheep, and has the additional advantage of being effective against rumen flukes. Resorantel appears to exert its effect on the parasite by impairing the final stages of glucose degradation and blocking the synthesis of ATP.

Bithionol

This drug is used for the treatment of tapeworms in poultry, dogs and cats. It is highly effective against taeniae species in cats but is less effective against *D. caninum*. In chickens it is effective against *Raillietina* species. In addition to its anthelmintic actions bithionol also possesses bacteriostatic and anti-fungal actions. Bithionol is believed to act by interfering with glucose metabolism.

Felix mas

This is an extract of the male fern and is an old, if not obsolete taeniacide. It is a thick dark green liquid whose active principle is filicic acid. The main importance of this drug now lies in its toxic effects. These include jaundice, gastro-enteritis, optic neuritis, and may also include coma, convulsions and heart failure.

SUGGESTIONS FOR FURTHUR READING

Arundel J H 1970 Control of helminth parasites of dogs and cats. Australian Veterinary Journal 46:164
Bueding E 1969 Some biochemical effects of anthelmintic drugs. Biochemical Pharmacology 18:1541
Gibson T E 1969 Advances in veterinary anthelmintic medication. Advances in Parasitology 7:349
Hatton C J 1965 A new taeniacide, bunamidine hydrochloride. Veterinary Record 77:408
Mansour T E 1979 Chemotherapy of parasite worms: new biochemical strategies. Science 205:462

Rew R S 1978 Mode of action of common anthelmintics. Journal of Veterinary Pharmacology and Therapeutics 1:95

Standen O D 1963 In: Experimental chemotherapy, Vol 1. Schnitzer R J, Hawking, F. (eds) Academic Press, New York

Van den Bossche H 1976 In: Biochemistry of parasites and host-parasite relationships. North Holland, Amsterdam, p 553

25

Chemotherapy of helminth infections

DRUGS ACTING AGAINST ROUNDWORMS

The large number and the diversity of species of roundworm pathogenic to the various domesticated animals poses particularly difficult problems in choosing an anthelmintic. A mixture of nicotine
and copper sulphate was used for many years in sheep with good
effect, against the parasite *Haemonchus contortus* which lives in the
abomasum. However, only worms in the abomasum are affected by
nicotine and copper sulphate. Phenothiazine was introduced in the
late 1930s and provided a drug with a greatly increased range of
activity and safety.

Worms infesting the lungs and causing bronchitis presented a
particularly important problem as they are unaffected by the older
anthelmintics including phenothiazine, however, they are susceptible to diethylcarbamazine. The introduction of methyridine was
a further advance since it represented a group of drugs which could
be given by mouth or by injection and was effective against worms
in both the alimentary tract and lungs of ruminants. Unfortunately,
it possessed some undesirable actions. These drugs have now been
replaced by compounds which are safer and have a wider range of
activity. Some of the more recently introduced anthelmintics such
as cambendazole are active against a number of species of both
roundworms and tapeworms. Ivermectin is a drug active against
roundworms in the alimentary tract and lungs as well as certain
ectoparasites such as lice.

Cholinomimetic anthelmintics

Acetycholine is an excitatory transmitter in nematodes. The action
of acetylcholine is to produce depolarisation and contraction of the
muscle. The acetylcholine receptors are located all over the surface
of the muscle cells as well as the neuromuscular junctions. It is not

surprising that certain cholinergic agonists have been used as anthelmintics. A successful anthelmintic which has this mode of action must be very selective in its effect. It should act on the parasite with little effect on the host. The cholinomimetic anthelmintics include levamisole, pyrantel tartrate, morantel tartrate, bephenium hydroxynapthoate, and thenium.

Levamisole

This anthelmintic has an activity against a wide variety of nematode species which infest domesticated animals. It is the L-isomer of tetramisole, and is effective against nematodes of chickens, sheep, cattle, pigs, horses, dogs and cats. A single dose is usually effective. This drug can be given orally in the feed or by subcutaneous, intramuscular or intraperitoneal injection.

Tetramisole has been shown to have a depolarising effect on nematodes which results in a spastic paralysis. The worms are rapidly expelled and may appear alive in the faeces. Levamisole produces a depolarising blocking action in mammalian tissues in high doses.

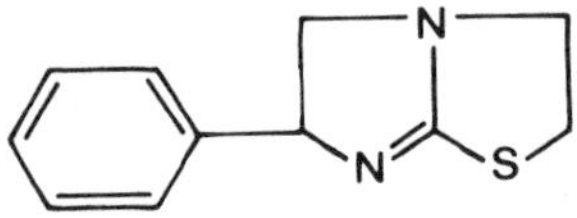

Fig. 25.1 The structure of levamisole.

Levamisole is less active against immature worms than adults in contrast to thiabendazole. The main advantage of levamisole is that it can be used to treat nematode infestations of both the gastrointestinal and bronchial tracts. Levamisole has no action against tapeworms or flukes and is ineffective against the small strongyles of the horse. It is contra-indicated in the horse because of its lack of efficacy and the possibility of producing excitement, sweating, dyspnoea and nasal discharge. The toxic effects which have been observed following the use of levamisole at therapeutic doses in domestic animals include depression, salivation, defaecation and muscle tremors. Colic has also been noted. Liver damage makes the sheep more susceptible to levamisole toxicity. This is particularly important if levamisole is used concurrently with carbon tetrachloride.

Pyrantel tartrate

This anthelmintic has an activity against *Nematodirus, Cooperia, Trichuris, Ostertagia* and *Haemonchus*. It has a depolarising action and produces a spastic paralysis of the worm. When given by mouth about one-third of the dose is absorbed and approximately one-quarter is excreted in the urine; the remainder of the absorbed fraction is metabolised some to urea and carbon dioxide. It does not leave residues in the tissues and is fairly free from toxic effects even in pregnant animals. If Pyrantel is inadvertently allowed to enter the lungs serious consequences may ensue. There is a rise in blood pressure followed by a profound fall from which there is rarely recovery.

Morantel tartrate

This compound is the 3-methyl derivative of pyrantel. It is more potent than the parent compound and has a similar mode of action. It is now available in bolus form which is designed to produce long-term release from the rumen. This may facilitate the onset of resistance.

Bephenium hydroxynaphthoate

This compound has a specific action in *Nematodirus* infestations. It is active against both adult and immature forms. The drug is used to prevent and treat *Nematodirus* infestation and given for prophylaxis at intervals of three weeks. It is given as a drench with water and a dispersing agent. Bephenium also has an activity against *Cooperia, Trichostrongylus, Ostertagia* species as well as *Haemonchus contortus*. It is used in the treatment of dogs infested with hookworms.

Thenium closylate is a drug with marked activity against hookworms in dogs. It is, however, only slightly active against dog ascarids and is given combined with piperazine to treat weaned

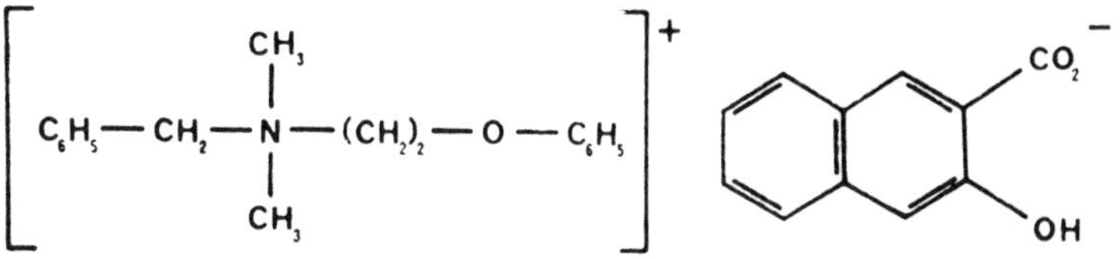

Fig. 25.2 Bephenium hydroxynaphthoate.

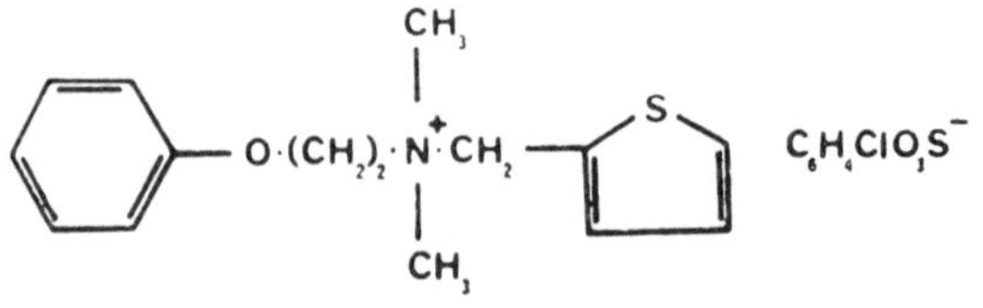

Fig. 25.3 Thenium closylate.

puppies and dogs infested with both hookworms and roundworms. This combination is usually given as a layered tablet with the thenium on the inside because it is a bitter-tasting compound. Food is withheld from the dog overnight and the dose is divided into two parts and given separately. Unweaned puppies should be removed from the bitch and fed protein hydrolysate until three hours after treatment. Toxic effects shown as a result of treatment with thenium include vomiting, diarrhoea and muscular weakness.

Organophosphorus anthelmintics

Cholinesterase is present in nematode parasites as well as in their mammalian hosts. Organophosphorus anthelmintics exert their action by having a selective effect on the cholinesterases of the nematode parasites. They therefore potentiate the effects of naturally released acetylcholine.

Haloxon is an organophosphorus compound with a high degree of anthelmintic activity against the nematodes of sheep and cattle. The adult forms of *Haemonchus, Ostertagia, Trichostrongylus, Cooperia, Strongyloides, Nematodirus* and *Bunostomum* are particularly susceptible. Haloxon is active also against *Capillaria* sp. in poultry, but not *Heterakis* infestations. This drug is effective against *Ascarids, Oxyurids, Tridontophorus sp., Trichonema* sp. and *Strongylus vulgaris* of the horse. It is less effective against the other horse strongyles but effective against bots (*Gastrophilus* sp.). *Ascaris suum* and *Oesophagostomum* sp. in pigs and *Ancylostomes* and *Ascarids* in carnivores are also eliminated by haloxon. The drug is palatable when given in a feed and can be administered to horses, pigs and poultry in this form. It has larvicidal activity.

Haloxon differs from closely related organophosphorus compounds in causing only slight depression of mammalian red cell cholinesterase. Toxic effects have appeared when ten times the therapeutic dose has been given. These effects consist of anorexia, diarrhoea and death after several days. A proportion of sheep and poultry treated with therapeutic doses of Haloxon may show ataxia. Atropine is not an effective antidote to the toxic effects of haloxon.

Geese are very susceptible to haloxon poisoning but fortunately 2-PAM is an effective antidote. Goose brain cholinesterase forms a stable phosphoryl derivative with haloxon and it is claimed that this is unique amongst vertebrates. This peculiarity of geese has caused fatalities from organophosphorus poisoning in wild species. Certain nematodes which are susceptible to haloxon have cholinesterases which form stable compounds with this drug whereas other nematodes which are insusceptible and mammals have cholinesterases which form unstable compounds with haloxon. This observation may explain a selective action of the drug and its freedom of toxic effects in the host.

Dichlorvos

This organophosphorus compound is active against Bots and Nematodes in the horse. It acts also against *Ascaris, Trichuris suis,* and *Oesophagostomum* spp. in pigs as well as *Ascaris Ancylostomes* and *Trichuris* in the dog. It has some insecticidal properties.

Metriphonate

An organophosphorus compound with anthelmintic and insecticidal properties. The insecticidal properties are seen after local application or oral administration of this drug. Metriphonate is rapidly broken down on the skin as well as in the body so that its duration of action is short. It can be used for the treatment of warble fly except during the months of December, January and February when the warble larvae are situated in the spinal cord. Drenching with metriphonate is an effective treatment for nematode infestations in cattle. *Cooperia, Bunostomum, Trichuris, Haemonchus* and *Oesophagostomum* sp. are susceptible. It is of little use in the treatment of nematodes of the sheep and goat because the effective dose in these species approaches the toxic dose. Toxicity is due to the inhibition of cholinesterase but recovery takes place in a few hours since metriphonate is relatively quickly metabolised. Atropine provides a specific antidote. The dose of atropine in the treatment of organophosphorus poisoning is 4–5 times the usual therapeutic dose.

GABA agonist anthelmintics

γ-aminobutyric acid (GABA) will hyperpolarise *Ascaris* muscle and produce relaxation. This evidence suggests that GABA may be an inhibitory neurotransmitter in nematodes. Some anthelmintics, notably, piperazine, appear to act by mimicing the action of GABA in the nematode.

Piperazine

The use of this drug was suggested by a pharmacist of Rouen for the treatment of *Ascaris* infection in man. It was used originally for the treatment of gout in man and appeared to be reasonably safe. It was found to be an effective anthelmintic against *Ascaris*, *Oxyurids*, *Oesophagostonum* and *Strongylus vulgaris*. However, it is ineffective against other horse strongyles and against *Haemonchus contortus*. *Trichostrongyles*, hookworms and tapeworms are unaffected by piperazine.

Piperazine is readily absorbed from the gut and between 30–40% is excreted in the urine in the first 24 hours. The remainder is metabolised. Piperazine depresses the motility of the worm by its GABA mimetic action so that it cannot maintain its position in the intestine. The worm is then expelled by the peristaltic movements of the gut.

Piperazine can be given by mouth as the adipate, citrate, hydrate, phosphate or as a complex with carbon disulphide. It is used against *Parascaris equorum*, *Trichonema* and *Oxyuris equi* in the horse, *Ascaris suum* and *Oesophagostomum* in pigs and *Ascaris* in the dog. Poultry infested with *Ascaridia* and *Capillaria* may be treated with piperazine hydrate in the feed or water. The activity of the various salts of piperazine are entirely due to the piperazine base. Horses are usually given the drug by stomach tube or in a bran mash; other animals receive it in the form of drenches, tablets, capsules or in the feed.

Diethylcarbamazine

This drug is a derivative of piperazine. It is one of the most active and least toxic piperazines to be used to combat infestations of microfilaria. After small doses of this drug 90% of the microfilaria rapidly disappear from the blood. However, a few microfilaria persist even after big doses are given. Diethylcarbamazine has little

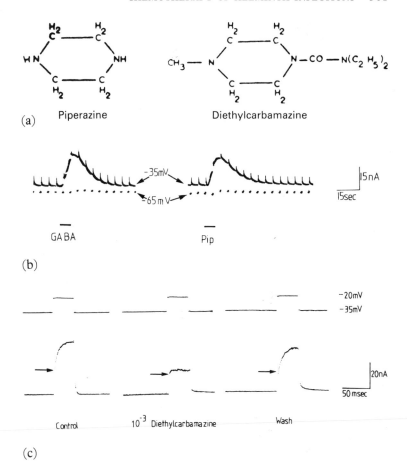

Fig. 25.4(a) Piperazine and diethylcarbamazine. (b) The effect of GABA and piperazine applied iontophoretically on the transmembrane current of Ascaris muscle. Both drugs produce an outward current at −35mV but have little effect at −65mV near the Cl⁻ reversal potential. (Modified from Martin 1982.) (c) The effect of diethylcarbamazine on the voltage sensitive current of *Ascaris suum* muscle. Top trace, membrane potential; lower trace, membrane current (Modified from Martin 1982.)

effect on the adult *Dirofilaria immitis* of dogs. When tested against other helminth parasites diethylcarbamazine was found to be about 100% effective against ascarids in dogs and cats. For this purpose it is given by mouth in gelatin capsules to avoid buccal irritation and it is unnecessary to starve or purge the host. The main disadvantage is its tendency to cause vomiting and loss of appetite. It is also active against hookworms and tapeworms. Given intramuscularly it is effective in the treatment of chronic parasitic bronchitis in calves and sheep. This is because it has an action against *Dictyocaulus viviparus* in calves and *D. filaria* in sheep.

Diethylcarbamazine is rapidly absorbed from the gut and is quickly metabolised to form 4 main metabolites. One of these metabolites is piperazine itself. It is of low toxicity although drug sensitisation has been reported in dogs treated with diethylcarbamazine.

The precise mode of action of diethylcarbamazine is not known. Diethylcarbamazine itself has an excitatory effect on Ascaris muscle strips due to blockage of a voltage-sensitive potassium conductance. It does not have an action on the GABA receptor unless it is metabolised to piperazine.

Ivermectin

This drug is a macrocyclic lactone derived from mycelia of *Streptomyces avermitilis*. It has a wide range anthelmintic activity. Parasitic nematodes are quickly immobilised at low doses and it has been suggested that its anthelmintic activity is the result of effects on the nematode nervous system. Further it may be that its mode of action involves a reduction in membrane resistance due to the opening of membrane chloride channels possibly including those regulated by γ-aminobutyric acid at the inhibitory synapse. In fact picrotoxin will antagonise the effects of ivermectin. Ivermectin is used for the treatment and control of gastro-intestinal nematodes, warbles, lungworms, mange, and sucking lice in beef and non-lactating dairy cattle. It is given by the subcutaneous injection of a small volume behind the shoulder. The withdrawal period of ivermectin is 21 days for cattle. It should not be used in cattle producing milk for human consumption or in dairy cows within 28 days prior to calving. It has also been used in horses and pigs. Gross overdosage causes paralysis in most animals.

The benzimidazole anthelmintics

Thiabendazole

This agent is effective against a wide range of nematode parasites and has a high degree of safety and efficacy. It is larvicidal and inhibits helminth egg production. It has little residual action and its use has been recommended on a continuous basis being injected every 6 weeks in the spring and summer. The high degree of effectiveness of this drug against adults and larvae may (by preventing the development of immunity), make the host more susceptible to reinfection.

Thiabendazole is quickly absorbed from the gastro-intestinal tract and widely distributed throughout the body tissues. It is quickly metabolised into 5-hydroxythiabendazole and excreted in the urine and faeces as the glucuronide or the sulphate. Within three days of administration approximately 6% of the dose is excreted in the urine and 20% in the faeces. 30 days after administration no residues of thiabendazole or metabolite is detected in the tissues.

Large doses of thiabendazole in sheep may cause anoxia, salivation, depression, incorrindation and even ataxia. Doses large enough to cause death showed evidence of liver and kidney damage. Large doses given orally may cause irritation of the reticulum and omasum. There is some evidence of teratogenicity when large doses are given to pregnant ewes.

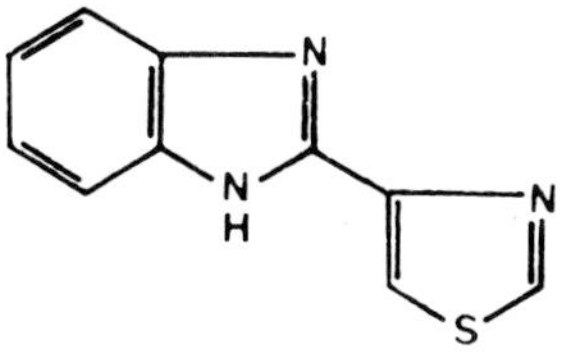

Fig. 25.5 Thiabendazole.

Otherwise, thiabendazole is safe and shows very low toxicity. It has been suggested that the mode of action of thiabendazole involves a specific effect on the energy systems of the parasite leaving the host animal systems unaffected. It has been found that the fumerate reductase of the parasite *Haemonchus contortus* is inhibited by thiabendazole. This enzyme is involved in the production of NADH in the parasite but not in the host animal. The activity of fumerate reductase in tolerant *Haemonchus contortus* is unaffected by thiabendazole. Although this is one explanation of the effect of the benzimidazoles there are others.

A wide range of benzimidazole compounds are used as anthelminitics, fungicides and anti-neoplastic agents. For example, benomyl and thiabendazole are used as fungicides; albendazole, cambendazole, fenbendazole, mebendazole, oxibendazole, oxfendazole, thiophanate, febantel, flubendazole and thiabendazole are used as anthelmintics; oncodazole was first investigated as an anti-neoplastic agent. The similarities between the structures of these drugs suggests a common mechanism of action. Benomyl interferes with the mitosis in fungi and mammalian cells. Mebendazole causes degenerative changes in the intestinal cells of parasitic nematodes, an effect attributed to interaction with cytoplasmic microtubules. Oncodazole interacts with microtubules in vivo and in vitro inhibiting the assembly by binding to the colchicine sensitive site of tubuline. It has been suggested that the action of the benzimidazoles is due to the conversion inside the cell to methylbenzimidazole-2-yl carbamate which may be the effective agent. Thiabendazole is not converted in this way but may still react with the same site on the microtubule system. Consistent with this latter mechanism is the fact that *Haemonchus contortus* and *Trichostrongylus colubriformis* have shown not only resistance to thiabendazole but a cross resistance to all the other benzimidazole anthelmintics.

After thiabendazole had been discovered various modifications of the molecule were tested for anthelmintic action. There are now a wide variety of benzimidazoles available as mentioned above. All benzimidazoles are sparingly soluble in water. This limits absorption from the gastro-intestinal tract. Peak levels of mebendazole occur in about 3 hours after administration. The peak levels of parbendazole occur 12–24 hours after dosing. The metabolism of these benzimidazoles varies with the product. Cambendazole is rapidly metabolised to a number of degradation products. Mebendazole, on the other hand, is poorly absorbed and is mostly excreted unchanged in the faeces. Residues for up to 1 week after dosing are seen with most benzimidazoles. This necessitates a withdrawal period before slaughter.

Albendazole: used as a multipurpose anthelmintic with a wide range of activity for the control of internal parasites in sheep and cattle. It is effective against gastro-intestinal worms, lungworms, tapeworms, and even adult liver flukes at higher doses. It is teratogenic and should not be used in pregnant animals.

Cambendazole: used against gastro-intestinal worms of the horse, cattle and sheep, lungworms of cattle and sheep, and active against the tapeworm *Monesia expansa*. It is also effective against the gastro-intestinal worms of the pig. It is teratogenic.

Fenbendazole: used as a broad spectrum anthelmintic for the treatment of immature and mature stages with an effect on nematodes of the gastro-intestinal and respiratory tracts of horses, cattle, other ruminants, dogs and cats. An interesting use of fenbendazole is for the treatment of pregnant bitches to reduce pre and postnatal transfer of helminth infection to their puppies.

Mebendazole: used as a wide-range anthelmintic against gastro-intestinal worms of sheep, dogs and cats as well as poultry. It is effective against worms, hookworms, roundworms, and tapeworms of the dog and cat. It is not recommended for use against fluke. Although this compound is quite safe and free from most toxic effects it is specifically recommended for use during pregnancy.

Oxibendazole: used as a worm drench for cattle and sheep as a wide range anthelmintic for the treatment and control of mature and immature gastro-intestinal worms, lungworms and also tapeworms. This parbendazole derivative is teratogenic.

Febantel: used as a wide range anthelmintic for the treatment of the gastro-intestinal worms of horses, cattle, sheep and pigs. It is also effective against lungworms of pigs, cattle and sheep and against tapeworms. It is activated by metabolism, to fenbendazole and oxyfendazole.

Oxfendazole: used as a wide range anthelmintic for the treatment and control of mature and immature gastro-intestinal roundworms, lungworms and tapeworms of cattle and sheep. High doses are teratogenic.

Thiophanate: used as a wide range anthelmintic against parasitic gastro-enteritis in cattle, sheep and goats and a parasitic bronchitis in sheep and goats although not a bendimidazole it is metabolised to ore.

Parbendazole: used for the treatment of gastro-intestinal roundworms in pigs, cattle and sheep. It is usually given in the feed. It is teratogenic.

Like thiabendazole, the other benzimidazoles leave significant tissue residues following treatment. This requires clearance times prior to slaughter. In addition to these clearance times the major contra-indication for the use of other benzimidazoles is during early pregnancy. It is recognised that parbendazole and cambendazole exert a teratogenic effect on the pregnant ewe during the 2nd and 4th weeks of gestation. This period coincides with the time of the normal embryonic limb development and is around the 20th day of pregnancy. The principal malformations occurring following treatment during the 21st to 24th days of pregnancy involve rotational and flexing deformations of the limbs and over flexion of the carpal joints. There may also be abnormalities of the ribs in addition to the abnormalities of posture and gait. The incidence of abnormalities is between 20 and 50% in animals treated around the 22nd day of pregnancy. No abnormalities are seen if the drug is administered as early as the 10th day of pregnancy but this treatment significantly reduces the lambing rate. Albendazole has a similar effect in sheep and cattle and is not recommended for use during the first month of pregnancy.

Phenothiazine

Phenothiazine is still an effective anthelmintic against some gastro-intestinal worms of cattle, sheep, horses, pigs and poultry. In horses phenothiazine given in combination with piperazine has been shown to be particularly effective against *Trichonema*, *Strongylus vulgaris*, and *S. endentatus*. Phenothiazine is also used in combination with various organophosphorus compounds in the treatment of nematode infestations of sheep. This combination allows a smaller dose of organophorphorus compound to be used without reducing the efficacy of the mixture and thus reducing the risk of toxicity.

Certain strains of *Haemonchus contortus* develop a resistance to phenothiazine. However, this resistance is less serious than originally thought since the use of newer micronised preparations of phenothiazine are still effective.

Phenothiazine is given by mouth as a compressed tablet or suspended in water with a suitable dispersing agent. The introduction of nematocides effective against a greater variety of species has largely replaced phenothiazine. There is some evidence that certain parasites have a special affinity for phenothiazine and absorb it through their cuticle. Phenothiazine inhibits glycolysis and egg-laying of worms. This last feature of the drug may produce an apparent cure if the absence of worm eggs is used as a criteria. Phenothiazine can be used to reduce the larvae on pasture by keeping the host animal on a continuous small dose. This drug can be used continuously for long periods without untoward effects. Toxic signs are more likely to occur in young animals. Sheep are more resistant to toxicity than the horse. In the horse haemoglobin urea and jaundice may be seen. Phenothiazine excretion imparts a red colour to the urine and milk and this should not be mistaken for haemoglobin. Milk is preserved because of the antiseptic action of phenothiazine. Phenothiazine is metabolised to a sulphoxide which is a photodynamic agent. The consequence of this in calves is the production of photosensitisation. The affected animals show a keratitis and corneal ulceration. This condition is seen in calves rather than in sheep because the sulphoxide is not completely metabolised in the liver.

DRUGS ACTING ON FLUKES

Carbon tetrachloride

Carbon tetracholoride has long been known to be an effective drug against adult liver flukes and its efficiency against immature flukes increases as the dose rate is increased.

Pharmacologically, carbon tetrachloride resembles chloroform. After absorption from the alimentary canal it is excreted mainly by the lungs because it is volatile drug. Some is excreted in the urine, but only 50% of a single dose can be accounted for, as carbon tetrachloride. There is evidence of the excretion of carbon tetrachloride in the bile. Mature flukes are more susceptible than immature parasites. This makes it usually necessary to repeat the dose after an interval of one month to give the larvae time to mature. Carbon tetrachloride is generally considered too dangerous a drug to use in fascioliasis in cattle. However, it is effective against hookworm and ascarids in the dog.

In the United Kingdom it is usual to administer carbon tetrachloride in gelatin capsules. It may be given orally dissolved in liquid paraffin. Carbon tetrachloride has been given also by subcutaneous or intramuscular injection and it has been shown that this route of administration is highly effective. This may be due to the fact that the part of the liver affected by fascioliasis has a better developed arterial blood supply than other parts of the liver and this may allow more carbon tetrachloride to be carried to the fluke-infested parts when the drug is given parenterally than after oral administration. Injections are irritant.

Toxic effects are, unfortunately, not uncommon, even in sheep treated with this drug, and these may be aggravated under various circumstances. Debilitated animals are usually more susceptible. However, since fascioliasis causes debility, it is difficult to avoid treating debilitated animals. Feeding oil cake increases the risk of poisoning, probably due to the additional protein the damaged liver has to metabolise. Such supplementary feeding should stop ten days before the treatment. Calcium deficiency accentuates carbon tetrachloride poisoning. The signs of acute poisoning are those of hypocalcaemia, and treatment, the parenteral administration of calcium borogluconate. Lactating and pregnant ewes are also rather susceptible to tetrachloride poisoning, probably because of the increased demands on their calcium reserves. The chief toxic effect of carbon tetrachloride is the production of fatty changes in the liver.

In view of the various factors which may influence the toxicity of carbon tetrachloride it is generally considered advisable before treating a whole flock of sheep with this drug to carry out what is sometimes called 'trial dosing'. This procedure involves administering the drug to a small number of sheep from the flock and carefully observing these animals to see whether any untoward effects develop before proceeding to treat on a larger scale.

Carbon tetrachloride has been used experimentally to produce liver damage, hence this phenomenon has received considerable attention. It appears that various lipoproteins are formed in the liver and extruded into the plasma. The fatty changes which are observed in the liver after exposure to carbon tetrachloride are due to a block of the secretion of triglycerides by the hepatic cells which thus accumulate in the cell.

For many years it was thought that the toxicity of carbon tetrachloride was due to its solvent actions on the lipids of the cell membrane but as many other compounds which were just as good nonpolar solvents as carbon tetrachloride did not show the same degree of liver damage this hypothesis was not tenable. Evidence has accumulated which supports the hypothesis that the oxidation of carbon tetrachloride was involved in some way with its toxic action. It is known, for example, that certain antioxidants protect the liver against damage by carbon tetrachloride and it is now thought that the toxicity of carbon tetrachloride depends to a considerable extent on the cleavage of the carbon to chlorine bond. The hypocalcaemia which is sometimes a consequence of treatment with carbon tetrachloride might be due in part to the accumulation of calcium in the liver. The calcium content of the liver mitochondria may rise to many times the normal level after exposure to this compound.

Although carbon tetrachloride is a reasonably efficient fasciolicide its toxic effects have led to a search for fasciocidal drugs free from this disadvantage and in recent years a number of active agents have been introduced. The available evidence indicates that the new drugs are not completely effective against immature flukes nor are they substantially better than carbon tetrachloride against mature flukes. In the treatment of fascioliasis in sheep, the cost of the drug is an important consideration and it does not appear that carbon tetrachloride will be replaced completely in the near future.

Hexachloroethane is used to treat cattle infested with liver fluke, as it is less liable than carbon tetrachloride to produce toxic effects and is equally effective. The white crystals of hexachloroethane smell like camphor and are given by mouth, usually suspended in water with a suitable dispersing agent. However, only mature flukes are affected by hexachloroethane.

It is slowly absorbed and excreted. A substantial proportion is excreted in the exhaled air and also in the bile; some is excreted in the urine. Tetrachloroethylene and pentachloroethane are two of the main metabolites of hexachloroethane in the sheep. Substantial amounts can be detected in the tissues 10 days after administration. Although hexachloroethane is less toxic than carbon tetrachloride it also causes appreciable liver damage in therapeutic doses.

Various other untoward effects sometimes occur and some animals show signs of intoxication and muscular incoordination. These toxic effects are amenable to treatment with calcium borogluconate given parenterally. Hexachloroethane taints the milk and may also cause loss of appetite and diarrhoea. A high protein diet predisposes the animal to these various toxic effects. Flukes in the rumen, abomasum and duodenum of cattle are also susceptible to hexachloroethane.

Hexachlorophane was introduced as a remedy for fascioliasis some years ago. It is given in an oily base by subcutaneous injection or orally dissolved in oil, as an aqueous suspension or in propylene glycol. The subcutaneous injection of this drug often gives rise to a large painful swelling. The effectivity of this drug against immature flukes is not substantially better than that of carbon tetrachloride and in cattle it does not appear to be a great improvement on hexachloroethane, although it has the advantage of not tainting the flesh or milk. Hexachlorophane has caused death due to biliary occlusion and occasionally produced signs of intoxication. This drug is probably excreted in the bile but more knowledge is required about its fate in the body and in particular what residues are likely to remain. It is a potent bactericide and is used in surgery to disinfect the hands.

Tribromosalicylanilide has been found effective against liver fluke in sheep. It is dispensed as a wettable powder and given as a drench. In a critical test in which groups of six sheep were used, both for the control and for the various treated groups, this mixture appeared slightly better than carbon tetrachloride. However, in these tests carbon tetrachloride appeared to be less efficient than in tests carried out by other workers and the efficiency of the bromosalicylanilide was not substantially better than that shown by other tests with carbon tetrachloride. The evidence, therefore, as far as this drug is concerned, is not completely satisfactory although it is probably more efficient against immature flukes than is carbon tetrachloride.

Oxyclozanide is a relatively recent introduction into the field of fasciocidal remedies. This drug is chemically related to hexachlorophane and appears to act by uncoupling oxidative phosphorylation. The main advantage of oxyclozanide over carbon tetrachloride or hexachlorophane is that it appears to be less toxic. The main toxic effect described as arising from this drug has been a slight scouring. Oxyclozanide does not taint milk although the milk yield is reduced, particularly when scouring occurs. Oxyclozanide appears to produce a lymphocytopaenia.

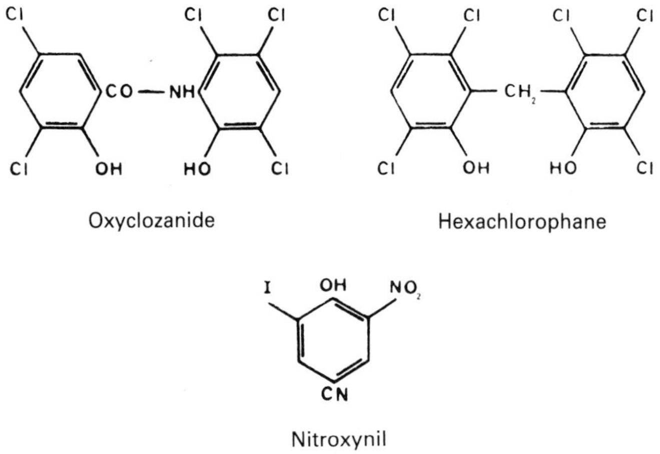

Oxyclozanide   Hexachlorophane

Nitroxynil

Fig. 25.6 The structural formula of three fasciolicidal drugs.

Residues of oxyclozanide have been detected in the tissues of sheep fourteen days after the administration of a single dose. It is recommended that animals treated with this drug should not be slaughtered until at least fourteen days have elapsed since the last dose.

Clioxanide (2-acetoxy-4-chloro-3,5 diiodobenzanilide) is another salicylanide fasciolicides whose efficacy against immature flukes is greater than 90%. It is usually given as a drench and is suitable for use in both sheep and cattle. There is some evidence that the route of administration is important in that when given by abomasal injection it is ineffective. Like rafoxanide it is effective against *Haemonchus contortus*.

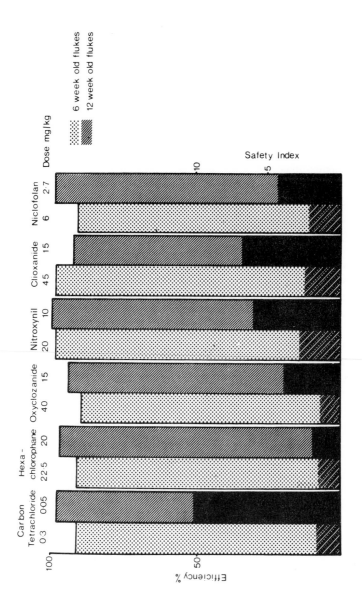

Fig. 25.7 The comparative efficiency of anthelmintics against fasciola hepatica in sheep. Safety index is the rates between maximum tolerated dose and adrenal dose and is shown by the darker hatching on each column. Adapted from Boray & Happich. *Australian Veterinary Journal* 1968 44:72.

A similar effective remedy for fluke is the drug brotianide.

Rafoxanide (3,5-diiodo-3-chloro-4-(p-chlorophenoxy) salicylanilide) is used against liver fluke in cattle when it has efficacy of about 98% against adult flukes but only 50% against the immature tissue forms of the parasite. It is advisable to repeat the dose after an interval of 3–6 weeks. Milking cows should be excluded from treatment and those animals intended for slaughter must not be killed until at least 28 days have alapsed since the last dosing. This drug is also effective against larvae of the nasal bot fly in sheep (Oestrus ovis).

Nitroxynil is a substituted phenol used in the treatment of fascioliasis which is more active after intramuscular or subcutaneous injection than after oral administration. Like the other fasciocidal agents it is more effective against the older fluke than the less mature. Deaths have occurred in sheep when twice the effective dose has been given. There is slight local reaction at the site of the injection and, as this drug is a yellow dye, the wool at the site may be stained.

In experimental animals nitroxynil has been shown to raise the blood pressure, increase the respiratory rate and cause a rise in body temperature. Since chemically it is a close relative of dinitrophenol which has well-known stimulating effects on metabolism, nitroxynil may act similarly by uncoupling oxidative phosphorylation. Over a month must elapse for this drug to be completely excreted in both sheep and calves. Moreover, in the first few days after administration, some is excreted in the milk.

Niclofolan has similarities in structure to nitroxynil and is also a fasciolicidal drug. It is suitable for use in cattle and has an efficacy of about 90% against mature flukes and 60% against immature flukes. The milk is free from the drug after 4 days and the tissues after seven.

Diamphenethide (2,2-bis(p-acethylaminophenoxy) diethyl ether) is another drug introduced for the treatment of fascioliasis. Whilst it appears to be more effective than niclofolan against immature flukes it is less effective against the mature parasite in sheep.

Triclabendazole is a bendazole with a potent effect against both immature and mature flukes but not nematodes. It is used in cattle and sheep.

FASCIOLIASIS THERAPY

After careful and critical experiments Boray and his colleagues found many drugs tested were efficient and reasonably safe against mature flukes. However, although all the drugs were efficient against immature *F. hepatica* as early as 4 weeks after infection the doses required were potentially toxic. These investigators considered the most critical periods as the 6th and 12th weeks after infection and concluded that in both acute and chronic fascioliasis, safety was increased by the use of clioxanide, niclofolan and nitroxynil. Their studies did not include rafoxanide or diampheneth-ide but it is unlikely that this would have changed their conclusions substantially.

Molluscicides

The control of fascioliasis usually involves in addition to the use of the specific drugs already discussed, an attempt to eliminate the snail intermediate host. Copper sulphate has long been used for this purpose and is highly effective in very low concentra concentrations. A concentration of 25 kg/ha is recommended. Other chemicals used for this purpose are trityl-morphine and sodium pentachlorophenate which are also effective. The spraying should take place in August or early September.

SUGGESTIONS FOR FURTHER READING

Boray J C, Happich F A 1968 Standardized chemotherapeutical tests for immature and mature Fasciola hepatica infections in sheep. Australian Veterinary Record 80:218

Boray J C, Happich F A, Andrews J C 1967 Comparative chemotherapeutic tests in sheep. Veterinary Record 80:218

Gibson T E 1962 Veterinary anthelmintic medication. Commonwealth Agricultural Bureau, England

Gibson T E 1965–1966 Anthelmintics. Vet. A. 7:291

Gibson T E 1966–1967 Anthelmintics. Vet. A. 8:264

Hawking F 1979 Diethylcarbamazine and new compounds for treatment of filariasis. Advances of Pharmacology and chemotherapy 16:130

Mansour T E 1979 Chemotherapy of parasite worms: new biochemical strategies. Science 205:462

Martin R J 1982 Electrophysiological effects of piperazine and diethylcarbamazine on ascaris suum somatic muscle. British Journal of Pharmacology 77; 255–265

O'Brien J J 1970 Toxicological aspects of some modern anthelminitics. Australian Veterinary Journal 46:297

Sheth U K 1975 Mechanisms of anthelmintic actions. Progress in Drug Research 19:147

Standen O D 1963 Chemotherapy of helminth infections. In: Schnitzer R J, Hawking F (eds) Experimental chemotherapy, Vol 1. Academic Press, New York

Van den Bossche H, Rochette F, Horig C 1982 Mebendazole and related anthelminths. Advances in Pharmacology and Chemotherapy 19:67–129

26

Pharmacology of ectoparasiticides for animal treatment

An ectoparasiticide is a substance which destroys ectoparasites. Those used for animal treatment may be destructive to insects, insect larvae and acarids. Ectoparasiticides which are absorbed through the parasite cuticle act as contact poisons, and those which are ingested are stomach poisons.

A great variety of chemical substances are used to kill ectoparasites. Unfortunately, the pests may become resistant to the action of any one of them. Toxicity to man, domesticated animals and wildlife also limits their usefulness.

Resistance

Resistance to an ectoparasiticide frequently arises through natural selection. A few ectoparasites, in possession of genes conferring resistance, survive exposure to the compound, others succumb. Over several generations, the survivors produce a population which resists destruction. This resistance is inheritable, and is the only kind which is known to occur in ectoparasites. The resistance of the population is lost slowly in the absence of the ectoparasiticide, as susceptible pests replace the resistant strain.

The spontaneous mutations which confer resistance are diverse. This is well illustrated by the organophosphorus compounds, where resistance to any one compound is accompanied by extensive cross resistance to others. The patterns of cross resistance are diverse, however, so that multiple mechanisms of resistance must be involved.

Selective toxicity

Selective toxicity of the ectoparasiticides depends mostly upon their relatively enormous uptake by ectoparasites. All ectoparasiticides are absorbed through the chitinous cuticle at a greater rate than

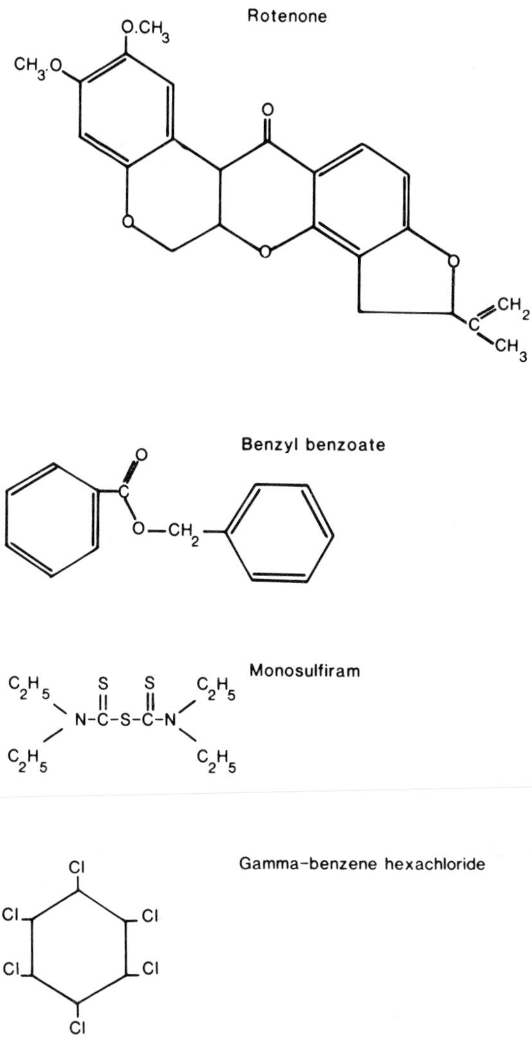

Fig. 26.1 Some ectoparasiticides used in the treatment of mange.

through the skin. Moreover, the ratio of surface area/mass is greater in ectoparasites than larger animals. As most ectoparasiticides poison neural structures, and these, in insects and acarids, are located just beneath the cuticle, it follows that selective uptake can account for the selective toxicity of these substances. Indeed, when given by intravenous injection the ectoparasiticides are all highly toxic in mammals and birds.

The risk of poisoning wildlife with ectoparasiticides is often considerable. Bees and fish absorb them readily. Birds and mammals eat seed treated with ectoparasiticides, which are absorbed from the intestines. Contamination extends through the biological food chain as predators take their prey.

Organosulphur compounds

Lotions or ointments containing sulphur are still occasionally used in the treatment of mange. The lotions often contain potassium carbonate or some other alkaline substance, as sulphur seems to be more effective at a high pH. *Mesulphen*, a yellow oily organosulphur compound, is used in an emulsion in the treatment of sarcoptic mange. Another organosulphur compound, monosulfiram, is more widely used.

Monosulfiram (Tetmosol)

This is a yellowish brown powder with the odour of sulphur (Fig. 26.1). It is insoluble in water, and is available either as a 25% w/v solution in alcohol or in a soap at a concentration of 5% w/v. These preparations are used to eliminate fleas, lice, ticks and certain mites from small animals. Both fleas and lice may be the secondary host for the dog tapeworm, *Dipylidium caninum*.

For the treatment of sarcoptic mange, the dog is cleaned with soap and hot water and roughly dried. The alcoholic monosulfiram solution freshly diluted with water (1 : 10) is scrubbed into the warm skin.

By mouth, monosulfiram may cause gastro-intestinal disturbances and drowsiness.

Naturally occurring substances, and derivatives

Benzyl benzoate

This exists as an oily liquid or colourless crystals, and is a constituent of Tolu balsam. It is toxic to mites. Benzyl Benzoate Application BP or an alcoholic solution of the substance is used in the treatment of sarcoptic, otodectic, psoroptic or chorioptic mange in the dog, horse or pig; and scaly leg in the fowl. Benzyl benzoate is contra-indicated in cats, because they are liable to lick the substance from their fur. By mouth, benzyl benzoate causes vomiting

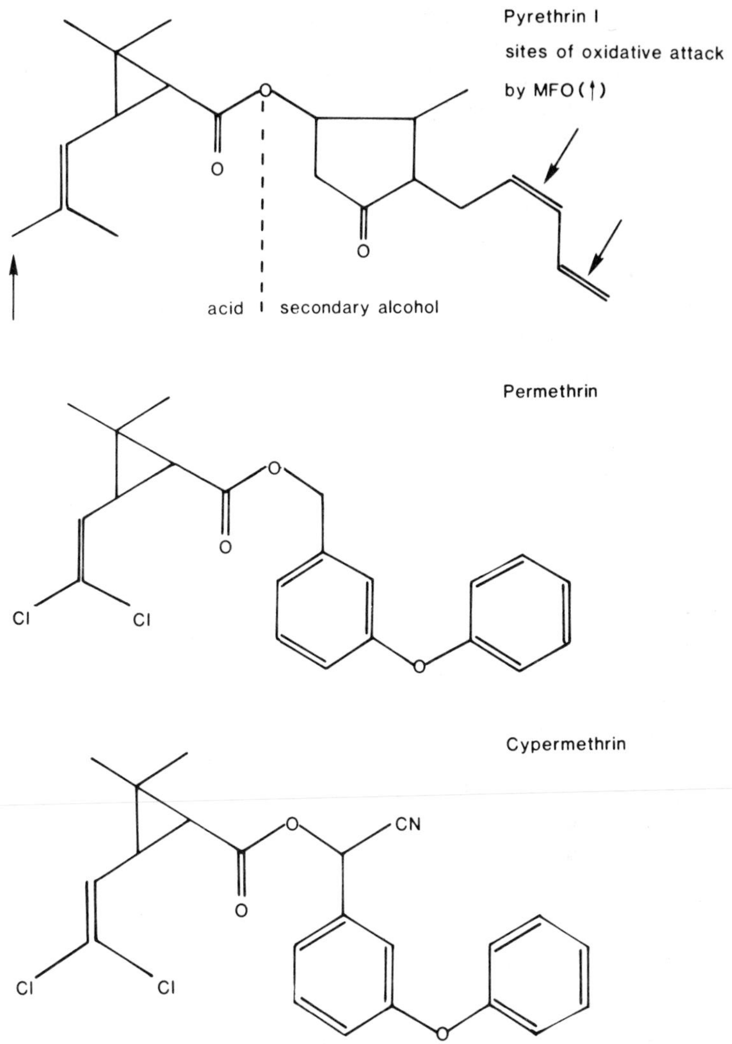

Pyrethrin I

sites of oxidative attack
by MFO(↑)

acid ⋮ secondary alcohol

Permethrin

Cypermethrin

Fig. 26.2 Chemical structures of a pyrethrin and two pyrethroids.

and purging, and, if sufficient is absorbed, stimulation of the CNS followed by cardiac and respiratory depression. It is very irritant, and should not be allowed to come in contact with the eyes.

Pyrethrum

Pyrethrum flower is the dried flower heads of *Chrysanthemum ci-*

nerariaefolium. The plant is indigenous to Yugoslavia, and was cultivated in Kenya and Japan for its insecticidal esters, the *pyrethrins.*

These are used in the control of flies and fleas. They are unstable substances, but powdered pyrethrum or an extract of pyrethrins in kerosene have a good shelf life provided they are kept in well filled containers and protected from light. A solution of pyrethrins (0.2% w/v) can be sprayed around milking sheds and on each cow as it comes in for milking. Poultry and small animals are dusted with pyrethrum.

These preparations are safer than most other insecticides, as in mammals and birds the pyrethrins are both poorly absorbed from the alimentary tract and rapidly metabolised by mixed function oxidase (MFO), which hydroxylates the molecule at multiple sites (Fig. 26.2). In common with other ectoparasiticides, however, they are toxic to bees and fish. The selective toxicity of the pyrethrins is mainly due to their rapid uptake through insect cuticle and fish gills followed by relatively slow clearance from these animals. They are nerve poisons, and rapidly knock down insects in flight. The affected insects lose their co-ordination, and either die or recover quickly, according to the amount of pyrethrins applied.

Pyrethrin 1, allethrin (a synthetic pyrethroid) and dicophane produce similar effects in the neurilemma, inhibiting the fluxes of Na and K associated with an action potential. The influx of Na ions develops more slowly and is prolonged, the efflux of K is inhibited. In consequence, the negative after potential is prolonged, and a single stimulus produces repetitive firing in the nerve. Insect and vertebrate nerves are similarly affected by allethrin.

The pyrethrins are inactivated by hydroxylation, rapidly in birds and mammals, more slowly in insects. This transformation is inhibited by substances containing the methylene dioxyphenyl group, e.g. piperonyl butoxide (Fig. 26.3). Piperonyl butoxide has a weak insecticidal action, and acts as a synergist when added to a pyrethrin preparation. The activity of the mixture far exceeds the sum of those of its components. Preparations containing synergised pyrethrins, e.g. Pybuthrin, are very effective remedies for infestations of flies or fleas, and are safer than most other insecticides.

Synergism would also occur between piperonyl butoxide and certain other ectoparasiticides which are hydroxylated to inactive products by MFO, e.g. carbaryl and some organophosphorus compounds. These substances would most likely become very toxic when synergised, however, and they are not used together with piperonyl butoxide.

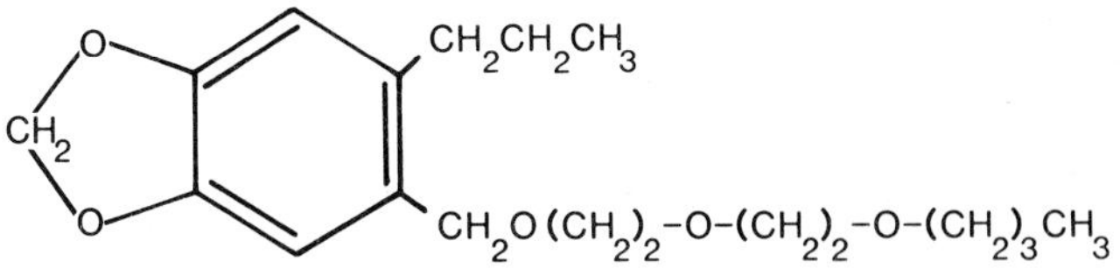

Fig. 26.3 Piperonyl butoxide, a pyrethrum synergist.

The pyrethrins are unstable in the environment, being inactivated by light, moisture and air. Whilst this contributes to their safety, it makes their insecticidal action brief. Thus synthetic pyrethroids have been made, which are both potent insecticides and stable in the environment.

Permethrin (Stomoxin) and *cypermethrin* (Rycopel) are used for killing flies on cattle and horses. Permethrin may be used on lactating cows. A PVC tag medicated with cypermethrin is available for attachment to the bovine ear. In a treated herd, the insecticide is transferred from tag to skin by direct contact, providing protection from flies for 5 months.

The pyrethroids are fat soluble and stable in the environment. Thus, unless they are rapidly cleared from cattle, their application is liable to produce a residue in meat and milk. Cypermethrin must not be sprayed around milking sheds, and animals must not be killed for human consumption until 48 hours after the last application.

The sites for enzymatic hydroxylation seem less numerous in the pyrethroids than in pyrethrin 1 (Fig. 26.2). It seems likely, however, that an ester link to a primary alcohol, as in permethrin, is vulnerable to hydrolysis by tissue esterases. If so, hydrolysis may be a route for the clearance of permethrin in domesticated animals. The substitution of the cyanide group in cypermethrin produces a secondary alcohol moiety, however, as in pyrethrin 1. Ester links to secondary alcohols are not readily hydrolysed in vivo.

Derris

This drug consists of the dried rhizome and roots of *Derris elliptica* and related species, which are indigenous to south east Asia. These climbing plants contain toxic crystalline resins, which are valuable insecticides, larvicides and acaricides. The most important constituent, rotenone (Fig. 26.1), is insoluble in water, soluble in organic solvents and unstable following extraction. Rotenone is readily oxidised in air and light, and rapidly inactivated by weak alkali.

Derris is reduced to a fine powder and adjusted to the required strength by mixture with other samples with a lower or higher rotenone content. The powder is dusted on animals to eliminate ticks, fleas and lice. A mixture of derris resins and dispersing agent can be made up to an aqueous suspension for washing or dipping animals. This was the most widely used remedy for the elimination of warble fly larvae from cattle, before the advent of the organophosphorus compounds.

Rotenone is used for the treatment of demodectic mange in the dog. In this condition it is difficult to bring a sufficient amount of acaricide in contact with the mites. *Demodex canis* infests the hair follicles and sebaceous glands, and produces a hyperkeratosis of the skin. In some cases the hair follicles rupture and abscesses form. Before the first application of acaricide the animal's coat is clipped and the skin cleaned, by removing crusts and washing with a medicated shampoo. Alcoholic rotenone (0.75% w/v) is applied to a third of the animal's skin daily, for a week. This treatment cures the condition in over 90% of cases, and compares very favourable with the only alternative acaricide available for demodectic mange, fenchlorphos. In a few cases the mites are not totally eliminated by the rotenone treatment, and these animals can be kept in satisfactory condition by maintenance treatment.

Rotenone inhibits the electron transport chain in mitochondria and depresses respiration, both in vertebrates and ectoparasites. The selective toxicity of rotenone is due to its selective uptake by the pests. The ectoparasites are immobilised, and die without exhibiting the inco-ordination produced by the neurotoxic ectoparasiticides. The action of rotenone is more rapid and transient than that of dicophane, and slower and more prolonged than that of pyrethrum.

Contact with rotenone as a dust or spray may cause irritation of the eyes, and numbness of the lips, tongue and throat. Side effects are extremely rare, however, when rotenone is used as recommended. Rotenone is not well absorbed from the skin or intestines, the latter possibly because of inactivation in the alkaline intestinal juice. Overdosage in dogs produces nausea and vomiting. Rotenone is very unstable in the environment, and is not toxic to wildlife, except fish and bees (and see general precautions, p. 393).

Ivermectin

The avermectins are macrocyclic lactones produced by *Streptomyces avermitilis*. Ivermectin is dihydroavermectin B_1.

Ivermectin (0.2 mg/kg) is administered parenterally in cattle and orally in horses and sheep, for the elimination of nematodes and many acarids and insects. It seems to act mainly as a stomach pesticide, and in cattle is more effective for the elimination of blood sucking lice than biting lice. It eliminates stomach bots from horses, nasal bots from sheep and warble fly larvae from cattle.

Although ivermectin does not produce prompt death or detachment of ticks, it has an adverse effect on their engorgement, moulting and reproduction. Ticks transmit British redwater and louping ill, and gamma-benzene hexachloride or an organophosphorus compound will probably eliminate these pests more readily than will ivermectin.

In cattle, the mites which cause sarcoptic or psoroptic mange are no longer recoverable from skin scrapings after ivermectin has been given by subcutaneous injection. Oral ivermectin is less effective for the treatment of bovine mange. In pigs however, *Sarcoptes scabei* is very susceptible to ivermectin by mouth. Ivermectin will probably become available for use in pigs and dogs, and may be very useful for the control of mange in these species.

Experimentally, avermectin B_1 blocked transmission at neuromuscular junctions in lobsters, and synapses between interneurones and motor neurones in the nervous system of *Ascaris suum*. These inhibitory effects of avermectin were antagonised by picrotoxin, which is an antagonist of a putative transmitter, gamma-aminobutyric acid (GABA). These observations suggest that the failure in transmission was due to stimulation of GABA receptors, either by GABA itself or by avermectin. GABA binds to a preparation of synaptic membranes made from mammalian brain, and it is presumed that the binding occurs at GABA receptors. GABA binding in the preparation was stimulated by ivermectin (0.5 μM). Thus it seems that avermectin did not combine with the receptors in competition with GABA. Ivermectin may stimulate GABA receptors indirectly, and this is presumed to be the mode of action of ivermectin.

Ivermectin has a good margin of safety, but overdosage may produce mydriasis, tremor and death. In cattle, toxicity and death occurred when the animals were given 40 times the therapeutic dose, but 30 times the normal dose did not produce signs of toxicity. Ivermectin is not teratogenic.

In cattle, sheep, pigs and rats, a hydroxylated metabolite of tritium-labelled ivermectin was found in the liver and body fat, together with traces of the unchanged drug. The radioactivity was all extractable into organic solvents, indicating that little was bound to macromolecules. The faeces were the main route for the excretion of ivermectin, even when it was given subcutaneously.

It is recommended that ivermectin should not be given to animals producing milk for human consumption, and that at least 14 days should elapse between treatment and slaughter for human consumption.

Chlorinated hydrocarbons

Dieldrin, aldrin and toxaphene were once widely used as seed dressings, and for the control of insect pests on crops and animals. These substances are both fat soluble and resistant to degradation, and their use led to pollution of the environment and an ever accumulating tissue residue in animals. In consequence wildlife was poisoned, and losses amongst birds and fish were considerable. In Britain, the use of chlorinated hydrocarbons has been controlled since 1965. Certain formulations of dicophane, gamma benzene hexachloride and bromocyclen are the only chlorinated hydrocarbons which may now be applied to animals.

Dicophane (DDT)

This is an odourless, white crystalline substance which is soluble in organic solvents and insoluble in water. It kills flies, fleas, lice, ticks and keds, but is ineffective against mites. DDT is a stable substance, and when applied to skin produces a long residual ectoparasiticidal action.

On skin, DDT is not irritant and its absorption depends upon the formulation used. It has been used as a dusting powder, or, mixed with a wetting agent, as a dispersable powder which may be made into an aqueous wash or dip containing DDT at a concentration of 0.2–0.5% w/v. Very little absorption of DDT occurs when the skin is dusted or wetted with an aqueous preparation, and these treatments do not produce poisoning in mammals. Oily solutions of the chlorinated hydrocarbons should not be applied to

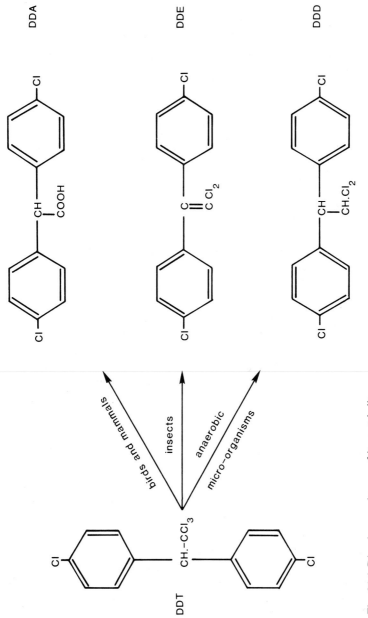

Fig. 26.4 Dicophane and some of its metabolites.

animals, however, as sufficient ectoparasiticide is absorbed from them to produce harmful effects.

Caution is required in the treatment of young animals, in which the enzymes which degrade DDT are poorly developed. DDT is contraindicated in the cat, and birds may be highly sensitive to its harmful effects.

In mammals, about 75% of absorbed DDT is metabolised, and the metabolite, bis-(p-chlorophenyl)-acetic acid (DDA) (Fig. 26.4), is excreted in the urine and bile. The unmetabolised DDT is taken up by the body fat, and slowly excreted in milk fat and urine. It is a health hazard, both to the animal and the public.

DDT produces chronic changes in liver, kidney, adrenal glands and heart. In hepatocytes, DDT causes a proliferation of the endoplasmic reticulum and induction of many of the enzymatic activities associated with this structure. This affects the metabolism of drugs and hormones, and may account in part for the failure of reproduction in wildlife exposed to DDT. Dicophane both releases adrenaline from the adrenal glands and sensitises the heart to its action, so that ventricular fibrillation may ensue.

Signs of nervous stimulation occur when a considerable amount of DDT has been absorbed. The signs of acute toxicity include muscular twitches, inco-ordination, convulsions and death. Barbiturates and calcium borogluconate are useful in controlling the signs.

Following absorption through the insect cuticle, DDT acts upon the underlying nervous system producing excitability followed by inco-ordination, paralysis and death. DDT affects the form of the action potentials in nerve, causing a prolongation of the falling phase of the spike. The prolongation of the negative after potential makes it outlast the refractory period of the axon, and repetitive firing occurs.

In the tissues of mammals, DDT is inactivated by oxidative dechlorination. This metabolic route is absent in insects with the exception of certain lice. Many insects contain a dehydrochlorinase, which transforms DDT to an inactive metabolite (DDE). Insect resistance to DDT is not uncommon, and is sometimes associated with an increase in DDT dehydrochlorinase activity. Resistance is often due to other mechanisms, however.

Anaerobic micro-organisms dechlorinate DDT by a reductive mechanism. The product, DDD (Fig. 26.4), is insecticidal. Soil micro-organisms can affect this transformation and DDD accumulates in wildlife. It is found at high concentration in the adrenal glands, where it produces degenerative changes.

Gamma-benzene hexachloride (gamma-BHC, Lindane)

This is one of the isomers of hexachloro-cyclohexane. Preparations of the mixed isomers have a musty odour and high chronic toxicity, due to the presence of the beta-isomer which is selectively absorbed from the intestines and very slowly cleared from the body. The separated gamma-isomer is less persistant in the body and less toxic (Fig. 26.1).

Gamma-benzene hexachloride is a white crystalline powder with a slight odour. It is soluble in alcohol and organic solvents, and insoluble in water. It is a more potent ectoparasiticide than DDT, and is an effective remedy for many mite infestations. The action of gamma-BHC is quicker in onset and less persistent than that of DDT.

A dust containing 0.6% w/w gamma-BHC or an aqueous wash or dip (0.016–0.05% w/v gamma-BHC) is an effective treatment for louse and tick infestations in cattle, pigs, sheep, poultry or horses. Cream of gamma-benzene hexachloride B Vet C is available for the treatment of small animals. Aqueous preparations of gamma-BHC (0.1% w/v) are effective in the treatment of sheep scab, poultry mites and sarcoptic mange in cattle, pigs, horses and dogs, but are less effective against demodectic mites.

All kinds of ectoparasite develop resistance to gamma-BHC. Some also develop cross-resistance to DDT, others not. In the absence of resistant strains, gamma-BHC is a good, cheap all-purpose ectoparasiticide.

The toxicity and contra-indications for gamma-BHC are similar to those for DDT. Gamma-BHC has been banned in the USA, Canada, Australia and New Zealand, because of the risk associated with residues in meat and milk.

Bromocyclen (Alugan)

Bromocyclen is a chlorinated hydrocarbon. It is available as a dusting powder, and as a dispersible powder from which an aqueous wash, dip or spray can be prepared. The indications for its use are similar to those for gamma-BHC. Bromocyclen is contra-indicated for poultry, and caution is necessary in the treatment of cats. Ectoparasite resistance to bromocyclen is a common problem.

Organophosphorus compounds

The residual action of some of the chlorinated hydrocarbons in sheep fleece was particularly useful in providing long lasting protection from ectoparasites. Unfortunately however, the stability of these compounds led to their widespread persistence in the environment, and their application is now restricted in order to limit pollution.

Organophosphorus compounds have replaced chlorinated hydrocarbons for the elimination of many ectoparasites from large animals. Some of the first organophosphorus compounds were developed as nerve gases for use in chemical warfare, but, provided suitable precautionary measures are observed, some are safe enough as pesticides. Both the ectoparasiticidal action and the acute toxicity of organophosphorus compounds are due to cholinesterase inhibition.

A general formula for an organophosphate is shown in Figure 26.5. A variety of side chains (R) may be substituted in the molecule, and in some compounds, one or two of the atoms of oxygen

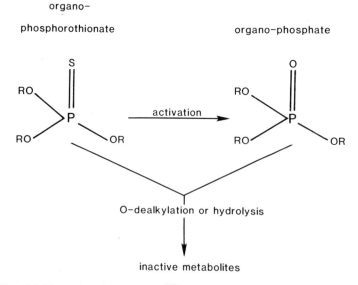

Fig. 26.5 Illustration of the in vivo transformation of organophosphorothionate to organophosphate, and degradation of these substances.

Table 26.1 Some organophosphorus ectoparasiticides for use in animals

Approved use**		Compound**	Formulation	Amount	minimum interval before slaughter or milking	
Bots	Horse	Dichlorvos (Astrobot)	Resin pellets, paste	3.66 g/100 kg	—	—
		trichlorphon (metriphonate, Neguvon)		3.5 g/100 kg	—	—
Warble fly larvae, lice	Cattle	Trichlorphon (as above)	Pour-on-soln.	0.6–0.8 g/100 kg	2 weeks	6 h
		*Fenthion (Tiguvon)	Pour-on-soln.	0.5–1.0 g/100 kg	3 weeks	6 h
		*Phosmet (Dermol, Orbiscet)	Pour-on-soln.	1.3–2.7 g/100 kg	2 weeks	6 h
Mange mites, lice	Cattle, pig, horse	*Dimpylate (Diazinon, Ficare)	Wash or spray	0.015% w/v	7 days	6 h
Mange mites, flies	Cattle, pig	Crotoxyphos (Rycovet, Flymort 24)	Wash or spray	0.5–1% w/v	2 days	avoid
Ticks, lice	Sheep	Crotoxyphos (as above)	Spray	0.2% w/v	—	—
Maggot fly	Sheep	Chlorfenvinphos	Spray	0.2% w/v	7 days	—
Blowfly, ticks, keds	Cattle, sheep, goats.	*Coumaphos (Asuntol)	Dip or spray	0.05% w/v	3 weeks	6 h
Lice	As above	Coumaphos (as above)	Dip or spray	0.025% w/v	3 weeks	6 h
Demodectic mites,	Dog	*Fenchlorphos (Ectoral, Ronnel)	Wash + tablet	1% w/v and 55 mg/kg	—	—
Fleas	Dog, cat	Fenchlorphos (as above)	Wash or tablet	0.75% w/v or 55 mg/kg	—	—
Mange mites, fleas, ticks	Dog	*Cythioate (Cyflee)	Tablet	3 mg/kg	—	—
Fleas	Dog	*Iodofenphos (Nuvanol)	Wash	0.5% w/v	—	—

* A phosphorothionate
** Recommended in data sheet

in the phosphate group have been replaced by sulphur, carbon or nitrogen.

O'Brien (1967) noted that many of the safest organophosphorus compounds were precursors of active metabolites. He indicated that the requirement for activation produces a delay in toxicity, which provides an opportunity for other enzymes to degrade the compound before it is activated. The microsomal enzymes which inactivate organophosphorus compounds, by O-dealkylation or hydrolysis, seem to be more active in mammals and birds than in ectoparasites. Perhaps therefore, the ratio of activation/inactivation for these pesticides, is greater in ectoparasites than in vertebrates.

Eleven organophosphorus compounds used for eliminating ectoparasites from animals are shown in Table 26.1. It is interesting to note that seven of these compounds are phosphorothionates, which do not inhibit cholinesterase directly. In vivo, phosphorothionates are transformed to oxygen anolgues which inhibit cholinesterase. Thus, following absorption, phosphorothionates are activated by metabolism. Trichlorphon, also, is activated by metabolism (Fig. 26.6).

Organophosphorus compounds are fat soluble and rapidly absorbed through the cuticle, whereupon they inhibit the cholinesterase in the nervous system. The nervous system of ectoparasites contains many cholinergic neurones. In consequence, unmetabolised acetycholine accumulates in the ectoparasite, producing disfunction and death. Some organophosphorus compounds seem to kill ectoparasite eggs, which are without cholinesterase. This may be a case of delayed toxicity, however, due to inhibition of cholinesterase as it develops in the embryo. Application of the organophosphorus compounds did not inhibit oxygen consumption or embryonic development in the eggs until the time of hatching, when the embryos failed to emerge.

Ectoparasite resistance to the organophosphorus compounds is increasing. There are many mechanisms of resistance (and see resistance, p. 374), some more important than others for a particular pesticide. For example, mites resistant to dimpylate may possess a cholinesterase which is insensitive to the inhibitor, or an arylesterase which metabolises it.

Formulations of organophosphorus compounds for oral administration include a paste and resin pellets, which are given to horses for the elimination of bots (Table 26.1). When a solution of organophosphorus compound in an organic solvent is poured on the skin, the active constituent is well absorbed. Pour-on solutions are

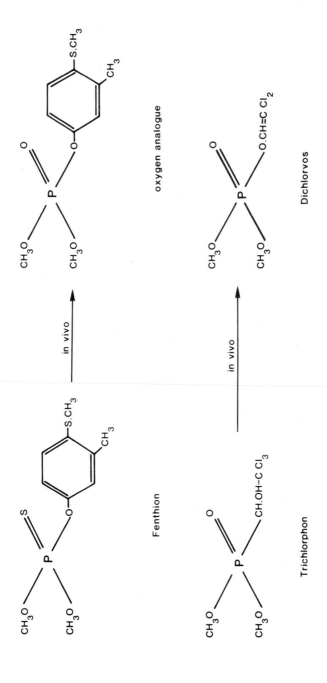

Fig. 26.6 Two examples of the metabolic transformation of organophosphorus compounds to active metabolites.

used for the elimination of warble fly larvae and mange mites. An aqueous solution or suspension of an organophosphorus compound may be used as a wash, dip or spray for the elimination of flies, fleas, lice, ticks or keds. These pests can also be removed from dogs and cats by the appropriate compound in a tablet. While the latter is convenient for the owner, the ectoparasites are not affected until the animal has been bitten. Impregnated plastic collars, from which dichlorvos or dimpylate are slowly released, are used to eliminate ectoparasites from small animals.

Some of the recommended uses of the organophosphorus ecto-parasiticides are listed in Table 26.1. In certain instances a compound may be toxic to additional species of ectoparasites, and yet not be recommended for their elimination. For example, **trichorphon** is toxic to many ectoparasites, but because it is rapidly metabolised in the body and not persistent on the skin, it is only recommended for the elimination of warble fly larvae and bots which multiply neither in nor on the host. Warble fly larvae migrate through the tissues of cattle between the beginning of December and mid-March, and at this time treatment must be withheld lest larvae be killed in the vicinity of the spinal cord.

Dichlorvos is also rapidly cleared from the body by metabolism, and is recommended for the elimination of bots and nematodes from horses. It is toxic in chickens, however, which must not be allowed to ingest the medicated resin pellets passed in the horse faeces.

Dimpylate is used to control mange in cattle and pigs, although it is contraindicated in young calves and piglets. **Fenchlorphos** is used for treatment of demodectic mange in dogs. A combination of topical and oral treatment with fenchlorphos is recommended, an application of a 1% solution over the entire body every fourth day, and 55–77 mg/kg/day orally, preferably in divided doses. This regimen produces side effects typical of organophosphorus poisoning in about 10% of treated animals. Scott, Schultz and Baker (1976) used topical fenchlorphos only, and found the improvement in demodectic mange to be as satisfactory as that in dogs treated both topically and orally. Moreover, topical treatment alone produced a lower incidence of signs of acute toxicity.

Several organophosphorus compounds are recommended for the elimination of biting and blood sucking lice from large animals, including lice resistant to gamma-BHC. It is recommended that treatment with **phosmet**, **crotoxyfos** or **dimpylate** should be repeated after an interval of 10–14 days. A single treatment with **coumaphos** is sufficient in cattle however, and protects sheep from lice for up to 20 weeks. Coumaphos is very persistent on the skin or fleece and in the body fat, and the minimum allowable interval between treatment and slaughter for human consumption is 3 weeks.

Organophosphorus compounds are absorbed through the skin and mucous membranes, and great care must be exercised in handling concentrates to avoid inhalation of any dust, mist or spray. Workers must wear protective clothing, and when using these compounds regularly, should have their blood cholinesterase checked (and see general precautions, p. 393).

Side-effects are infrequent when organophosphorus compounds are used as recommended. In cases of overdosage or undue exposure to these compounds, symptoms of cholinergic poisoning occur. These may include salivation, constriction of the pupil, muscular tremors, colic, diarrhoea and respiratory failure. Atropine sulphate (0.1–0.2 mg/kg) should be injected repeatedly until the muscarine actions of acetylcholine are antagonised, as indicated by a dilatation of pupil, tachycardia and decreased salivation. The effect of an organophosphorus compound may persist for several days, and if signs of the poisoning reoccur it is necessary to atropinise the animal further. Pralidoxime (20 mg/kg) may produce additional benefit by reactivating cholinesterase at neuromuscular junctions in skeletal muscle, and this is suggested in the data sheets for phosmet and cythioate.

Organophosphorus compounds are contraindicated in any animal treated with another drug that stimulates cholinoceptors or inhibits cholinesterase or is inactivated by tissue esterases. Neither should these substances be used in an animal suffering from a disorder of respiration or of the alimentary tract, until the condition has been rectified.

Although some organophosphorus compounds accumulate in the body, there is little information on their chronic toxicity. Scott et al (1976) reported liver damage in dogs treated with fenchlorphos, but could not exclude the possibility that the solvent or other medication was responsible.

Carbamate

Carbaryl is an ester of methylcarbamic acid which is sparingly soluble in water. It is rapidly absorbed through ectoparasite cuticle and skin, whereupon it inhibits cholinesterase reversibly. In vertebrates, carbaryl is inactivated by mixed function oxidase which hydroxylates the molecule (Fig. 26.7).

Carbaryl is selectively toxic to ectoparasites. When toxic amounts are absorbed in vertebrates, the signs of poisoning develop rapidly and minimise the risk of further poisoning. The signs are similar to those produced by the organophosphorus compounds, but only last for 3–4 h and are readily abolished by atropine. Oximes are ineffective as antidotes, as they do not reactivate carbamylated cholinesterase.

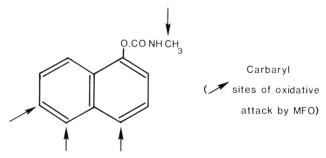

$O.CO\,NH\,CH_3$

Carbaryl

(⟋ sites of oxidative

attack by MFO)

Fig. 26.7 Carbaryl, a competitive inhibitor of cholinesterase.

A shampoo containing carbaryl is used for the elimination of fleas, mange mites, lice and ticks from dogs and cats. Rapid metabolism of carbaryl accounts for the safety of the preparation, which is contraindicated in animals which are less than four weeks old or pregnant. The animal owner is advised to wear rubber gloves, although carbaryl is safer than organophosphorus compounds, the medicated shampoo being a general sales list medicine.

Carbaryl (Sevin) has been mixed with chicken feed, for the elimination of fowl mite and chicken mite.

Propoxur (o-isopropoxyphenyl methylcarbamate) is one of the active constituents of a powder (Negasunt), which also contains coumaphos and sulphanilamide. This preparation is supplied as a larvicidal and bacteriostatic wound dressing.

Carbamates combine with cholinesterase more rapidly than do organophosphorus compounds, and so protect the enzyme from phosphorylation. In general, the duration of cholinesterase inhibition produced by a mixture of a carbamate and an organophosphorus compound, is less than that produced by the organophosphorus compound alone. Thus it is unusual to find both a competitive and a non-competitive inhibitor of cholinesterase in the same preparation.

Diamide

Amitraz, a diamide, is an active constituent of Mitaban Liquid Concentrate. There have been encouraging reports upon the use of this preparation for treatment of demodectic mange in dogs. For example, 4–8 applications of amitraz 0.025% w/v to the whole body of affected dogs at 14 day intervals, produced recovery in 86% of treated animals (Muller, 1982). Moreover, most of the other 14% of dogs could be kept in good condition by maintenace treatment.

The mode of action of amitraz is unknown. Application of amitraz (0.025% w/v) produces sleepiness in about 10% of the dogs, which lasts from a few hours up to 2 days. At half the recommended concentration, amitraz loses some of its acaricidal action.

General precautions

The ectoparasiticides are fat soluble, and may be absorbed through skin. Operators should wear a face shield, gloves and other protective clothing when spraying or dipping animals. If an ectoparasiticide should contaminate the skin, it must be washed off immediately with soap and water. When the eyes are affected, medical advice should be sought after thoroughly rinsing them with water.

In many instances the data sheet specifies a minimum interval which must elapse between treatment and slaughter for human consumption. This must be observed, otherwise a residue of the pesticide will contaminate meat.

All the ectoparasiticides are toxic to bees and fish. Thus they should never be sprayed in the vicinity of beehives, and any unwanted ectoparasiticide or a used container must not be allowed to contaminate ditches, ponds or watercourses. The high toxicity of metriphonate and rotenone to fish, coupled with their instability in the environment, have led to their use in the removal of trash fish from lakes before restocking with game fish.

Ectoparasiticides should never be sprayed directly into the eyes. When the head region of an animal is to be treated, it is often advisable to protect the eyes with a bland ointment.

SUGGESTIONS FOR FURTHER READING

Brooks G T 1979 The metabolism of xenobiotics in insects. Progress in drug metabolism, Vol 3. John Wiley, Chichester.

Brown A W A, Pal R 1971 Insecticide resistance in arthropods. WHO monograph series, No 38. WHO, Geneva

Campbell W C, Fisher M H, Stapley E O, Albers-Schonberg G, Jacob T A 1983 Ivermectin: a potent new antiparasitic agent. Science 221: 823–827

Corbett J R 1974 The biochemical mode of action of pesticides. Academic press, London

Muller G H 1982 Amitraz treatment of demodicosis. Journal of the American Animal Hospital Association 19: 435–441.

O'Brien R D 1967 Insecticides: action and metabolism. Academic press, New York

Scott D W, Schultz R D, Baker E 1976 Further studies on the therapeutic and immunologic aspects of generalised demodectic mange in the dog. Journal of the American Animal Hospital Association 12: 203–213

Wouters W, Van Den Bercken J 1978 Action of pyrethroids. General Pharmacology 9: 387–398

27

Disinfectants

The terms disinfectant and antiseptic are usually regarded as synonymous; disinfectant is commonly employed when referring to a drug used to kill micro-organisms on inanimate objects and antiseptic when the drug is applied to the skin and living tissues. The agents considered here are those which may be applied locally to tissues in the treatment of infections caused by pathogenic micro-organisms. However, it is customary to employ disinfectants to reduce the potentially pathogenic micro-organisms present on the surgeon's or animal's skin prior to surgery and agents used for this purpose are considered.

Bacteria are destroyed by heat, light and osmotic pressure, moist heat being better than dry heat. Steam at 115° C for thirty minutes destroys all life including spores. The disinfectant properties of sunlight are due to its ultra-violet rays. The disinfectant action of osmotic pressure is used to prevent the decomposition of jam, strawberries and salted fish.

There are a large number of chemical compounds used as disinfectants. The number is large because no single substance is a suitable disinfectant for all purposes. An ideal disinfectant should have a high activity against all organisms, and this activity should persist on dilution. The ideal disinfectant should not injure tissues, otherwise healing might be delayed by attempts to disinfect a wound. Disinfectants should be efficient in the presence of organic matter and should penetrate tissue crevices and infected debris; no disinfectant will penetrate sweat glands. Other properties desirable in a disinfectant include solubility in water, stability and cheapness. Disinfectants should not corrode metallic objects and should be chemically compatible with other drugs. It may be an advantage if the disinfectant discolours skin when used to prepare the site of a surgical operation.

The effectiveness of a disinfection is usually tested by finding the dilution which has the same effect as a 1% solution of phenol on a test organism. If the disinfectant under test killed the bacteria in a concentration of 0.1 per cent whereas with phenol 1.0% was required, the disinfectant would be said to have a phenol coefficient of 10.

The test organism is usually *Salmonella typhi*, although sometimes *Bacillus subtilis* is used because this latter organism sporulates and thus presents a more severe test organism. The result of this comparison is called the Phenol or Rideal Walker Coefficient of the disinfectant under test. The determination of the Phenol Coefficient was studied by Chick and Martin, who found that it was affected by factors such as temperature, duration of action, species and number of bacteria and the presence of organic matter. They devised a more elaborate test in which autoclaved faeces were added to the disinfectant under investigation, but this did not remove all the sources of error and the ideal test remains to be discovered.

Table 27.1 The Phenol Coefficients of some common disinfectants.

Compound	Phenol coefficient
Phenol	1
Chlorocresol	12
Phenylmercuric nitrate	250
Cetrimide	150
Benzalkonium chloride	130

Tests such as those described give only a rough idea of the potency of a disinfectant and are most useful when comparing disinfectants of a similar chemical series, for example the phenols. An example of the results of such tests are shown in Table 27.1. They give no indication of the suitability or otherwise of the disinfectant for application to tissues. The activities of disinfectants are sometimes compared by means of the D value. This is taken as the time required for a particular concentration of the disinfectant under test to kill 90% of the test organisms.

The effect of organic matter on a disinfectant is important as some disinfectants such as the halogens are inactivated by it. The activity of most disinfectants is also influenced by the pH of the solution. The concentration at which a disinfectant acts influences the choice, since any substance which kills bacteria is likely to have some damaging action on tissue cells. For example, the caustic action of strong acids and alkalies makes them useless as disinfectants to apply to tissues. Some tissue damage is caused by phenol and cresol when used in bactericidal concentrations, and superficial damage is produced by the disinfectants which precipitate proteins, as these substances do not discriminate between bacterial protein and tissue protein. Alcohol, formaldehyde and mercuric chloride are examples of the latter type of disinfectant. It is desirable, therefore, for a disinfectant to act in low concentration, and in this respect the salts of heavy metals are better than the derivatives of coal tar such as phenol.

It is important to appreciate the time taken by a disinfectant to kill bacteria. The quickest-acting are the oxidising and reducing agents and the halogens. In contrast the heavy metals are amongst the slowest, for example, 0.5% mercuric iodide or chloride does not kill staphylococci in 15 minutes. The dyestuff disinfectants act slowly.

The bacterial cell membrane acts as an osmotic barrier and the osmotic pressure within the organism is quite high. The bacterial cell wall of Gram-positive organisms is comparatively rigid and more resistant to rupture than that of Gram-negative organisms. The cell wall is also the location of many important enzymes hence damage to the membrane can result in the inhibition of important enzymes and/or changes in the permeability of the wall causing leakage of metabolites and thus interfering with the metabolism of the organism.

Halogen disinfectants

Chlorine and *iodine* are widely used as disinfectants. Chloride and iodide ions have no antibacterial action. Chlorine has a phenol coefficient of 200 and is used to sterilise water. It is quickly inactivated by organic matter and alkaline solutions, whereas ammonia increases its activity. The disinfectant action of chlorine is due to the formation of hypochlorous acid. Bleaching powder disinfects by releasing chlorine and a solution of bleaching powder and boric acid, 'eusol', is sometimes used to clean and disinfect wounds. The boric acid buffers the solution, preventing it becoming too acid. These simple sources of chlorine have been replaced by substances such as *chloramine-T* and *dichloramine-T*, which liberate chlorine slowly until they come in contact with protein.

The chloramines are less potent than chlorine but exert a more prolonged action. In addition to its oxidising action on bacterial protein, chlorine probably also acts by halogenating amino groups on bacterial protein. Chloramine T can be used to irrigate wounds and does not retard healing. Dichloramine T is much less water soluble and is used in ointments. *Iodine* is as efficient a disinfectant as chlorine, has a counter-irritant effect and is a good disinfectant for catgut. Iodine acts quickly but is quickly inactivated by tissue and other protein. Solutions of iodine in alcohol and potassium iodide are used to disinfect the skin for this purpose it is as good or better than most other disinfectants. These solutions impart a yellow colour to the skin which disappears as colourless iodides are formed.

Iodophors are substances in which iodine forms a complex with a suitable carrier so that free iodine is liberated in solution. These preparations are used mainly as skin antiseptics although it has been shown that a 1% solution of iodine in 70% ethanol is better. When applied to wounds and abrasions iodophors are less painful than simple solutions of iodine. Undecoylium chloride-iodine is such an agent which has potential value as a skin antiseptic. A widely used iodophor is povidone-iodine. The iodine concentration is so low that skin staining is slight and the immediate bacteriocidal action is only moderate compared with that of iodine solutions.

Heavy metal disinfectants

Simple salts of *mercury*, and *silver*, are used as disinfectants. Their action is mainly bacteriostatic. They act slowly and in high dilution, probably by reacting with sulphydryl groups on bacterial enzymes. *Mercuric chloride* has the greatest immediate action and was a widely used skin disinfectant. The *nitrate* and *oxide of mercury* are used as disinfectants in the form of ointment. Mercurous nitrate gives an active, irritant, antiseptic effect whilst the oxide of mercury is so mild an antiseptic as to be quite suitable to apply as an ointment to the eye. The repeated use of mercury eye ointment may cause inflammation. An ointment of the red iodide of mercury is a very active blister or counter-irritant. Various organic compounds of mercury act as disinfectants without liberating mercury ions. *Thiomersalate* (merthiolate) and *phenyl mercuric nitrate* are active substances suitable to use as disinfectants on the skin, wounds and instruments. The latter compound of mercury is sometimes used as a preservative in solutions intended for injection.

The salts of silver used as antiseptics fall into two groups, those liberating free silver ions and the non-ionising preparations. The latter are non-corrosive, non-irritant and non-astringent. The silver salt liberating free silver ions which is usually employed is silver nitrate but it tends to be rather irritant. The non-ionising preparations are compounds of silver with protein; these are non-corrosive, non-irritant and non-astringent.

Oxidising and reducing disinfectants

Various oxidising agents have disinfectant properties. Chlorine, although an oxidising agent, has already been discussed. *Hydrogen peroxide* releases oxygen when in contact with the enzyme catalase. The effect is increased by the presence of copper or iron. It kills most bacteria, *E. coli* being killed in sixty minutes by a one-in-ten dilution of a ten-volume solution of hydrogen peroxide. The mechanical effect of the bubbles of oxygen released by hydrogen peroxide when applied to tissues is valuable in breaking up scabs and in removing dressings. Liberated oxygen, unfortunately, does not affect all organisms.

Potassium permanganate is an oxidising agent whose germicidal powers are selective. The purple crystals of this substance give a pink-coloured solution in water. It is used as a deodorant.

Formaldehyde is an irritant gas which, as a 40% solution in water, is called *Formalin* and kills most organisms when diluted one part in eighty parts water. It is unaffected by organic matter and disinfects by combining with amino groups on the surface of the bacterial cell. Formalin is used to make toxoids from bacterial toxins. In acid solutions formaldehyde is liberated from *hexamine*. When this drug is given by mouth it is excreted in the urine, and, provided the urine is acid, disinfects the urinary tract.

Disinfectant acids and alkalies

Caustic soda and *quick-lime* are used to disinfect buildings but corrode tissues.

Mandelic acid is a bactericidal agent in acid media and is sometimes used as a urinary antiseptic, for which purpose it is given by mouth either as the calcium salt or as *methenamine mandelate*. It exerts its action in the urinary tract and bladder provided the urine has an appropriately low pH.

Nalidixic acid is derived from naphthyridine and when given by mouth is excreted mainly in the urine where it is active against many Gram negative bacteria. It is useful in treating urinary infections but those due to *Pseudomonas* are usually resistant. It may cause vomiting and occasionally jaundice.

Phenol and derivatives

By using phenol as the principal agent in antiseptic surgery, Lord Lister ensured this drug's popularity for many years, despite many surgeons and their patients developing phenol poisoning. It is no longer used except as a comparison for other disinfectants.

Phenol acts quickly: a solution of 2% phenol kills *S. typhi* in 10 seconds. Concentrations below 0.5% have no disinfectant properties and bacteria can grow in them. Phenol is more soluble in fats than water and probably acts on bacteria by dissolving in the lipoids of the cell surface. Sodium chloride increases the disinfectant power of phenol solution by making the phenol less water-soluble and so increasing the rate of solution in the cell lipoid. Alcohol, by increasing the solubility of phenol in water, has the opposite effect. Phenol probably kills bacteria by combining with their protein. It is unaffected by organic matter. The main disadvantages are its toxicity and loss of activity on dilution. *Staphylococci* are resistant to the actions of phenol.

Phenol is absorbed from mucous membranes, wounds and intact skin. It is partly oxidised in the body to hydroxyphenols and hydroquinone. Phenol is excreted in the urine as these oxidation products and in combination with sulphuric and glucuronic acids which give the urine a dark colour. Strong solutions are caustic and cause necrosis of all tissues with which they come in contact.

Phenol stimulates the central nervous system the affected animal showing muscular tremors and eventually convulsions. This is followed by depression and death results from respiratory failure. Dogs and cats are particularly susceptible.

The addition of a methyl group to phenol gives *cresol* of which there are three isomers. These are less water-soluble than phenol and more powerful disinfectants. A mixture of cresols dispersed in water with the aid of soap, 'Lysol' is useful for disinfecting instruments. It is less toxic than phenol, more powerful and unaffected by organic matter; however, it is unsuitable for application to living tissues.

Chlorocresol is made by the introduction of chlorine into the cresol molecule. This gives a disinfectant similar to cresol but ten times more powerful. It is sometimes used as a preservative in solutions intended for injection. *Chloroxylenol* dispersed in water with soap makes a very effective disinfectant, less irritant than cresol in soap and suitable for application to the intact skin. This solution has a phenol coefficient of three and is effective in a dilution of 1 : 50.

Disinfectant dyestuffs

Various dyestuffs are important for their disinfectant properties. Basic dyes are more active antiseptics than acidic dyestuffs. The dyestuffs used as disinfectants are usually derivatives of triphenylmethane or of acridine. The triphenylmethane dyes act by interfering with the glutamic acid metabolism of the micro-organism whereas the acridines inhibit synthetic processes of the micro-organisms by intercalating with the DNA molecule.

Brilliant Green and *Gentian Violet* are triphenylmethane derivatives which both stain and kill Gram-positive bacteria but are inactive against Gram-negative organisms. Serum decreases the activity of these dyes and streptoccoci resist Gentian Violet.

Acriflavine is a mixture of variable composition derived from acridine and existing as a water-soluble orange powder. It has a phenol coefficient of several hundred and is not inhibited by serum. Acriflavine acts slowly in low concentration and does not affect phagocytosis. However, prolonged applications of this drug delay healing.

Proflavine hemisulphate is the most important acridine disinfectant, being a pure substance of constant composition and less irritant than acriflavine, a 1/1000 dilution has no effect on the exposed rabbit brain. The solution of this salt is acid and requires to be neutralised. It is active in the presence of pus. The acridines appear to act as cations which compete with hydrogen ions for receptors in the tissues of bacteria.

Although *fluorescein* is not an antiseptic dyestuff it is a useful diagnostic agent. When applied to the eye, as a 2% solution, ulcerated areas are stained green and foreign bodies surrounded by a green ring. The viability of a strangulated intestine can be determined by the presence of fluorescence in that the dead cells do not take up the dye. This is useful to indicate the extent of resection required. Brain tumours fluoresce more than normal brain tissue following the administration of this dye. The dye appears in the urine for up to 2 days after administration and is apparently of very low toxicity.

OTHER ORGANIC ANTISEPTICS

The nitrofurans are a group of compounds which possess antibacterial activity against a wide range of organisms. *Furazolidone* has particularly marked activity against *Salmonella* sp. and *Shigella* sp.

Nitrofurazone is bactericidal to both Gram-positive and Gram-negative organisms; both *Furazolidone* and *Nitrofurazone* have activity against coccidia (p. 330).

The nitrofurans are used for their antiseptic properties either by local application or given systemically. The latter route is used mainly for the treatment of infections of the urinary tract. Their activity as local antiseptics is reduced in the presence of plasma. Resistance to the nitrofurans is rare: however, they may exhibit some toxic effects such as depression in growth, neurotoxic actions and inhibition of spermatogenesis.

In the body these compounds are metabolised by reduction of the nitro group and subsequent acetylation. They inhibit a number of enzymes such as pyruvic oxidase and aldehyde dehydrogenase.

The nitrofurans are preferentially reduced by the microorganisms and thus deprive the bacterial cell of the energy required for its growth.

Nitrofurazone is a potent bacteriostatic in a concentration of 1 : 200 000; higher concentrations are bactericidal to both Gram-positive and Gram-negative organisms.The activity of this drug is reduced by the presence of plasma and blood. The bacteria which are resistant to the sulphonamides and antibiotics usually remain sensitive to nitrofurazone.

Propamidine isoethionate, a drug used in treating babesiasis, is also a useful antiseptic for application to open wounds and burns as a jelly or cream. It is not antagonised by para-amino benzoic acid. Propamidine causes the release of histamine.

Disinfectant detergents

Chlorhexidine as the hydrochloride or gluconate is a potent bactericide against both Gram-positive and Gram-negative organisms, Gram-positive being more susceptible and is unaffected by serum or other body fluids. Spores and acid-fast bacteria are unaffected. Chlorhexidine appears to act by causing the leaking of intracellular material from the bacteria. It is a cationic substance and, therefore, incompatible with soaps and similar anionic agents. An aqueous solution of 0.02 to 0.05% is used to disinfect wounds and burns and a 0.5% solution in alcohol to disinfect the skin before surgical operations and to disinfect instruments. This substance is used as a pessary or in suspension as a uterine antiseptic.

A number of anionic and cationic detergents have antiseptic

properties and, as with the dyestuffs, the cationic compounds are the more active.

Soaps are bactericidal to some organisms but not to others, *Staphylococcus aureus*, for example, is not affected. Washing with soap alone, therefore, cannot be relied on to sterilise skin. Soaps are the sodium or potassium salts of large anions. The chlorides or bromides of certain large cations have detergent properties similar to soap, and are better disinfectants.

Cetrimide is a cationic detergent. It is obtained by replacing three hydrogen ions of ammonium bromide with three methyl groups and the fourth hydrogen by a long chain of — CH_2 —. This compound is used to cleanse the skin and is also antiseptic but not strongly so; it is bactericidal to Gram-positive micro-organisms but relatively ineffective against Gram-negative bacteria. It is non-irritant and does not stain. The skin may become sensitive if detergents are used continuously because they remove the normal fats. It is essential to rinse well with water between using ordinary soap and cationic detergent as they are incompatible. The hydrophobic ion of the quaternary ammonium detergent has a positive charge, whereas that of the soap has a negative charge and so they neutralise each other.

Benzalkonium chloride is a cationic detergent with bactericidal properties similar to those of cetrimide. This activity is reduced by serum, and spores are unaffected. It has the same incompatibilities and disadvantages as the other cationic detergents. The continuous use of the detergent type of antiseptic may cause defatting of the skin which may give rise to irritation and render the skin more susceptible to infection. Protection may be provided by application of a cream containing a suitable oil or fat. Ointments and creams containing various antibacterial agents are often applied to the udders of milking cows. There is little evidence that these preparations have any useful antiseptic action.

FUNGICIDES

Fungi are killed by many bactericides, but often these drugs lack other desirable therapeutic actions. The fungi causing ringworm are sometimes treated with solutions or ointments of *phenylmercuric nitrate* or *acetate*, *dichlorophen* or *iodine*, *iodides* have no direct disinfectant action but *potassium iodide*, given by mouth, or *sodium iodide*, by intravenous injection are the traditional remedies for *actinobacillosis* and *actinomycosis* in cattle. However, these remedies have been replaced by various preparations of penicillin. In general and provided problems of toxicity are not involved, it is better to treat fungal infections by using systemic fungicides than by local applications of fungicidal agents.

Griseofulvin is an antibiotic which, when given orally, is an effective treatment for ringworm. It is ineffective as a local application. The drug causes inhibition of fungal mitosis. This appears to be brought about by disruption of the mitotic spindle by griseofulvin interacting with polymerized microtubules. Griseofulvin is well absorbed from the gut and evenly distributed in the tissues. It appears to be nearly completely metabolised in the body in that less than one per cent of the total dose is excreted unchanged in the urine. Very large doses of griseofulvin cause the arrest of mitosis in the bone marrow and testes although no such effect has been observed when the drug is given at normal therapeutic levels. In man, gastro-intestinal upsets have been caused. It does not appear to be effective in all cases of ringworm, although some cases may require prolonged treatment. It is available as tablets or in the form of a feed additive. Pregnant animals should not be treated with this fungicide.

Nystatin is an antibiotic with activity against yeasts and fungi; it is poorly absorbed from the gut and finds its main use as a local application, being incorporated in dusting powders, creams and ointments. The drug's antifungal activity depends on it binding to a sterol in the membrane of the fungi. This appears to cause the formation of pores resulting in the leakage of various small molecules from the fungi. In veterinary medicine it is most useful in the treatment of mastitis caused by yeasts for which purpose nystatin is given as a preparation injected into the teat canal.

Undecylenic acid was discovered as a result of a systematic investigation of the antifungal activity of fatty acids. It is used as an ointment with zinc undecylenate; the latter compound may be used alone as a powder.

Clotrimazole (I) (o-Chloro α-α-diphenylbenzyl) is a drug which is effective against *Candida*, *Trichophyton mentagrophytes* and *Aspergillus*. It may be applied topically, given by mouth or parenterally. *Miconazole* is a β substituted phenethyl imidazole compound which is active against *Trichophyton*, *Microsporum* or *Candida* infections. This substance may be applied topically or given by mouth. It appears at least in the case of yeasts to inhibit the intake of nucleic acid precursors.

Natamycin is administered as a spray for its fungicidal and sporicidal activity. Since it is not absorbed through the skin there is no problem of residues. It is used mainly in the treatment of Trichophyton in cattle and Trichophyton or Micosporum infections in horses.

Enilconazole is active against dermatomycoses and ringworm in cattle, horses and dogs. It is used as a wash or spray.

Etisazole is used as a local application for the treatment of ringworm in horses, dogs and cats.

SUGGESTIONS FOR FURTHER READING

Alexander F, Davies M E 1979 A comparison of the antibacterial properties of some udder creams and ointments. Veterinary Record 104:253

Bean H S 1967 Types and characteristics of disinfectants. Journal of Applied Bacteriology 30:6

Bond J M 1966 Antibiotics used in the chemotherapy of bacterial and fungal infection. In: Schnitzer R J, Hawking F (eds) Experimental chemotherapy, Vol 4. Academic Press, New York

Gibbs B M, Stuttard L W 1967 Evaluation of skin germicides. Journal of Applied Bacteriology 30:66

Hugo W B 1967 The mode of action of antibacterial agents. Journal of Applied Bacteriology 30:17

Kelsey J C, Maurer I M 1967 Choice of disinfectants for hospital use. Mon. Bull. Minist. Hlth. 26:110

Ryley J F, Wilson R G, Gravestock M B, Poyser J P 1981 Experimental approaches to antifungal chemotherapy. Advances in Pharmacology and Chemotherapy 18:50

28

Tumour chemotherapy

Although even in man the treatment of neoplasia with drugs is incompetely effective, certain advances have been made. Antineoplastic agents are of interest to veterinarians not only because of their potential application to similar diseases in animals but in part because spontaneous tumours in animals have provided experimental material with which to study such drugs. Moreover, these drugs usually have other actions. Amongst the other effects of antineoplastic agents are carcinogenesis, mutagenesis and immunosuppression.

A major obstacle to the production of an antineoplastic agent lies in the fact that malignant cells are almost indistinguishable from normal cells. An interesting exception is the finding that certain leukaemic cells are deficient in the enzyme necessary for the synthesis of the amino acid L-asparagine which is essential for nucleic acid formation. These tumour cells fail to survive in the presence of the enzyme L-asparaginase which deprives the cells of the essential asparagine.

It is convenient to classify the chemotherapeutic drugs used against tumours as alkylating agents, antimetabolites, antibiotics; alkaloids, hormones, and certain miscellaneous substances.

The alkylating agents include the nitrogen mustards such as mustine and cyclophosphamide, ethylenimines, and alkyl sulphonates such as busulphan. These drugs interfere with cell division in all rapidly proliferating tissues. Various cells differ greatly in their susceptibility to these substances. Their actions resemble in many ways those of ionising radiations and are sometimes termed radiomimetic. The haematopoietic system is particularly sensitive to the actions of alkylating agents. Within a few hours of administration mitosis in the bone marrow and lymphoid tissue ceases, the lymphocytes are especially sensitive and this action accounts for the immunosuppressive action of these compounds.

Antimetabolites are analogues of normal metabolites and act by competition usually interfering with nucleic acid synthesis. The folic acid antagonist methotrexate has been used in leukemia and also as an immunosuppressive agent in organ transplant operations. The pyrimidine analogues such as fluorouracil have been shown to produce a temporary regression of solid tumours in man and are also of value in man in the treatment of proliferative skin diseases. The purine analogues such as mercaptopurine are of value in treating leukemia in man and also have immunosuppressive activity. Certain antibiotics react with DNA and prevent the synthesis of RNA. Actinomycin D is typical of this group of drugs.

The vinca alkaloids occur in the periwinkle plant (*Vinca rosea*). Vincristine is a typical member. This alkaloid exerts a cytotoxic effect on a number of tumours and is remarkable in having a low toxicity for normal cells.

The hormones used in tumour chemotherapy are those of the adrenal cortex, oestrogens, androgens and progestagens. The adrenocorticosteroids produce remission in certain leukaemias. Oestrogens are used in the treatment of anal adenomata in dogs in which condition they are reasonably effective, these substances are also useful in reducing tumours of the prostate in dogs. Androgens have been used in the treatment of mammary neoplasia in women. However, oestrogens have been shown to increase the incidence of mammary carcinoma in mice and it has been observed that the administration over a period of synthetic oestrogens to bitches caused an increased incidence of cystic adenomata and adenocarcinomata; these tumours regressed when the treatment was stopped. Progestagens have been found useful in certain uterine tumours in women.

The anti-androgen cyproterone (see p. 223) has been used to treat prostatic hypertrophy in dogs.

A few reports of the use of various antineoplastic agents in domesticated animals have appeared. A nitrogen mustard, triethylenethiophosphamide, has been used in the treatment of bovine lymphatic leukaemia. Unfortunately the treated cases progressed in a manner little different from that of the untreated animals. However, a transmissible venereal tumour in dogs when treated with cyclophosphamide together with brudnisole showed complete regression. Lymphomata in dogs when treated with cyclophosphamide showed remission of the tumours in males but in females it was without effect.

The combination of three or four antineoplastic agents has shown promise in the treatment of lymphosarcoma in dogs and cats. One of the more successful regimes included the use of vincristine, prednisone and cyclophosphamide. Osteosarcoma in dogs showed some regression following the intra-arterial administration of triethylene glycol diglycidyl ether (ethoglucide).

Mitogillin a polypeptide produced by *aspergillus restrictus* has produced regression in several tumours in dogs. The growths included mastocytoma, squamous cell carcinoma and mammary gland adenocarcinoma.

Carcinogenicity testing

It is now essential for all new drugs to be tested for carcinogenicity. This is done by administering the drug to a small rodent over a long period preferably its life span and determining whether the incidence of tumours is greater in the treated animals than a control group which has been properly selected. A similar test is usually carried out on a species other than a rodent. To try to obviate in part such long and expensive procedures, commercial establishments sometimes use a test which depends on the close correlation between the occurrence of micronuclei and polychromatic erythrocytes from the bone marrow and mutagenicity. This test is usually carried out on mice. Drugs may also be tested to see whether they induce mutations in certain strains of *Salmonella typhimurium* injected into the peritoneal cavity of mice. Carcinogenic compounds are usually also mutagenic and these relatively simple and inexpensive tests allow a potential carcinogen to be eliminated very early in the stage of developing a new therapeutic agent. Since many of the antineoplastic drugs are themselves carcinogenic it is important that the clinician using them should avoid the ingestion, inhalation or skin contamination of or by these agents.

Immunosuppressive drugs

These substances are of interest as research tools, for their use in organ transplant operations, because of their possible use in diseases due to immunological reactions and their potential role in tumour chemotherapy. The immune response usually begins with the phagocytosis of antigens by macrophages. This leads to the coating of the macrophage membrane by antigen molecules. These antigenic determinants bind to antigenic receptors of corresponding antigen-sensitive small lymphocytes causing these to differentiate and proliferate. Small lymphocytes arising from bone marrow differentiate into cells producing humoral antibody, and lymphocytes derived from the thymus differentiate into cells responsible for cellular immunity. Immunosuppressive drugs must act on one or more steps in these processes. Certain agents such as the corticosteroids, X-rays and anti-lymphocytic serum produce a very marked depletion of the total pool of lymphocytes. Most immunosuppressive drugs interfere with cell multiplication or protein synthesis.

Non-specific immunosuppression is produced by alkylating drugs, antimetabolites, antibiotics and certain alkaloids which have been discussed for their role in tumour chemotherapy and carcinogensis. Immunosuppression is also produced by the administration of various antisera such as antilymphocyte sera and by removal of lymphoid tissue. The latter includes thymectomy, splenectomy, fistulation of the thoracic duct and, in birds, removal of the bursa of Fabricius.

It is of interest to note that the anthelmintic levamisole not only stimulates the immune response increasing the activity of macrophages but can also act as an immunosuppressive drug.

The use of immunosuppressive agents is fraught with hazards. All non-specific immunosuppressive drugs impair the body's defence against infections and appropriate antibacterial drugs must be used to combat these infections. Cytotoxic drugs not only depress bone marrow but are usually carcinogenetic. These agents also show mutagenicity and teratogenicity and therefore should not be used in pregnancy.

SUGGESTIONS FOR FURTHER READING

Gerebtzoff A, Lambert P A, Miescher P O 1972 Immunosuppressive agents. Annual Review of Pharmacology 12:287

Holcenberg J S, Camitta B M 1981 Cancer chemotherapy and immunopharmacology. Annual Review of Pharmacology and Toxicology 21:231

Owen L N 1976 Therapy of neoplasia in domestic animals. Advances in Veterinary Science 20:223

Owen L N 1979 Cancer chemotherapy. Vet. Ann. 19:204

Sartorelli A C, Creasey W A 1969 Cancer chemotherapy. Annual Review of Pharmacology 9:51

Segaloff A 1980 Cancer chemotherapy and immunopharmacology. Annual Review of Pharmacology and Toxicology 20:429

Young C W, Burchemal J H 1971 Cancer chemotherapy. Annual Review of Pharmacology 11:369

Index